Dementia: Its Nature and Management

**FRANCIS CLOSE HALL
LEARNING CENTRE**
Swindon Road Cheltenham
Gloucestershire GL50 4AZ
Telephone: 01242 714600

UNIVERSITY OF
GLOUCESTERSHIRE
at Cheltenham and Gloucester

Dementia:
Its Nature and
Management

Morris Fraser

*Consultant in Psychogeriatrics, University College Hospital,
London and Friern Hospital*

A Wiley Medical Publication

JOHN WILEY & SONS
Chichester · New York · Brisbane · Toronto · Singapore

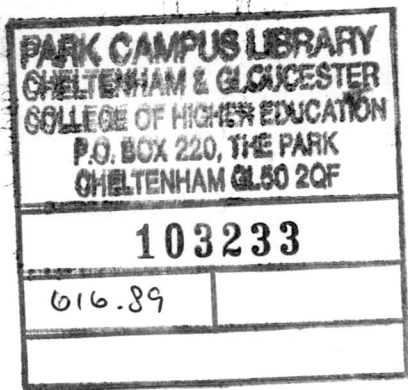

Library of Congress Cataloging-in-Publication Data:

Fraser, Morris.
   Dementia: its nature and management.
   (A Wiley medical publication)
   1. Senile dementia. 2. Dementia. I. Title.
II. Series. [DNLM: 1. Dementia. WM 220 F8415d]
ISBN 0 471 91548 3

British Library Cataloguing in Publication Data

Fraser, Morris
   Dementia: its nature and management.
   I. Dementia
   I. Title
   616.89   RC524
ISBN 0 471 91548 3

Printed and bound in Great Britain
by the Bath Press, Avon.

Contents

Preface

Early in 1986, a radio programme provided a vivid account of the life of Bedřich Smetana, the Czech composer. In his later years Smetana suffered a number of small strokes and gradually lost his memory. The programme ended with an eye-witness description of the old man, in his best suit, being helped down the steps of his house by his daughter and then being half-lifted into a carriage which drove him to Prague Lunatic Asylum, where he died in 1884.

The listener was meant to consider this very sad and shocking, which it was. But it is even more sad and shocking that, more than a century later, large numbers of elderly people with dementia still have nowhere to go but to the county lunatic asylum, whatever it may now be called. This is not purely a social policy defect — though it is certainly that — but it is also an outcome of the fact that doctors still have great difficulty in understanding and treating dementia. It is usually said, indeed, that dementia is untreatable. This is only partly true, but it is nevertheless the case that the number of people suffering from the various kinds of dementia is on the increase, not because these conditions are 'spreading' like an epidemic (a word often inappropriately used in phases such as 'the silent epidemic'), but because more people now survive into the high-risk period for dementia, which can strike at any time from middle age onwards. It is also true, though it is slightly less well known, that dementia is now a less immediately fatal condition, and that sufferers commonly 'live' for long periods following diagnosis. And most adults, if they think about their old age, almost certainly fear dementia even more than they do death. The word conjures up, not inaccurately, the image of months or even years spent in a mental or geriatric ward, confused, drooling and incontinent. 'If I ever get like that,' I am often told, 'please God they won't keep me alive.' But doctors, surely, are meant to preserve life . . .

This is only one of the dilemmas that the mental illnesses of late life present; there are many others, to be examined later. But the purpose of the following chapters is not to deal in hopes and fears about dementia, both of which tend to be exaggerated, but simply to ask: what can be done about dementia in the 1980s and 1990s? Certainly more knowledge and more resources are needed, but we do not make the best use of what is already known and the resources that already exist. The book, then, falls naturally into two parts. The first few chapters examine the results of the main investigations into the causes, diagnosis and treatment of dementia, and the remainder deal with the ways in which our present-day knowledge can be utilized in order to treat sufferers. However, in the light of this knowledge, 'treatment' has to be interpreted broadly; it might mean giving a drug or it might equally well mean providing a good and humane environment. And the second form of treatment may be as slow of delivery as the first. The old sanitoria did not begin to empty until chemotherapy effective against the tubercle bacillus became available in the 1950s; in the same way, the huge mental hospital population of more than 40 years ago began to decrease only following the introduction of ECT, the phenothiazines and the antidepressants, not because of any noticeable enlightenment in social policy and attitudes (much as we now like to believe so). And the process is still incomplete. Will the demented be more fortunate?

There are signs that they might be. But there is in any case no need to await a 'miracle cure' for dementia. Given what we already know, determination on the part of clinicians to translate theory into practice, and vastly improved co-operation between the medical and social services, the management of dementia could be revolutionized now.

Acknowledgements

In addition to the specific acknowledgements included as appropriate later, I would particularly like to thank Dr Doris Hollander for Figures 7–10 and Dr Ginny Wright for Figures 15 and 16.

CHAPTER 1

The origins

Dementia is not a diagnosis, but a group of conditions whose only common feature is a state of chronic confusion evident in both patient and doctor. Each views the other through a moderately dense fog of incomprehension, raised on one side by brain disease and on the other, for the most part, by serious misconceptions about the nature of the dementing illnesses, about how they are diagnosed and classified, and about how they are best treated — this often to the point where the very status of dementia as a 'medical' condition is not acknowledged. As a result, few patients are less happily situated than the sufferer from dementia who has, for example, been admitted into an acute ward in a general hospital or who has, even worse, been decanted by 'the community' into a casualty department. He is likely to fare indifferently in his new surroundings. In due course, pronounced not 'ill' enough to be in hospital but too confused to be sent home, he will probably attain membership of a novel diagnostic category which, though now large, is not dealt with in any standard textbook; he will be a 'bed-blocker'. Or a 'geriatric cuckoo', a droplet in the 'rising tide', or the target for some other item from the wide vocabulary of disparagement that has come to attach to the elderly confused.

The solution, should the patient arrive at the head of the almost inevitable waiting list (on which patients commonly celebrate first, second or third anniversaries), will be transfer either to the 'dementia ward' of a distant mental hospital or, if he is clean, decent and properly subdued by tranquillizers, to a local authority home for the elderly — that is, in the jargon of the day, to Part 3 accommodation. Now his situation may well improve. He is likely to be looked after in generally agreeable surroundings by staff who are employed exclusively in the care of the elderly and in general deeply devoted to their task. Indeed, were there enough suitable establishments throughout the country, 'bed-blocking' could be eliminated at a stroke, pressure on families and domiciliary services would be immeasurably eased, and the dementing population could partake *en masse* of what a recent parliamentary reply called the 'greenhouse philosophy' — that is, where the elderly are kept warm, fed, and watered until they die' (Holt, 1984). A greenhouse is certainly a pleasant and sunlit place, but

1

the reference was of course derogatory; the flaw in both the greenhouse philosophy and the dismissive medical view is their common assumption that severe mental decline in old age is both inevitable and untreatable. Neither is the case, and this is why the present book has been written.

Almost everything which follows will be based on a small number of key propositions about dementia. All will need to be supported and elaborated at a later stage, but they will be set out fairly briefly to begin with.

First, dementia does not represent part of the normal ageing process. The *normal* experience is that the individual retains adequate mental capacity to serve him throughout his physical life-span. Naturally there is always some terminal decline in cognitive ability, but the difference between normal ageing and dementia is that in the latter *the brain degenerates in advance of the body* — that is, in the virtual absence of a parallel ageing process in other organs. Therefore, dementia represents a process neither of normal ageing nor of accelerated ageing. There may be some abnormal organ ageing outside the brain in the dementias of early onset, but the rate of overall ageing is certainly nothing like that seen, for example, in Down's syndrome where, in addition to Alzheimer-like dementia, there is extensive degeneration of connective tissue throughout the body, with death usually occurring before the age of 60. In dementia, by contrast, life in general is not shortened drastically, and prolonged survival in a brain-damaged condition is now the rule rather than the exception.

Second, dementia is not only selective to the brain but damage is anatomically and biochemically *selective within the brain*. The term 'global' as sometimes applied in the past to dementia can no longer be considered accurate. In Alzheimer's disease, the most common form of dementia, the functions most severely impaired are memory, personality, language and the more subtle motor and sensory abilities, whereas gross motor and sensory functions are preserved relatively intact. Thus the cruel paradox is that massive cell death occurs in almost all brain areas except those which will, by continuing to function, ensure the patient's survival. Dementia is thus characteristically a condition that causes severe handicap and long-term dependency rather than premature terminal illness. Indeed, there is now no other condition that makes so many people totally dependent on others for such a large part of their lives.

Third, dementia is treatable. This proposition is a little more contentious, but it is capable of at least partial support. To begin with, however, dementia needs to be defined, and an outline classification has to be introduced.

Dementia is acquired brain disease which is both diffuse and chronic. The category thus excludes congenital disorders, acute confusional states (which are generally secondary to extracerebral disease), and focal conditions such as tumour or stroke. It includes, to take two examples, multi-infarct dementia and dementia of Alzheimer's type. Although the disorders which may be properly described as 'the dementias' are numerous, the great majority of cases fall into only these two subcategories. Of all dementias, about 55 per cent are of Alzheimer's type, 15–20 per cent are of multi-infarct type and 15–20 per cent represent these two types combined. The remaining types are relatively uncommon, but they include some that can be successfully treated and even completely cured (unlike Alzheimer's disease) and, more important, so also can many conditions that *present* as dementia. Of 50 cases of suspected dementia referred to a specialist outpatient clinic (Van der Cammen *et al.*, 1987), a positive diagnosis of the condition could be supported in only 28. Five patients were suffering from affective disorder; among the other causes of confusion, some treatable, were two patients whose cognitive impairment was entirely the result of overprescription of tranquillizers and who recovered when the drugs were withdrawn. Of the patients positively diagnosed as demented, four were considered to be suffering from the multi-infarct type, which often responds at least in part to remedial or preventive measures.

The present book deals largely with Alzheimer's disease (AD), first because it is still considered almost inaccessible to effective therapy, but also because of the immensity of human suffering that results from the disease and its complications.

In the first-ever debate on senile and presenile dementia in the British House of Commons (at 4.30 a.m.) Mr Richard Holt (1984) read a number of letters from constituents who had relatives suffering from the disease; he included a letter written to one of them, presumably from a doctor, which said bluntly: 'I am sorry, but your wife has Alzheimer's disease. Unfortunately there is no cure. A lot of care will be needed.'

In his reply, the Under-Secretary of State detailed some measures that the Government were taking in order to improve the care of the demented and to encourage medical research into the syndrome, but conceded that dementia was an increasingly grave health and social problem, and that the possibility of a cure was, as matters stood, 'only a hope'.

The age of the patient described above is not stated, but it is likely that she was aged under 65. There has been an unfortunate convention, in the UK especially, that AD is referred to as 'senile dementia' if the onset is after the age of 65, although it has been recognized for at least sixty years that senile dementia and AD are morphologically and biochemically similar and probably identical. 'Alzheimer's disease' is therefore best applied to the morphological form described by Alzheimer in 1906 regardless of age of onset; the term 'senile dementia' should gradually be abandoned, since it appears to draw a distinction between a form of dementia which is premature and one which is not. *All dementias are premature.* A difficulty nevertheless arises in that some morphological features of AD are apparent in 'normal' elderly people, and that their number increases with age. Will we all become AD sufferers if we live long enough?

Perhaps — but this is not an argument against the disease model or against treating. There is debate among gerontologists, to be examined later, about whether, with the conquest of physical disease, the human life-span can be extended indefinitely (probably with an increasing number of people becoming demented) or whether it will conform increasingly closely to a 'rectangular'

4

pattern (p. 35). The latter model is marginally the more convincing, but the issue is still highly theoretical. A physician in the year 2000 will in all likelihood be writing a book which is completely different from this one; however, as matters stand, the task of a doctor treating dementia is, as far as possible, *to maintain adequate cognitive function throughout the individual's physical life-span*, not primarily to extend his life-span, although in the event a longer life will be an incidental benefit for most patients treated successfully.

But this is still only a distant prospect and, of course, the reason why such major attention is now focused on dementia is precisely because the conquest of other forms of disease has made for an increased survival rate of the population in general and thus to a corresponding increase in the population at risk for dementia. The actual prevalence rate of the disease has not increased, but the factors that have made for increased survival of the general population have also made for increased survival of the demented as a subgroup; over the course of the last 20 years, the two-year survival of people diagnosed as demented appears to have increased by approximately one-third (p. 33). Yet, although the condition is now immensely consumptive of health and social resources, it is still one of the few disease processes on which medicine has made almost no impact. On the positive side (quoting again from the parliamentary reply), 'there seems to be no difficulty in interesting able psychiatrists to take up the psychiatry of old age'; indeed, dementia has begun to engage the attention of psychiatrists, neurologists, biochemists, geriatricians and other researchers to an unprecedented degree. A reason for this (in addition to pure necessity) is that a number of consistent biochemical changes in the brains of demented patients have now been identified, and, as there is evidence that at least some of these may occur in advance of the structural damage, it appears quite rational to hope that correctible elements in the condition may exist and that their discovery may not be far off. The lure of a possible biochemical cause for the symptoms of dementia is of course a strong one. Many disorders which were not long ago widely destructive of the central nervous system will now respond almost completely to a simple treatment — usually either an antibiotic or some form of replacement therapy; examples are diabetes, tuberculosis, pernicious anaemia, parkinsonism, syphilis and, probably the most dramatically effective in normal clinical practice, the replacement therapy of hypothyroidism in adults and children.

Might Alzheimer's disease in the same way result from a simple biochemical defect and thus prove to be as treatable in due course as, say, Parkinson's disease? Strictly speaking the answer has to be in the negative, because in established AD cell death has already occurred on a scale far exceeding that in any of the above examples and, as brain cells are post-mitotic, the damaged tissue cannot be replaced. Any kind of intervention in the biochemistry of the disease is thus likely to be effective only in patients in whom there has not been appreciable cell damage, and it is doubtful whether we have at present reliable means of identifying this group. This is probably why attempts at treatments which appear to be rationally based biochemically have proved disappointing so far; our methods of diagnosing early or 'preclinical' dementia are only now being developed.

Fortunately — and this is the fourth proposition — even as matters now stand the clinical condition of demented patients can be vastly improved by measures that do not amount to radical intervention in brain chemistry; work to be described in later chapters will show that the demented rarely present primarily because of their cognitive loss, but more commonly because of problems that have become superimposed on the dementia and which in themselves are likely to be treatable. A patient, for example, may be living alone and unsupervised, and thus be a prey to malnutrition, hypothermia or accidents; there may be an infection, or the dementia may have caused a serious emotional reaction in the patient or a relative. Further, a systematic approach can help with symptoms of the dementia itself (e.g. incontinence or wandering), and there are now drugs available which may even improve cognition somewhat, though all still have to be much more thoroughly evaluated.

The final proposition is that *continuing or 'terminal' care provision for the most severely demented, either at home or in hospital, can and should be in no way inferior to the terminal care provision now available to other groups of patients.* This state of affairs has by no means been achieved, but it is achievable.

Still, for the clinician, admission of his patient to a continuing care ward (a term, incidentally, preferable to 'long-stay ward' or 'dementia ward') represents at least partial defeat. We now return to the model of dementia — specifically AD — as a disease which may be treatable, and examine the main theories of causation.

INHERITANCE PATTERNS

There is some evidence of genetically determined vulnerability to AD.

The first large familial study was by Sjörgen *et al.* in 1952. Some small pedigree studies had been published in the 30s and 40s; these generally reported instances of families in which there was an unusually high prevalence of dementia; Sanders *et al.* (1939), for example, published a pedigree with 17 affected members in four generations. But the issue of inheritance was still confused by problems of diagnosis and terminology, in particular by the question of whether a distinction could be drawn between AD and 'senile dementia'. The study by Sjörgen *et al.* was partly addressed to this question; it was hypothesized that if the two conditions were a single entity they should be genetically uniform; that is, each should 'breed true'.

The authors identified patients with AD from hospital case records, confirming the diagnosis clinically in 62 patients; 18 of this group were histopathologically confirmed at post-mortem. The average age at onset was 61 years. From extensive field studies they identified 30 secondary cases among close relatives of 20 of the probands. Twenty-six of these were, however, deceased: from the case records a diagnosis of Pick's/Alzheimer's disease was made in 11 cases (the

Table 1. Risk of Alzheimer's disease/senile dementia

Study	Siblings	Parents	Children	Gen. population	Theory	Comment
Sjögren et al. (1952)	3.8% 16% one parent affected 2.5% neither affected	10%		0.1%	Polygenic inheritance	Includes Pick's disease patients; autopsy confirmation only in minority
Larsson et al. (1963)		10.8%		Males 3.2% Females 3.5%	Autosomal dominant with partial penetrance	Heavy dependence on records; no autopsy confirmation
Heston et al. (1981)	19.5% 45% one parent affected 17.6% neither affected		22.7%	6.4%	Autosomal dominant in severe cases	All probands and many secondary cases confirmed at autopsy
Heyman et al. (1983)		25%			Autosomal dominant in familial cases	All probands and most secondary cases thoroughly diagnosed clinically
Breitner and Folstein (1984)		50% in language-disordered cases		8% (controls)	Autosomal dominant with complete penetrance by age 90	All cases thoroughly diagnosed clinically

Study	Siblings	Parents	Dizygotic twins	Monozygotic twins	Theory	Comment
Kallman (1950) (twin families)	6.5%	3.4%	8%	42.8%	Polygenic inheritance	Weak diagnostic criteria

authors were unable to make a distinction), 3 were rather unsatisfactorily diagnosed as 'dementia presenilis', and in the remaining 12 a diagnosis 'only' of senile dementia could be made. The authors calculated the risk of AD/PD within the ages 40–70 years as being some 10 per cent for the parents of probands and about 3.8 per cent of siblings. For siblings where one parent was also affected the figure was about 16 per cent, and for those where neither parent was affected it was about 2.5 per cent (Table 1). It was calculated that the risk from ages 40 to 70 in the general population was of the order of 0.1 per cent; it was concluded only that inheritance was multifactorial.

These results cannot be taken as dependable since the study, along with many others, presupposes the existence of a 'senile dementia' entity with an independent pathology. The patients in this group are poorly described in the Sjörgen study (all of the cases in this diagnostic category had in fact died and the authors were dependent on case-notes), in contrast to the AD patients who were thoroughly examined clinically and diagnosed on the basis of memory loss together with aphasia, apraxia and agnosia. In this study, as in others, it is difficult to believe in a substantial elderly confused population free from these defects, and more easy to believe in one not examined for them specifically. Subsequent and thorough studies of cognitive impairment in dementia have indicated that memory loss as an isolated feature is rare (Lauter and Meyer, 1968; Breitner and Folstein, 1984; Van der Cammen et al., 1987); there is almost always some degree of dysphasia and dyspraxia in addition. By excluding the senile dementia group, therefore, Sjörgen et al. arrived at what is probably a considerable underestimate of the hereditability of AD.

Larsson et al. (1963) identified 719 cases diagnosed as senile dementia in Swedish hospitals between 1935 and 1950. They excluded patients whom they considered to be suffering from AD on three criteria: aphasic disturbance, rapid progression to profound mental deterioration and comparative early onset. The proband population for the study was 377; among close relatives (parents, siblings and children), 60 secondary cases were traced. They calculated that the morbidity risk in this group was 10.8 per cent up to age 80 as compared with a general expectancy of 3.2 per cent for males and 3.5 per cent for females. The suggestion was that the disease was in the main conditioned by a major dominant gene. The authors stated that no instances of AD were found in any of these relatives, and on this basis concluded that there 'definitely' cannot be any unitary genetic origin for AD and senile dementia. However, this massive study was based on surprisingly weak clinical foundations. There was no histopathological confirmation of the diagnoses, and the authors do not appear to have examined any of the 'senile dementia' patients themselves — in order, for example, specifically to exclude the clinical features that they take to be indicative of AD. Where the secondary cases are concerned, among 40 whose ages are recorded, 5 were aged under 65; 1 of these, for example, 'was taken ill at age 52, was hospitalized at age 55, and died within 3 months.' Diagnosis was 'dementia cerebri' and post-mortem examination showed 'slightly flattened' gyri.

We are not told what pathological process is postulated for these younger patients; the evidence disproves a diagnosis of AD neither in this group nor in any other of the secondary cases or the probands (age 56–92 at onset). Unfortunately, Larsson et al. is still cited (e.g. by Roberts, 1984) as 'the principal evidence' that AD and senile dementia are separate conditions.

Leaving terminology aside, however, the study does broadly indicate a clear familial bias in susceptibility to dementia. There was, by contrast, no significantly increased risk among the first-degree relatives for schizophrenia, manic–depressive psychosis, mental handicap or suicide. Breitner and Folstein (1984) calculate that, if AD and senile dementia are placed in a single category, the findings of Larsson et al. can be reconciled with a mendelian dominant pattern of inheritance.

Heston et al. (1981) found 87 secondary cases among parents, siblings and second-degree relatives of 125 autopsy-proven AD patients who had died between 1952 and 1972. Twenty-four of the secondary cases were autopsied and in all of these the clinical diagnosis was confirmed. The probands were found to have relatively severe disease ('a common finding in medical genetics'), with a mean age at onset of 67.4 (men) and 64.8 (women) and at death of 75.3 (men) and 72.5 (women). The risk by age 75 was about 19.5 per cent for siblings, 22.7 per cent for parents, 7 per cent for second-degree relatives, 17.7 per cent for controls who had other forms of brain disease and 6.4 per cent for the general population. The greatest risk was to siblings of probands who had one affected parent; this was considered to be in the range of an autosomal dominant trait; that is, 50 per cent. At the other extreme, the risk to siblings of probands in whom illness began after the age of 70 was scarcely different from that of the control group.

Whalley et al. (1982) identified 74 probands with autopsy-proved AD who had died between 1959 and 1978, and found 8 patients with presenile dementia among 322 first-degree relatives, all from different pedigrees. They excluded 4 patients with diagnostic terms on their death certificates considered to be vague, but the risk by age 80 was still considerably increased as compared to the expected number of 0.3 in the general population.

The authors, however, calculate that this falls short of the number required to support a mendelian dominant hypothesis and favour a polygenic model. But their findings do rely on what was written on a mere handful of death certificates and, as the authors found during an earlier part of their study, such records are unreliable and tend to under-record AD. The expected number of AD in the general population is almost certainly also an underestimate, based as it is purely on the number of patients dying in mental hospitals.

Heyman et al. (1983) identified 66 AD patients and found a 25 per cent incidence of dementia among first-degree relatives. Diagnosis and exclusion of non-AD brain disease was thorough, although neuropathological confirmation was obtained in only 3 probands and 2 siblings. The majority of their cases were sporadic, but it is suggested that the figures support a hypothesis that familial aggregations of AD could be accounted for by the existence of a single gene with typical autosomal dominant inheritance.

The evidence from some of the above work is re-examined by Wright and Whalley (1984); they find that the highest hereditability estimates are for early-onset illness in the relatives of early-onset probands and that the hereditability of 'all types' of AD is higher for early-onset probands. From scrutiny of the 30 or so published reports of autopsy-proven AD, they conclude that there was segregation in a manner consistent with autosomal dominant inheritance. The hereditability of 'all types' of AD might be consistent with a polygenic model, but there was a clear pattern of association between early-onset illness and a more extreme deviation, a greater genetic risk and, probably, a major gene defect. They thus postulate a subgroup of 'familial AD' which is most plausibly explained on the basis of a single mendelian gene. There remains, by implication, a non-familial AD group, but this group is more difficult to define, the illness being of late onset and, as a result, obscured by additional brain or extracerebral disease; the group is considered to be numerically small.

Breitner and Folstein (1984) identified a group of 62 patients who were demented; in 78 per cent there was also language disorder and apraxia; they interviewed all siblings and children (at least two relatives had to be aged over 60) and also those of an equal number of non-demented age-matched controls. It was found that the relatives of the agraphic or aphasic probands were at a 50 per cent risk of developing AD by the age of 90; in the age-matched controls the risk was only 8 per cent. No cases of AD were identified among relatives of non-aphasic/agraphic probands. These results are striking, and the authors conclude that AD is a dominant genetic disorder with age-dependent penetrance. It is also concluded that the entity 'familial AD', which includes agraphia/aphasia and has previously been considered rare, is in fact the most common type of dementia. This is consistent with the view of Lauter and Meyer (1968) who, after a careful examination of 40 patients with the diagnosis 'senile dementia', found only 3 without dysphasia or dyspraxia; 26 were dysphasic and 30 dyspraxic, and 20 showed disorders of spatial orientation. Breitner and Folstein write, in conclusion, that it should become possible in due course to discard the term 'senile dementia' in favour of 'Alzheimer's disease' and other terms equally descriptive of specific clinical entities.

There is only one major *twin study*. Kallman's (1950) study of 108 twin families (index patients all over 60) provided risk factors of 3.4 per cent for parents, 6.5 per cent for siblings, 8 per cent for dizygotic twins and 42.8 per cent for monozygotic twins. A polygenic hypothesis is favoured, but 'senile psychosis' is poorly defined, and the few clinical examples quoted include paranoid and affective disorders.

There have been other and more brief reports on twins. Sharman *et al.* (1979) reported presumably monozygotic twins concordant for AD, but the clinical manifestations were atypical (with upper motor neurone signs and involuntary movements), and there have been two reports of discordant monozygotic twin pairs (Davidson and Robertson, 1955; Hunter *et al.* 1972). In the last paper there was 10 000:1 probability of uniovularity and autopsy-proven AD in twin

1, but there was no evidence of clinical deterioration in twin 2 by age 66 (when she died of bronchial carcinoma). If AD were transmitted as a mendelian dominant, there would have been a strong likelihood of penetrance in twin 2 by that age; Hunter *et al.* suggest that exogenous factors may play a considerable part, and that closer studies of such factors in individual AD patients might well prove fruitful. However, since twin 2 had only just entered the senium at the time of her death, the finding does not by any means provide strong evidence against mendelian dominant transmission.

Alzheimer's disease and Down's syndrome

There are close similarities between the morphological changes of AD and those that become evident in the brains of Down's syndrome patients. The typical neuropathological features of AD — neuronal degeneration, plaques and tangles — appear in virtually all patients with Down's syndrome aged over 40 (Ellis *et al.*, 1974; Ball and Nuttall, 1980). Malamud (1972) examined 134 Down's syndrome (DS) patients aged from 11 to 70, and found that the risk of Alzheimer-type neuropathology began in adolescence, advanced rapidly and reached 100 per cent by age 45. These findings were replicated by Sylvester (1983). In fact, pathologists have been unable to distinguish between tissue from AD brains and DS brains with AD-type changes using both light and electron microscopes (Ellis *et al.*, 1974). Heston (1984) reviews a number of studies and notes that no exceptions have so far been found to the general rule that all AD patients over the age of 65 exhibit Alzheimer-type neuropathology.

In brains of DS patients there are other changes similar to those found in AD; for example, deficiencies in acetylcholine synthesis (Yates *et al.*, 1980) and aluminium accumulation (Crapper *et al.*, 1978).

It is not altogether clear whether intellectual and neurological defects similar to those of AD occur in parallel with the morphological changes. Wisniewski *et al.* (1978) examined 50 unselected DS patients aged from 5 to 72 and found significant mental and neurological deterioration in those aged over 35. In terms of cognitive function, there was recent memory loss, aphasia, agnosia, loss of vocabulary and emotional flattening or lability. Neurologically, frontal release signs were common, together with snout, palmomental and grasp reflexes (p. 109). These changes appear to have been consistent across the older group. Other studies, reviewed by Wisniewski *et al.*, report similar changes, mainly in the area of cognitive decline. Hewitt *et al.* (1985), on the other hand, were able to demonstrate significant mental decline in only 9 of 23 DS patients aged over 50, although it is not clear whether the precise cognitive and neurological signs characteristic of AD were sought. These studies were all cross-sectional, having the defect common to all such studies that the ageing patients increasingly represent a survivor population, with the likelihood that morbidity is underestimated. Only one prospective study appears to have been reported, and this confirms a progressive decline in learning ability with age in DS patients (Dalton *et al.*, 1974). The severity of Alzheimer-type changes seen at autopsy was found to correlate positively with the degree of cognitive deterioration (Crapper *et al.*, 1978).

The parallel between AD and DS is imperfect, the main differences being that in DS there is of course a degree of primary impairment and also that in DS patients there are widespread connective tissue changes such as cataracts, pigmentation, loss and greying of hair, diabetes, vascular disease and decline in immune function which, taken together, make the condition conform much more closely to an 'accelerated ageing' model. But the brain changes in the two conditions are sufficiently similar to have stimulated a number of studies based on cross-susceptibility hypotheses. DS is, in fact, the only known condition in which all the brain changes of AD occur together.

In their 1981 study of 125 patients with AD, Heston *et al.* found a substantial excess of DS patients among relatives (11 cases among 3044 relatives, a risk of 0.36 per cent as compared to a general risk of 0.14 per cent). It is of interest that DS was found only among relatives of the youngest probands (i.e. those with the most severe disease). Heyman *et al.* (1983) found a DS prevalence rate of 3.6 per 1000 among AD relatives, against an expected rate of 1.3 per 1000; Ball and Nuttall (1980) found a somewhat smaller excess. Heston *et al.* suggest that the genetic material on the abnormal long arm of the 21st chromosome pair is likely to contain a gene product aetiologically important in AD, and that a specific gene abnormality may be common to both conditions.

Whalley *et al.* (1982), in their study of 74 AD probands, did not find any cases of DS among 329 first-degree relatives. Their view is, however, that neither their own sample size nor that of Heston *et al.* was sufficiently large to yield a conclusive answer in favour of a genetic association between AD and DS. It is pointed out, also, that the mean age of the mothers of the DS children in the sample of Heston *et al.* (34) is considerably higher than the national average (28.2) and also that, if a genetic mechanism applied, risk would have been greater in first-degree relatives; this did not appear to be the case.

Whalley *et al.* offer an alternative hypothesis: the extra genetic material associated with trisomy 21, by disrupting the genetic balance of cells, makes for an imbalance among gene products that protect against DNA-damaging agents — with a resulting increase in susceptibility to viruses, toxins or autoimmune processes. AD might in the same way result from a genetically determined vulnerability to external agents, and it is thus not necessary to postulate a common genetic defect for AD and DS. This is an exceedingly cautious reading of the evidence, but the area is still one of deep uncertainty especially since, more recently, the idea of a common origin has again been given impetus. 'Protein A4' is the major sub-unit of the amyloid of both plaques and tangles. Kang *et al.* (1987) have identified a gene which encodes for the A4 sequence on chromosome 21, and which does not appear to be located on any other chromosome; it is suggested that in both AD and DS there is a gene dosage effect with overproduction of A4 leading in turn to interference with neurotransmission, since A4 closely resembles cell-surface receptor proteins. It is therefore thought possible that further work with genetic probes based on

12

protein A4 could lead to the isolation of abnormal gene products and perhaps to treatments for both conditions (Ferry, 1987). But this remains optimistic; it is still not altogether clear whether A4 is specific to AD and DS; if not, other explanations of abnormal protein deposition are possible (p. 76).

To summarize thus far — where AD is concerned there would appear to be a fairly clear overall pattern that, the more rigorously the condition is defined clinically, the more closely does the pattern of inheritance conform to that of a mendelian dominant with fairly complete penetrance by the age of 90, although additional, possibly exogenous, factors may play a part in gene expression. The abnormal gene could, for example, be the major element determining vulnerability to a toxic or infective agent common in the environment. It is possible that attempts to identify such agents will prove more fruitful than will the elaborate DNA recombinant techniques used to probe for abnormal genes. But it has also been suggested that transmission of AD could be merely 'quasi-mendelian', due to the operation of an infective agent with a long incubation period; in the opinion of Wright and Whalley (1984) this possibility still cannot be ruled out and it is true, of course, that so far no specific chromosome defects have been associated with cases of 'pure' AD. Alternative — though possibly overlapping — aetiological models are therefore possible: in particular, theories in the 'slow virus' category have had some currency in recent years.

INFECTIVE HYPOTHESES

The infective-agent model of AD rests not on the conventional evidence for infectious disease (e.g. transmissibility, fever, raised white cell count) but on adducing a number of similarities between AD and other CNS conditions that are known to be of infective origin. These are: Creutzfeldt–Jakob disease, Kuru and scrapie.

Creutzfeldt–Jakob disease (CJD)

This was first described in 1920 by Creutzfeldt who observed a rapidly progressive dementia associated with motor disorder in a 22-year-old woman, with onset of symptoms at age 16; four similar cases in middle-aged patients were described by Jakob in the following year. Annual incidence is about 1 per million, with equal sex incidence and onset usually in the fourth or fifth decade. The symptoms, not altogether consistent from patient to patient, arise from damage both to the cerebral cortex and to adjacent structures, especially the subcortical nuclei, the cerebellum and the spinal cord. The characteristic clinical pattern is one of intellectual deterioration associated with upper or lower motor neurone signs and myoclonic jerking, but there is also likely to be cerebellar ataxia, and there may in addition be signs indicative of damage to the parietal or visual cortices. Death usually occurs within a year of onset.

Morphologically, there is widespread vacuolation and death of nerve cells in the affected areas, giving rise at post-mortem to a sponge-like appearance; the category title 'acute spongiform encephalopathy' has been applied to CJD and a small group of other conditions where there are similar changes, notably kuru and scrapie. The alternative is 'transmissible spongiform encephalopathy', since proven transmissibility is the additional factor common to all of the group. It was in fact the identification of kuru (described below) that led to frozen biopsy tissue from a CJD patient in England being sent to Gajdusek and Gibbs in the USA; they inoculated the tissue into a chimpanzee in the same way as they had earlier inoculated kuru tissue, and 15 months later the animal died; its brain showed the same spongiform changes as CJD and kuru brains (Gibbs et al., 1968).

There have been at least 68 instances of experimental transmission of CJD between primates. In about 8 of these cases, however, the disease proved not to be further transmissible; the clinical correlates of transmissibility were a shorter duration and a typical EEG (periodic, generalized, repetitive, bilaterally synchronous triphasic waves at 1–2 c/s); there were no clear neurological indicators (Traub et al., 1977).

CJD appears also to have been transmitted between humans. In 1974 a man of 55 developed CJD 18 months after he had received a corneal transplant from a patient who had died from the illness; the brains of both patients showed 'spongy' change at post-mortem (Duffy et al., 1974). There was a subsequent report (Bernouilli et al., 1977) of two patients who developed the symptoms of CJD, with histological confirmation in one, after the insertion into their brains of electrodes which had previously been inserted in the brain of a 69-year-old woman with proven CJD.

Masters et al. (1979) observed an unusually high frequency of previous cranial or ocular surgery among people who developed CJD, and occurrence of the disease has also been described following the administration of human growth hormone (Powell-Jackson et al., 1985). Corsellis (1979) has reviewed the minimal evidence of geographical clustering of the disease and concluded that there is no firm evidence that CJD is spread other than iatrogenically. However, the question was subsequently reopened by the reporting of three apparent conjugal cases (Will and Matthews, 1982). It is suggested that an unusually virulent strain of the agent could be responsible for such cases, which are unlikely to have occurred by chance (Matthews, 1985).

Where experimental animals are concerned, however, the disease has been transmitted only by inoculation, never by other forms of contact or genetically (Goudsmit et al., 1980).

Kuru

This resembles CJD in being a rare brain disease in man which has been transmitted experimentally to animals. It was first described by Gajdusek and Zigas in 1957, and has only been known to occur in the Fore tribesmen of New

Guinea (in whose language the name means 'trembling sickness'). It is also a rapidly progressive condition in which there is widespread spongiform change throughout the brain; the cerebellum generally shows the most severe damage. An additional feature, in three-quarters of all cases described, is the presence, mainly in the cortex, of plaques similar to those seen in AD, consisting of a solid amyloid core surrounded by a 'halo' of radiating fibrils.

Cell-free brain extracts from affected patients have transmitted the illness to chimpanzees, and between chimpanzees. Spread from man to man is believed to have been partially genetic, but also by way of ritual feasting on dead relatives. The practice has now died out, but it was considered notable that the illness affected women and children almost exclusively, since in the feasting ritual the women and children ate the brain and viscera, while the adult males ate the muscle only. Lishman (1978), who reviewed some of the above evidence, has pointed out that the cannibalism hypothesis remains unproven; kuru has never, for example, been transmitted to chimpanzees by ingestion.

Scrapie

This is an infectious CNS disease of adult sheep and goats which has been experimentally induced by inoculation and transplant in a number of other small mammals, especially mice. The condition has a restricted host range and it does not occur in man, but its importance is that it was the first transmissible encephalopahy to be identified and studied in detail; it was the scrapie model which led to the kuru transmission studies and subsequently to the demonstration, described above, that CJD was likewise experimentally transmissible. Gajdusek deservedly won the Nobel Prize for Medicine for his painstaking and hazardous work with the transmissible encephalopathies; the fascinating story is told in June Goodfield's *From the Face of the Earth* (1985).

Features of some strains of scrapie further resemble kuru in that they include amyloid plaques with radiating fibrils similar to those seen both in kuru and in AD (Outram, 1980). It has been suggested that CJD, kuru and scrapie are so closely related that the last might cause disease in the human through handling sheep or eating mutton, but investigations among butchers, shepherds and consumers of sheep (Masters *et al.*, 1979) and groups who eat sheep's eye-balls (Kahana *et al.*, 1974) have not yielded positive results.

Certain other rare conditions fall into the 'spongiform encephalopathy' group, and morphological changes in the animal hosts are probably indistinguishable (Goudsmit *et al.*, 1980). In the past few years there has been considerable debate over, first, the nature of the infective agent responsible for this group of diseases and, second, the question of whether AD, in view of several points of resemblance, might be caused by a similar agent.

Several viruses (the rubella virus, for instance) are already known to cause encephalopathies in man. Viruses differ from bacteria principally in their size and in their requirement of host cell enzymes for reproduction, but the agent responsible for the spongiform encephalopathies differs again from viruses in that it is not visible under the electron microscope (it appears, from irradiation target studies, to be much smaller than a virus (Rohwer, 1984)), in that it resists inactivation by agents to which viruses are susceptible, such as formaldehyde and ultraviolet light, and in that it has not thus far been shown to contain any nucleic acid (Prusiner, 1982b). Prusiner (1982a, b) has proposed the existence of a novel infective agent, a 'prion' (*prote*inaceous *in*fectious particle) in which genetic information may be coded by protein alone. From purified preparations of scrapie agent, a single major protein, PrP, which is required for infectivity, has been isolated; the preparation has also been found to contain numerous rod-shaped structures which were considered to be aggregates of prions. These rods in addition show biological characteristics of amyloid, and it is suggested that the amyloid deposits in the spongiform encephalopathies, and also in AD, may be paracrystalline arrays of prion rods. Prusiner found, further, that purified fractions from the brains of two patients with CJD contained protease-resistant proteins that reacted with antibodies formed against scrapie prions, and drew attention to the similarity between the 'prion rods' of rodent scrapie and those that have been experimentally induced in rodents by inoculation of human CJD tissue (Masters *et al.*, 1981). Prusiner's group (Bockman *et al.*, 1985) also report independent work (DeArmand *et al.*, unpublished) that shows specific binding of prion antiserum in rodent CJD amyloid plaques.

The suggestion is, therefore, that the amyloid or 'senile' plaques characteristic of AD may in fact be aggregates of the pathogenic agent itself.

Somerville, in a detailed critique of 1985, discounts this possibility on the grounds that the evidence is indirect and depends on too many unproven assumptions, and also on the more specific grounds that scrapie-associated fibrils (possibly containing the infectious agent) and amyloid fibrils from the same brain are ultrastructurally distinct. It is likely, he believes, that the amyloid deposits which form plaques in AD originate from partial degradation of the host protein by the disease process, of which they are simply a byproduct — as in all other forms of amyloidosis.

Therefore the infective model of AD is based only on certain resemblances which on present evidence are superficial. There are in fact more differences than similarities between AD and conditions known to be transmissible; for example, although spongiform encephalopathy has been described in some otherwise typical cases of AD (Flament-Durand and Couck, 1979), it is an extremely rare feature; similarly, amyloid plaques are uncommon in CJD, having been described in only about 10 per cent of cases.

Other obstacles stand in the way of an 'infectious agent' hypothesis. Bendheim and Bolton (1985) list four criteria that must be satisfied in order to provide proof of an infective aetiology for a disease:

(a) The causal agent must be regularly found in the diseased tissue.
(b) It must be capable of isolation and propagation in an artificial medium or susceptible model host.

16

(c) The isolated agent should produce a similar disease when inoculated into the experimental host.

(d) The agent should be recoverable from the lesions produced in the host.

Clearly AD can be made to satisfy none of these criteria on our present knowledge of the condition, and a number of negative points are worth noting in particular. First, there is no evidence of person-to-person spread; epidemics of AD have never been described, and there is no geographical or familial clustering other than by way of genetic patterns; spouses of AD sufferers are not, for example, at increased risk (Sjörjen *et al.*, 1952). Epidemiological studies have failed to demonstrate an increased incidence of dementia among nurses, physicians, pathologists and other health care workers who have been in frequent contact with demented patients (Gajdusek, 1977). Second, attempts to transmit AD from humans to experimental animals have been uniformly unsuccessful. Traub *et al.* (1977) inoculated tissue from 220 cases of various types of dementia, including AD, into animals; 78 cases were transmitted, but in no case did AD transmit *as* AD, only as a spongiform encephalopathy similar to CJD and kuru. Goudsmit *et al.* (1980) inoculated brain tissue from 62 patients with AD into several species of primate. Two of the latter developed disease, also of the spongiform type; however, the original biopsy tissue failed to produce disease in other hosts, and the authors write that laboratory errors or mislabelling could not be ruled out. On the other hand, it is very possible that AD is specific to man or that any causative agent may have an incubation period that exceeds the life of a laboratory animal.

In summary, therefore, an association between AD and the transmissible encephalopathies is still unproven; resemblances between the diseases in the two categories are non-specific and occur in many forms of brain damage, including trauma (p. 68). There is thus far no additional evidence suggesting that AD might be transmissible.

AUTOIMMUNITY

Since AD is an age-related condition, it is likely that failure of immune competence plays at least some part in its pathogenesis.

Ageing affects the immune system in two ways. First, there is impairment of the defensive response to most diseases, especially to infections. There is increased liability to bacterial and viral disease, but there is also a progressive decline in the immune system's policing efficacy against other invaders such as toxins or cancer cells. There is failure of replication and repair of stem cells (which differentiate into T-cells, B-cells and macrophages), with a resulting loss especially of T-cells, the main vehicles of cell-mediated immunity. There is also an effect, to a lesser degree, on B-cells. These, like the T-cells, are lymphocytes; they differentiate into plasma cells which secrete humoral antibody (i.e. the immunoglobulins). Ageing appears to affect principally IgG and IgA (Kay, 1985). IgM level may also decrease, although results are conflicting (Cohen and Eisdorfer, 1980a). The role of IgM and IgG is in protective immunity from infection, and of IgA in the protection of mucous membranes (e.g. in the bronchial and gut walls).

With ageing there is, secondly, an increased incidence of autoimmune disease; that is, there is an increased risk of self-destruction as a result of a body's decreased ability to distinguish between 'self' and 'non-self'. The expectation of disorders such as systemic lupus erythematosus, rheumatoid arthritis and chronic thyroiditis increases with age, there is increased amyloid deposition (Burch, 1968) and there is decreased antibody response to immunization (Finkelstein, 1984); there is also a raised level of circulating autoantibody (Mackay *et al.*, 1977).

Disordered T-cell function may also play a part in autoimmune disease in the elderly. The interaction between T-cells and B-cells is complex, since the former can take both a helper and a suppressor role in the antigen–antibody reaction; there is evidence that in old age there is an increase in the number of suppressor T-cells (Callard and Basten, 1977).

The question is whether, in addition to the changes normally associated with ageing, some immune system defect more or less specific to AD favours the onset or advance of the disease. Evidence has been examined in three areas.

Brain-reactive antibodies

Nandy (1975) demonstrated the presence of antibody which bound specifically to brain tissue in ageing mice. This effect could be increased by damage to the blood–brain barrier; there is, however, no evidence that this is damaged in AD. Nandy (1978), in a study of brain-reactive antibodies in clinically diagnosed cases of senile dementia and age-matched people with normal mental function, found significantly higher levels of these antibodies in the demented group. It is pointed out, however, that antibodies against CNS structures have been found in a number of other conditions, such as multiple sclerosis and schizophrenia (Heath and Krupp, 1967), cerebrovascular disease (Motycka and Jezkova, 1975), SLE (Bluestein, 1978) and epilepsy (Diederichsen and Pyndt, 1968).

Amyloid

Amyloid is a dense filamentous material composed of protein which accumulates in a wide range of diseases. It is at least partly made up of immunoglobulin molecules and it is probably associated with autoimmune disease, though it may also be present in chronic infections such as tuberculosis.

The brain, mainly by way of the 'senile' plaques of dementia and old age, produces more amyloid than any other organ, although experimental amyloidosis cannot be induced as readily in the brain as it can elsewhere (Cohen and Cathcart, 1974). There are considered to be two types of amyloid — A and B; the amino-acid sequence of amyloid B is the more homologous with that of immunoglobulin, and it has been suggested that the amyloid core of senile plaques (composed primarily of amyloid B) represents antigen–antibody complexes catabolized by phagocytes and degraded by lysosomes (Glenner *et al.*, 1971, 1973). In addition to senile plaques, 'neurofibrillary tangles' exist in abnormal abundance in AD; these also contain protein similar in some respects to amyloid, and animal studies have shown that extracts from these 'tangles' (described in Chapter 3) are capable of raising antibodies against normal brain tissue and T-lymphocytes (Dahl and Bignami, 1978; Schlaepfer and Lynch, 1976).

Humoral antibodies

A number of investigators have measured circulating antibody levels in demented patients, though reliable ranges for the elderly are lacking. Kalter and Kelly (1975) found 'high normal' levels of IgM and IgA in 8 out of 16 patients with AD as compared with 8 patients with other brain diseases; Mayer *et al.* (1976) found no differences between serum immunoglobulin levels in patients with senile dementia, cerebrovascular disease, and elderly patients without brain disease. Cohen and Eisdorfer (1980b) found that 57 cognitively impaired elderly people had significantly elevated levels of serum IgG and IgA as compared with elderly controls. These changes were most marked in women. But immunoglobulin levels — especially the IgG level — have been shown, by means of longitudinal studies, to be positively associated with survival (Buckley *et al.*, 1974), and the cohort of elderly women in the study were of course survivors. In other words, all that can be concluded is that — as might be expected — one needs a higher-than-average level of circulating immunoglobulin to survive into old age with a diagnosis of dementia, as distinct from, say, succumbing to intercurrent infection in an institution. It is noteworthy, in fact, that 74 per cent of Cohen and Eisdorfer's demented subjects were institutionalized, as compared to none of the controls. Smith and Powell (1985) found a higher level of IgA in demented patients aged 90–95 as compared with younger demented patients; again, the 'survivor' factor cannot be ruled out.

There is a suggestion from a study by Buckley and Roseman (1976) that survival can be attributed to a *rising* level of antibody, as distinct from a level that was initially higher than that of non-survivors, but the question is still fairly open.

Eisdorfer and Cohen (1980b) found, in a group of 42 patients with senile dementia, that immunoglobulin levels were positively correlated with cognitive test scores; IgG level was the best predictor of cognitive status. It is suggested that aberrant immune function might be characteristic of dementia, but the most that can be said is that relatively high levels of immunoglobulin appear to be protective in the condition, in that they are associated with a lesser degree of deterioration. This is true of other conditions — for example, chronic respiratory disease and melanoma (Buckley *et al.*, 1974).

A further difficulty in implicating the immune system directly in the pathogenesis of AD is that changes in immunoglobulin levels have thus far not been demonstrated in the cerebrospinal fluid (Böck *et al.*, 1974; Jonker *et al.*, 1982). The possibility therefore remains that survival or less rapid decline is associated with factors *external* to the CNS — for example, resistance to intercurrent infection.

The evidence for an immune hypothesis in AD is therefore incomplete. The presence of amyloid has been adduced in support of both an autoimmune and a viral origin for the disease. The two are not of course mutually exclusive, but the origin of amyloid also remains deeply obscure; it is, however, well recognized to be a fairly non-specific feature of chronic brain disease.

TOXINS

Aluminium encephalopathy has been proposed as a partial model for AD.

The neurotoxicity of a number of heavy metals (e.g. lead, mercury and manganese) has now been recognized for some time, and each causes a characteristic set of changes within the CNS. None of these encephalopathies bears any close morphological resemblance to AD, but in the case of aluminium encephalopathy, by contrast, there are certain similarities to AD, both in terms of morphology and distribution, that have suggested a toxic role for aluminium in the AD process. Some studies of AD brains have appeared to implicate aluminium even more directly.

Aluminium encephalopathy has been described as a consequence both of occupational exposure (McLaughlin *et al.*, 1962) and of renal dialysis (Alfrey *et al.*, 1976). High levels of aluminium in the environment have also been associated with amyotrophic lateral sclerosis and a parkinsonism–dementia complex (Garruto *et al.*, 1985). In all of these there is a high brain aluminium content together with progressive and irreversible dementia, but the neurological damage is more widespread than that of AD, and the characteristic morphological changes of AD have not yet been described. For example, dialysis dementia and occupational aluminium encephalopathy do not show neurofibrillary change, although neurofibrils have been experimentally induced in animal brains by the intracranial injection of aluminium compounds (Crapper and De Boni, 1977). These occur only in some animal brains, excluding primates (McDermott *et al.*, 1979), but they have been induced in human fetal neurones. These latter are, however, dissimilar to the paired helical filaments of AD, consisting of single-strand filaments as in the animal models (Crapper *et al.*, 1978).

In a series of studies, Crapper *et al.* (1978) have found aluminium concentrations in some brain regions of both AD and MS patients of approximately 10–30 times normal values. These changes were evident mainly in the frontal and temporal cortices; they were not demonstrated in the hippocampus, as in some animal studies by the same group (Crapper and Dalton, 1973). The distribution of aluminium did not altogether coincide with that of filamentous change, and the content of the neurofibrils remains unclear; they may or may not themselves contain aluminium. But the group suggest, on the basis of further work, that aluminium may interact with DNA, resulting in faulty transcription of genetic material and faulty protein synthesis (Crapper and De Boni, 1980).

In a careful study which matches 10 brains from AD patients with 9 controls, McDermott *et al.* (1979) found that there was a high degree of variation in aluminium concentration both between individuals and between brain areas. The highest concentrations were found in the hippocampi of both control and AD brains. In the AD brains there was no significant difference in aluminium levels between regions high and low in neurofibrillary degenerative change. The most notable finding was that no significant difference was found in aluminium concentration between control and AD brains. They suggest that, as aluminium accumulates in the brain with age, the discrepancy between their results and those of Crapper *et al* (1978) could be due to a considerable difference in the age ranges of their respective control groups; in their own study the average age was 73 and in that of Crapper *et al.* (1976) it was only 47. Crapper more recently, in fact, found normal levels of aluminium in the brain of a patient with presenile dementia (McDermott *et al.*, 1979).

The possibility is therefore that aluminium, one of the most abundant elements in the environment, simply accumulates passively in ageing or damaged cells. Aluminium accumulation has been described in a number of brain disorders, including Down's syndrome (Crapper *et al.*, 1976), but also in conditions morphologically quite unlike AD, such as those described above together with hepatic encephalopathy (Thal, 1984), the striatonigral syndrome (Duckett and Galle, 1976) and in a case of chronic alcoholism associated with multiple sclerosis (Lapresle *et al.*, 1975).

Furthermore, neurofibrils do not appear to be specific to toxic encephalopathies induced by aluminium; they have also been described in rats poisoned with tetraethyl lead (Niklowitz and Mandybur, 1975).

Other substances, such as silicones, may accumulate in brain tissue damaged by AD (Austin *et al.*, 1973), although studies by Crapper *et al.* (1978) specifically excluded accumulation of other trace metals — lead, iron, manganese, zinc and cadmium — indicating that the aluminium accumulation in AD probably is not part of a general failure to exclude trace metals. It is suggested that, if aluminium is shown to be of cytotoxic significance in AD, then aluminium chelation therapy might play a part in management but, on the evidence thus far, a rare degree of therapeutic optimism would also be called for.

PSYCHOLOGICAL FACTORS

This is dense and virtually uncharted territory. Is dementia wholly or partly a psychosomatic condition? Does depression, disappointment, inactivity or stress make any contribution to the disease process?

'John's memory began to go just after his wife died. He has aged more in the past year than he did in the last ten; he has become an old man, senile. He can remember almost nothing now, and a lot of what he says doesn't make sense.'

'Dad has never been the same since he was made redundant. He became moody, started forgetting things, losing things . . .'

Histories like these are given sadly but fairly philosophically; there is a widespread belief that the brain atrophies with disuse, the doctors working with older people are regularly asked for confirmation of this . . . 'If I keep my mind active, will it prevent my becoming demented?'

Millard, a professor of geriatrics, reviews some of the treatments for a failing memory at present available and concludes that the best advice he can give to his mother is that she continue to do the crossword in her daily paper (Millard, 1984).

'Keep your mind active' is certainly a harmless and a suitably muscular precept for the medical consulting-room, but does it work? It is possible now to provide at least a partial answer, although there has been very little in the way of helpful research in the area. The 'life events' school of psychiatry has not yet turned its attention to organic brain disease and, in any case, it will be well understood that there is little common ground between doctors who work in the latter area and those whose vantage point is largely psychoanalytic. Wilson (1955), for example, writing that dementia 'has all the hallmarks of a psycho-somatic disorder', suggests that 'the blood vessel constriction may well be part and parcel of a restricted life which has become narrow and meaningless' — a theory that bears little relation to the pathology of AD as at present under-stood. Miller (1977) has critically reviewed a number of theories which in the same way propose that the changes of dementia either mirror external (adverse) events or represent one or another form of reaction to them. Morgan (1965) suggested that the memory loss of dementia was a 'defence against a personal and inevitable death'; the fact that recent memory is selectively impaired is held to support this view in that more recent experiences would remind the patient of increasing age, infirmity and approaching dissolution. Rothschild (1937, 1942) failed to demonstrate any difference between the brains of demented patients and those of normal elderly people and therefore regarded dementia as a functional disorder related to failure to adapt to normal ageing. Ferenczi (1922) saw in organic brain disease the features of an infantile state of narcissism and considered its symptoms to be psychotic reactions to underlying damage rather than direct manifestations of the damage. These and other vaguely psychodynamic theories about the symptoms of dementia often contain misconceptions about the morphological basis of the disease, but all are not necessarily as outlandish as they sound. Miller writes that no ex-perimental evidence can be adduced either to support or to refute such views, which is not entirely correct; for example, a hypothesis that a symptom was psychotic could be tested by the use of an antipsychotic drug. He does, however, make an extremely valid point that from the psychoanalytical

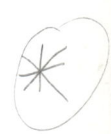

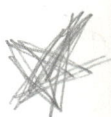

formulations can be derived 'the general notion that some of the signs and symptoms of dementia might be caused primarily by the disease process whilst others could be the consequence of the patient's reactions to these basic changes'. He adds that this idea has not yet been given any serious consideration, but the concept is in fact a familiar one to any doctor who deals with demented patients. Depressive and paranoid symptoms in particular may complicate the underlying memory loss, and the recognition and treatment of these symptoms (Chapter 6) represent a major element in the overall management of the demented.

Are certain types of individual especially prone to develop dementia, or do adverse life events initiate or hasten the process? Such evidence as exists is weak and generally negative. Oakley (1965) found, by means of a questionnaire administered to relatives, a significantly higher incidence of premorbid obsessoid features in a group of demented female patients as compared with age-matched controls. But the author recognized that apparent obsessional behaviour could well represent the first stages of a dementing illness, which is almost always insidious in onset. Amster and Krauss (1974) discovered that 25 demented patients had, in the previous five years, experienced twice the number of 'life crises' as had age-matched controls, but it is not clear whether these life events were truly independent of the illness or a consequence of the demented people's inability to cope with the management of their lives. Unfortunately, there is little information either about the diagnoses or about the nature of the life crises, so all that is established is a possible but unsurprising relationship between social stress and mental deterioration.

De Alarcon (1971) extensively reviewed the evidence for a causative association between various social stresses (isolation, bereavement, retirement) and mental illness in old age. Her conclusion was that, while such factors clearly make for hardship, unhappiness and withdrawal from others, there is no evidence that clearly defined mental illness followed these social stresses; in particular, she concluded, 'there is little firm evidence that retirement plays any part in producing or potentiating the onset of mental illness in old age'. This cannot be taken as a final judgement, based as it is on an extremely variegated group of patients, often with confused definitions of mental illness, and with statements which at times conflict; de Alarcon suggested that the belief that retirement has adverse psychological effects is based largely on sociological speculation, but added that her personal and professional experience indicated that affective illness of at least brief duration following retirement is fairly common. Clearly, a definitive study of the effects of retirement and other stress on the expectation of dementia and depression is still awaited; certainly, no compelling evidence exists where dementia is concerned.

But what about the other side of the coin? Can an active mind keep dementia at bay? Sadly, it does not appear so. During the past five years we (Van der Cammen *et al.*, 1987) have been operating a clinic for the investigation of memory disorders in patients past middle age, a specific purpose being the early detection of dementia. This work is described in more detail in Chapter 5.

One peculiar feature was our largely professional clientele, the unforeseen consequences of a number of factors — the nature of the hospital catchment area, self-referral and the means by which the clinic was publicized. A number of those we have seen were skilled, even distinguished, in their individual areas. The precise difficulties will not be described fully here on the grounds of confidentiality; it can simply be said that many were people continuing with intellectually stimulating and demanding work around or after the normal retirement age, who yet presented the classic symptoms of Alzheimer-type dementia. Very few conclusions can be drawn from observation of such an untypical population, but one is that continued intellectual activity after retirement age, whatever other benefits it may confer, is not an infallible safeguard against dementia. Preventive measures almost certainly lie elsewhere.

What is one to make of these widely diverse theories about the pathogenesis of dementia? The 'choline hypothesis' (p. 41), incidentally, is not being regarded as a causative theory but rather as a group of observations that associate AD with deficiencies in the central cholinergic neurotransmitter system; acetylcholine deficiency is not the cause of AD any more than dopamine deficiency is the 'cause' of Parkinson's disease. It is no longer generally claimed, either, that a slow virus infection, an autoimmune mechanism or an ingested toxin or any other factor represents the sole cause of AD; most authorities, by contrast, favour a catch-all hypothesis such as:

> '. . . the interaction of aluminium with other pathogenic processes including slow virus infection and immunological processes that may be responsible for amyloid formation' (Crapper et al., 1978).
> 'perhaps infection of the agent of the disease (if there is one) requires a particular genetic make-up, a concurrent immune disorder, or prior exposure to an environmental toxin' (Wurtman, 1985).
> 'It is apparent that practically no aetiologic agent can be excluded' (Torak, 1978).

Such views are mildly optimistic, suggesting a variety of starting-points for further research, especially into a number of types of therapy. An alternative but equally possible reading of all the evidence would be that certain unfortunate individuals are genetically programmed to undergo premature brain ageing (or a variant of brain ageing), that no intervening factors operate and that the condition cannot be arrested or alleviated in any way. This would arise from the meticulous genetic research described earlier, the paucity of other information and the apparent morphological continuity between some of the changes of AD and those of normal brain ageing; it is the most pessimistic hypothesis, but it ought to be faced. However, even the most relentless genetically determined conditions, such as Huntingdon's chorea, are subject to some degree of symptom control, and if AD in particular were vulnerable neither to such control nor to treatment and if it progressed independently of any outside influence, it would certainly be unique in the whole of medicine. There is evidence, to be examined in subsequent chapters, that it is not. Indeed, it is axiomatic in medicine that lack of knowledge about the precise cause of a disease is not a bar to effective therapy; diabetes, parkinsonism and hypothyroidism are classic examples.

In the next few years the search for a cause of AD is likely to proceed in many areas that are relatively inaccessible and mysterious to the average clinician; for example, in that of molecular biology. On the possible basis that AD involves abnormalities of gene expression, RNA sequences which code for various key peptides (which are often messenger substances) would be extracted from AD brains and controls. Any abnormal sequences would be recloned, labelled and employed as probes to investigate the expression of these sequences in the AD brain (Thoenen, 1982; Rosenberg, 1983). This technique could also be useful in identifying novel antibodies which might be raised in AD and which might interfere with the synthesis or activity of messenger peptides or other neurotransmitters (see also p. 11). As a result, more accurate diagnostic techniques might become available, but it is doubtful whether investigation of AD at molecular level will yield the sought-after 'therapeutic handle' for clinicians, at least in the near future. Effective treatment in the medium term is more likely to consist of intervention in the biochemical systems that are known to play at least some part in the shaping of AD pathology.

PREVALENCE

It is not possible to give prevalence figures for the various types of dementia that are altogether accurate. The main studies in the area have been reviewed and summarized many times (e.g. Bergmann, 1969; Royal College of Physicians, 1981; Gilleard, 1984), and the difficulties that arise in estimating prevalence are fairly familiar and often self-evident. These are, first, problems with terminology. Roth's 1955 classification of the mental disorders of old age was an essential starting-point, since it made available unambiguous diagnostic criteria which enabled the separation of functional and organic syndromes, and of 'senile' and 'arteriosclerotic' dementia. A number of studies, however (e.g. Gruenberg, 1961; Hartelius, 1972), treat the latter two as a single entity, which is uninformative, since the epidemiological pattern of the main subtypes of dementia is quite different; cerebrovascular disease, for example, is more common in males and is partially related to occupational exposure and cigarette smoking (p. 82). Again, 'Alzheimer's disease' and 'senile dementia' have only in recent years been accepted as synonymous (and still not by everyone), the former having been widely taken to refer to a relatively uncommon condition with onset usually before the age of 65. Kraepelin, possibly the true 'godfather' of Alzheimer's disease (he established and encouraged Alzheimer at Heidelberg), suspected the morphological identity of the two conditions in 1909 or earlier, while Alzheimer himself still believed that 'his' disease was rare and of vascular origin. This problem with nomenclature would not, however, distort the over-65 prevalence figures greatly.

Second, there is a diagnostic difficulty in that dementia exists in a continuum of severity; the elderly population cannot easily be categorized as affected or unaffected by a simple test or tests, as they might be in relation to, say, diabetes or infections. Agreed cut-off points in terms of mental function are lacking, and so vary from one study to another. The criteria of Kay *et al.* (1964a), subsequently adopted for most prevalence studies, are fairly broad and are weighted towards the more severe and established cases:

> 'Senile brain syndrome was diagnosed when there was evidence of progressive mental deterioration, characterized by 'organic' mental syndrome (disorientation, failure of memory and intellect), provided that it was not due to specific causes such as neoplasms, chronic intoxications or cerebrovascular disease.'

Early dementia, by contrast, remains diagnostically elusive.

Another complication is that nearly all prevalence studies have been cross-sectional rather than longitudinal. Tests of mental function in, say, octogenarians could be influenced by such historical factors as education, diet or exposure to certain diseases or occupational hazards that are now less common; there might therefore be an overestimate of the expectancy of dementia in a present-day younger population.

It is more likely, however, that expectancy would be *under*estimated. The present-day octogenarians are the survivors, and there is some indication that individuals resistant to the various life-threatening diseases of middle and older age might be resistant to dementia as well; the prevalence rate of dementia actually falls off slightly in nonagenarians (Larsson *et al.*, 1963; Torak, 1978). With the increasingly effective treatments available for other diseases, it is inevitable that more of the less fit will survive into old age, so the *proportion* of demented people in the elderly population is likely to increase.

The prevalence of moderate to severe dementia in the population aged 65 and over appears to be in the range 5.0–7.1 per cent (Table 2); the results from major studies show a fair degree of consistency. The prevalence of 'mild dementia' has been estimated at figures ranging from 5 to 53 per cent, but this entity has no formal status as a diagnosis and criteria are not agreed. All studies show a steeply rising age-incidence (e.g. Helgason, 1977), published data suggesting that there is an almost tenfold increase in the annual incidence of dementia from age 65–69 to 80 and over. No large prevalence studies of dementia have been published in recent years; it is possible that figures would prove smaller than those in Table 2, since more stringent diagnostic criteria would now apply. Kay *et al.* (1964a), for example, gave a figure of 10 per cent for dementing illnesses of all grades of severity in the over-65 population; in the 1970 study by Kay *et al.*, which included only those patients with a 'firm' diagnosis, the figure is 6.2 per cent.

The *lifetime expectancy* of developing senile dementia was calculated by Larsson *et al.* (1963) as 1.8 per cent for males and 2.1 per cent for females; the difference was considered to be due to relative female longevity.

Only a few studies make a separation between the subtypes of dementia. Of

Table 2.   Prevalence of moderate or severe dementia (%)

	Kaneko (1969)* N = 531	Neilsen (1962) N = 878	New York Study (1961)† N = 1503	Kay et al. (1970)* N = 758	Essen–Möller (1956)‡ N = 443	Clarke et al. (1984)* N = 1073
Age						
65+	1.9	2.1	3.7	2.4	0.9	
70+	2.7	4.0	5.4	2.9	5.1	
75+	11.3	7.8	9.3	5.6		
80+	9.9	12.6	8.8	22.0	21.8	1.6
5+	33.3	21.4	23.7			
All ages	7.1	5.9	6.8	6.2	5.0	

* Persons living at home only.
† Includes some functional psychoses.
‡ Age groups 60–69, 70–79, 80+.
(Based on table from the Royal College of Physicians Report of 1981. Reproduced by permission of the Royal College of Physicians of London).

a total of 687 patients in the Larsson et al. study, 227 (33 per cent) were diagnosed as suffering from definite or probable senile dementia, and 15 (2.2 per cent) from arteriosclerotic dementia. Diagnosis was made from case records, and the authors' criteria for cerebrovascular dementia suggest that it was underdiagnosed. But it was probably also under-represented in the population, which consisted purely of mental hospital admissions. The authors considered the population with the two types of dementia combined to have been negligible. Kay et al. (1964a) sampled 309 subjects from an over-65 population living at home and 134 from institutions. All patients were interviewed and examined. Of the subjects living at home, 10 per cent were considered to be suffering from an organic brain syndrome; 4.2 per cent were diagnosed as 'senile brain syndrome' and 3.9 per cent as 'arteriosclerotic brain syndrome'. Among institutionalized patients only 0.76 per cent were suffering from an organic brain syndrome; the figures for senile and arteriosclerotic dementia were 0.4 per cent and 0.2 per cent. 'Other severe brain syndromes' accounted for the remainder. There is no information on mixed types; patients were assigned only on the basis of main diagnosis.

Fisch et al. (1968) diagnosed 17 per cent of an over-65 population in New York as 'chronic brain syndrome', but, as this was an inner urban and low income group, it is likely that extracerebral disease and other brain conditions (including alcohol-induced disease) contributed to the total.

In our own study of 50 patients with memory disorder, all of whom were neurologically examined (Van der Cammen et al., 1987), a diagnosis of Alzheimer-type dementia was established in 25 patients, and of multi-infarct dementia in 2.

Hachinski et al. (1975) thoroughly examined a small group of 24 patients who had been referred for investigation for dementia and also measured regional

Table 3. Proportion of subtypes of dementia

Alzheimer's (senile) type	55%
Multi-infarct type (MID)	20%
Mixed AD and MID	20%
Other dementias	5%

cerebral blood flow. An 'ischaemia score' based on clinical features was bimodal, without any overlap, enabling patients to be assigned to a multi-infarct dementia group (10 patients) and a primary degenerative dementia group (14 patients).

Marsden and Harrison (1972) investigated 106 patients with suspected dementia: 84 were considered to be demented and, on clinical criteria, 8 patients were diagnosed as cerebrovascular dementia and 48 as probably of Alzheimer's type. In a clinicopathological study of 258 female patients (Sourander and Sjörgen, 1970), 132 were classified as Alzheimer-type dementia and 72 as cerebrovascular dementia.

A consecutive group of 73 demented patients aged over 65 were assessed pathologically by Tomlinson *et al.* (1970): 38 showed definite or probable senile dementia of Alzheimer's type, 12 showed definite or probable arteriosclerotic dementia and 12 were mixtures or probable mixtures of the two. The authors write that it is not always possible to be certain what pathological change is making the major contribution to the patient's symptoms. On the best evidence so far, then, it would appear that the distribution of the subtypes of dementia is as in Table 3.

There is some consensus (Corsellis, 1969; Tomlinson *et al.*, 1970) that the contribution of cerebrovascular disease tends to be overestimated in clinical practice. But multi-infarct dementia (as it is now more usually called) should be recognized where it exists since it is, generally speaking, more susceptible to treatment and prevention than is AD; careful history-taking and physical examination together with, perhaps, use of the Hachinski ischaemia score (Hachinski *et al.*, 1975), will lead to more accurate (though not watertight) assignment of demented patients to one or other of the two major subtypes.

Sex, social class and environment

There is invariably a preponderance of females in any demented population, though this largely reflects the larger number of elderly females in the population generally. A woman of 45 in the UK still has a life expectancy 21 per cent greater than a man of the same age (Faculty of Community Medicine, 1986). Heston *et al.* (1981) found the excess of females among 125 cases of autopsy-proven AD to be entirely consistent with the age-matched male-to-female ratio in the general population, and most other surveys have indicated that percentage prevalence of AD is about the same for both sexes (Larsson *et al.*, 1963; Torak, 1978; Kay and Bergmann, 1980). Only a few studies have

28

Table 4.   Sex distribution of senile and vascular dementia
(Prevalence rates among subjects aged 65+ living at home)

	Males ($N = 115$)	Females ($N = 194$)
Senile	2.6%	5.2%
Vascular	8.7%	1.0%

(Reproduced from Kay *et al.* (1964a) by permission of *The British Journal of Psychiatry*.)

suggested that there may be a slightly greater age-specific risk for females (e.g. Kay *et al.*, 1964a; Åkesson, 1969). There is general greement, however (e.g. Kay *et al.*, 1964a; Hagnell, 1970), that cerebrovascular disease is much more common in males (Table 4).

The preponderance of females is also explained by the fact that females with AD survive longer following diagnosis (Larsson *et al.*, 1963; Heston *et al.*, 1981; Barclay *et al.*, 1985: Table 5). The reason for this is open to speculation, but it is probably due to the fact that male demented patients tend to be in relatively poor physical condition generally. In one study of 100 consecutive patients referred to a psychogeriatric service from a district general hospital (Fraser and Healy, 1986), physical illness clustered strongly among males; other studies have revealed a similar pattern (New York Department of Mental Hygiene, 1961; Lowenthal and Berkman, 1967). Men who are now in their 70s and 80s worked in conditions very different from those of the present day, smoked too much and ingested too much carbohydrate — the latter often as beer — but perhaps relatively more than women in any case, since the latter were always 'figure-conscious'. It may be that some of these differences will

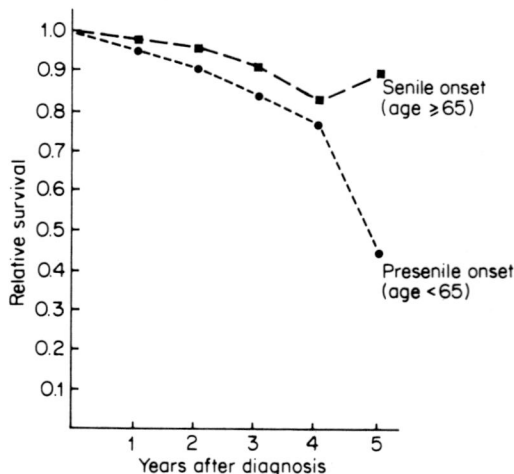

Figure 1   Relative survival in dementia (survival compared with that of age-matched controls). (Reproduced from Barclay *et al.* (1985) by permission of the publisher. © 1985 Elsevier Scientific Publishing Co., Inc.)

Table 5. Relative survival in Alzheimer's disease patients

Factor		N	Surviving 500 days (%)	Surviving 1000 days (%)
Age at onset	65−	56	83*	59*
	65+	143	89	59
Sex	M	71	84†	49‡
	F	128	99	96
Duration (years)	2−	57	91	57
	5+	47	80	54
All		199	88	65

* Difference non-significant (but see Figure 1).
† Difference significant at 1% level.
‡ Difference significant at 0.1% level.
(Derived from Barclay *et al.* (1985) and reproduced by permission of the publishers. © 1985 Elsevier Science Publishing Co. Inc.)

even out as dietary, occupational and other habits change, but some authorities believe not; many of the differences in habits persist, and new differences are emerging: men still drink and smoke more than women, and they also use more illicit drugs and drive more (Hazzard, 1984; Nathanson, 1984).

There is no clear evidence that social class, poverty, unemployment, isolation or malnutrition make for an increased risk of AD; although these factors have been found in association with dementia, they are more likely to be the result rather than the cause of it (Kay *et al.*, 1964b; Bergmann, 1977). Gruenberg (1954) found that there was a relatively high rate of first mental hospital admissions with senile and arteriosclerotic psychoses from inner city areas where there was overcrowding and poverty, but this does not, of course, reflect a relatively high prevalence of these conditions. More recent studies carried out in rural areas and suburbs, however (Hagnell *et al.*, 1981; Clarke *et al.*, 1979, 1984), have found a relatively low prevalence of dementia; the fact that the studies of the 60s and 70s were carried out in inner city areas might have been a distorting factor, and it is possible that the overall prevalence of dementia in the UK might not be as high as has been believed.

But the question is still open. Torak (1978) found that the prevalence rate of AD in an upper-middle-class community was similar to those reported from more heterogeneous populations, and concluded that 'optimal socioeconomic status and environment' does not appear to be a deterrent to the evolution of Alzheimer's disease'. In the same way, Larsson *et al.* (1963) found that there was no over-representation of patients from lower socioeconomic groups; occupational status (or previous occupational status) among 168 male patients with a diagnosis of senile dementia was distributed much as in the general population. Single females with dementia appeared to present a lower socioeconomic status but, as many had not been employed, the group as a whole was difficult to 'place'. The authors concluded that occupational status probably has no influence on the onset of senile dementia. Patients from lower socioeconomic groups were, however, much more likely to be admitted to hospital when they had developed dementia.

Where are the demented?

Kay *et al.* (1964b) found that fewer than one-fifth of their patients with a diagnosis of organic brain syndrome (including both arteriosclerotic and senile dementia) were in institutional care. However, half of the organic brain syndrome patients in the community showed severe deterioration to a degree usually found in demented hospital patients.

But severity of dementia does at least partly determine hospital admission, as one might expect. During a four-year period, 58 per cent of elderly patients with chronic brain failure were admitted to hospital at some time, as compared with 22 per cent of controls. Comparative figures for admission to a long-stay unit (geriatric or mental hospital or day placement) were 54 per cent as compared with 7.3 per cent (Bergman, 1977). Taking the figures together, elderly patients with chronic brain failure were two-and-a-half times as likely to be admitted to hospitals or homes, where they spent in all six times as long as those without chronic brain failure.

The Kay study found a considerable sex difference among dementing patients living alone. Whilst 24 per cent of the normal male elderly and 29 per cent of the normal female elderly lived alone, none of the dementing males and 53 per cent of the dementing females lived alone. Gaspar (1980), in a survey of 230 referrals to a dementia service, found that while only 16 per cent of the male dementia patients lived alone, 33 per cent of the female dementia patients did so; 56 per cent of the male patients lived with a spouse, but only 26 per cent of the female patients did so. Analysing these differences, Gilleard (1984) concludes that data on living arrangements of the demented elderly seem simply to reflect general demographic patterns. The 1980/81 General Household Survey indicated, for example, that 17 per cent of all elderly males lived alone, whereas 45 per cent of elderly females did so. Also, 70 per cent of elderly males lived with their spouses, as compared to only 37 per cent of females.

There is, in fact, no 'typical' carer, and the common stereotype of the single woman who has sacrificed marriage and career prospects to look after an elderly mother can be misleading. Of those who care for elderly relatives, 41 per cent are men — though it is also the case that men are more likely to receive outside help (Equal Opportunities Commission, 1984).

There is a high prevalence of dementia in wards for the physically ill elderly and in old people's homes. Dementia is present in at least one-third of patients under the care of geriatricians in long-stay wards, and it may often be the key disability determining the need for institutional care (Denham and Jefferys, 1972; Pasker *et al.*, 1976). Mann *et al.* (1984a) examined 438 residents of homes for the elderly in the London Borough of Camden and found that one-third were suffering from severe dementia and another third from mild or moderate dementia. In 1972 Meacher found that 16 per cent of residents in 11 old people's homes showed some form of confused behaviour; this figure cannot be taken to represent the proportion of residents who were suffering from dementia (which would almost certainly be greater), but there is little doubt that the numbers of demented residents in such homes has increased substantially in recent years. In 1979 Clarke *et al.* found substantial dependency among 2248 residents of local authority homes (at least 25 per cent were occasionally incontinent, for example), but there are no figures specifically for dementia.

There are certain national differences in the pattern of institutional care. Mann *et al* (1984b) examined the mental status of random samples of elderly females in residential care and in long-stay nursing care in London, New York and Mannheim (Table 6). The percentage of patients with established dementia in residential care was much higher in London than in the other two cities; this difference probably reflects the relatively poor nursing home provision for the elderly in the UK, especially for the elderly mentally ill. The next few years are likely to see at least some nursing home provision for the latter group; the figures for dementia in local authority homes are alarmingly high, given that such homes were not planned for people with severe mental infirmity.

It is nevertheless the case that the majority of those with dementia, even severe dementia, live at home and are cared for by their relatives. It is a common belief that present-day Western families do not care for their elderly as they did in the past, or as families in other cultures do, but there is a good deal of evidence that makes this belief difficult to sustain. Laslett (1977) examined the patterns of family life during the seventeenth and eighteenth centuries and found it difficult to confirm, for example, that jobs were given up any more readily in the past than in the present so that elderly relatives could be cared for; he reached a general conclusion that younger people in these earlier generations behaved towards their elderly 'very much as we behave now . . . no better and no worse'. Townsend (1957), in a study of the family life of old people in East London, found no evidence that the ties of kinship between the old and the young had altered. He wrote:

> 'The extended family is slowly adjusting to new circumstances, not disintegrating. To the old person as much as the young it seems to be the supreme comfort and support. Its central purpose remains as strong as ever.'

Rosenmayr (1983) has examined the status of the elderly in a wide range of historical cultures, from Ancient Egypt through Judaism, the Roman Empire, and the European Middle Ages, to the present. He concludes:

> 'The aged have never been valued separately from their usefulness to society. The aged who were rich in knowledge, power and property enjoyed high esteem. But it is nothing more than a retrospective myth that old people earlier in history generally enjoyed high esteem and good treatment.'

Coming to the present day, Jones and Vetter (1985) describe a detailed study

Table 6.   Patterns of institutional care
(Percentage of residents with established dementia)

	New York	London	Mannheim
Residential care	3.3	16.9	5.9
Nursing care	23.6	27.5	25.4
Totals	15.9	21.0	15.8

(Reproduced from Mann *et al.* (1984b) by permission of the authors and Springer-Verlag)

of 1079 old people in Cardiff aged over 70, and find no support for the view that families neglect their elderly relatives; the indications are that carers support elderly dependants at great cost to themselves and with inadequate support from community services; it is suggested that GPs, having the only available register of people over 65 living in the community, should monitor more closely the need for such support and its provision.

So what factors other than severity of dementia (with problems such as wandering or incontinence) determine admission to hospital or residential care? Clearly, one is that no family carers may exist — but even where they do, the acceptability of a patient at home is surprisingly independent of his level of disability; Eagles and Gilleard (1985) have found that 'social' factors could be more important than 'medical' factors in determining whether a demented patient was discharged from hospital; the relatives' attitude towards the patient mattered more than the patient's behaviour as measured objectively.

What has shaped these attitudes? No research has so far given a clear answer, but it is very often the case that in families with a permanently hospitalized demented relative there have been long-standing domestic or marital difficulties upon which the old person's illness has been imposed as the 'last straw'. A key relative may himself be ill or, sometimes, a parent may be recalled as harsh and tyrannical when the family was young. I have recently come across a family where the father appears to have behaved incestuously over 40 years ago and another where it was said that, in the remote past, the mother had spent the family's meagre funds on alcohol. In both cases a patient with only a moderate degree of dementia had to be hospitalized; these grievances were in due course acknowledged by the families with great bitterness. In the case of a childless couple, where a wife with mild dementia was hospitalized, mutual accusations of impotence and frigidity were resurrected after nearly 60 years.

All instances are not as extreme, but many such conflicts, greater or lesser, all of long duration, have become woven into the family mythology, and little can be done about them. The importance in discovering the hidden element among all the factors that have brought the patient into hospital is that the clinician can be enabled to plan rather more realistically for the patient's future, rather than to struggle incomprehendingly in a situation where goodwill and co-operation are unlikely to be forthcoming.

The changing scene

It is well known that the elderly population is increasing; current projections indicate that the over-65 population of the UK as a whole will increase only by a modest degree (about 7 per cent) over the next 25 years, and that there will be a decrease in the number of those in the 65–74 age-group, but there will be a 7 per cent increase in those aged 75–84 and a 34 per cent increase in those aged 85 and over (Office of Population Censuses and Surveys, 1983). There will, as a result, be a greater proportion of 'old old' in the community. On the global scale, epidemiologists have predicted that reduced mortality in both the early and late stages of the life-cycle will result in the histogram of life-spans becoming increasingly gaussian about a mode of 70–80 years (Shepherd, 1984).

Where dementia is concerned, it has been calculated on the basis of current prevalence figures that over the next 25 years the absolute number of those affected will increase by about 50 per cent in the developed industrial countries and will more than double in the developing world. In 20 years' time, three-fifths of all people aged over 60 will be in countries at present classed as 'developing' (WHO, 1969; Kramer, 1980; Cooper and Bickel, 1984).

Projections based on present-day prevalence rates may not be altogether accurate. As suggested earlier, very old people of today, having survived other pathological hazards, could be as a group relatively resistant to dementia; future generations of the very old might therefore contain a greater proportion of demented people, especially those with AD. So, for example, the prevalence rate for dementia in those aged 80 and over could rise from its present 20 per cent to 25–30 per cent. These percentages would be further inflated by the trend for people to live longer following a diagnosis of dementia. Blessed and Wilson (1982) (Table 7) reviewed 320 patients over 65 and over who had been admitted to a mental hospital during 1976. They compared outcome patterns for those for patients admitted during 1948/49 (Roth, 1955), and found that the two-year survival of patients admitted with dementia had increased by 14 per cent, this difference being largely accounted for by the increased long-term survival of very elderly females with Alzheimer-type dementia. It is likely, the authors conclude, that the condition is 'a less fatal disease than hitherto'. Their impression is that 'old people entering a mental hospital are likely to be older than their predecessors 25 years ago, more likely to suffer from an organic dementia, and more likely to survive in a state which demands continuing care in an institution'.

Christie (1982) also carried out a partial replication of Roth's 1955 study in order to examine the changing pattern of mental illness in the elderly over a 25-year-period; he found that the death rate of demented patients at two years following admission had fallen from 87 per cent to 55 per cent (i.e. an increase in the two-year survival rate of 32 per cent). Sex differences were not reported. Christie and Train (1984) subsequently compared the progress of 82 demented female patients admitted to the same hospital during the period 1957–59 with 107 similar female patients admitted during 1974–76, and found an overall

34

Table 7. Survival of hospitalized demented patients

Study	Year of admission	N	Survival at 6 months (%)	Survival at 2 years (%)
Roth (1955)	1948/49	76	42	18
Christie and Train (1984)	1957/59	82*	79	42
Christie (1982)	1974/76	107*	85	50
Blessed and Wilson (1982)	1976	320	71	32

* Female patients.

increase of 24 per cent in the mean duration of survival. The increase was greatest in patients aged over 85 with senile dementia. Eagles and Gilleard (1984) compared the outcome for demented elderly patients admitted to a short-stay unit during 1977–78 with those admitted during 1981/82. The median length of stay had increased by some 42 per cent and there was significantly greater disability on discharge in the second group, with a larger proportion of patients in the second group discharged to long-stay psychiatric care (an increase from 49 per cent to 76 per cent).

Given that dementia remains resistant to medical treatment, there is little to set against the gloomy figures summarized in Table 7. The future burden of care may be lightened in that, by the end of the century, more old people will have been married and a higher proportion of them will have had children (Leading Article, 1979a); single or childless status strongly determines admission to institutional care (Eagles and Gilleard, 1984). Shulman and Arie (1978) showed that admission rates of old people to psychiatric hospitals fell steadily during the years 1970–74, but the authors believe that this is not to be interpreted optimistically; the probable reason was a growing reluctance to admit the elderly demented to such institutions. There is every indication that the demented are increasingly finding their way into other forms of institutional care (p. 30), and an increasing responsibility is bound also to fall on domiciliary services, since even at present 80 per cent of all those aged 85 and over live in private households (Royal College of Physicians, 1981).

Will the human life-span continue to become ever longer, bringing about an almost limitless increase in the proportion of people at risk for dementia? Hayflick, a gerontologist, believes not (1983); although life expectancy has increased, he asserts, human life-span has remained virtually unchanged from the beginning of recorded history. The conquest of disease results simply in more people reaching what appears to be an 'immutable' upper age-limit. In the course of experiments carried out over 20 years, he observed that cultured human cells were capable of only a finite number of reproductive doublings, and concludes that both this loss of reproductive capacity and the loss of a range of functional capacities in non-dividing cells represent the central mechanisms

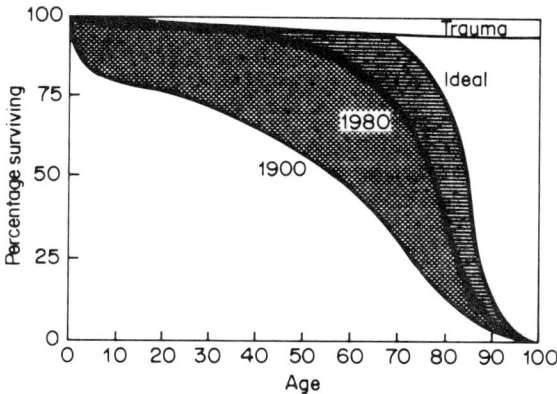

Figure 2   The increasingly rectangular survival curve. About 80 per cent (stippled area) of the difference between the 1900 curve and the ideal curve (stippled area plus hatched area) had been eliminated by 1980. Trauma is now the dominant cause of death in early life. (Reproduced from Fries (1980) by permission of *The New England Journal of Medicine*.)

of ageing. In a further series of investigations, he and his co-workers localized the age-clock first to the cell, then to the nucleus; even when old cells are transplanted into young tissue, or old nuclei into young cytoplasm, the nuclear 'death-clock' ticks inexorably on.

In an article which created considerable interest and debate, Fries (1980) set out the concept of 'rectangularization' as applied to the human life-span. From examination of mortality figures throughout the present century, he suggests that morbidity has progessively been compressed into the last few years of life, and predicts that this trend will continue (Figure 2). His radical conclusion is therefore that the medical conquest of disease would not result in an ever-older and more feeble population but would bring about a tendency towards one in which life remained fairly full until about the age of 85, when everything would 'come apart at once'.

This conclusion (based partly on Hayflick's work) has been challenged both on biological and on statistical grounds. Schneider and Brody (1983) cite work which indicates that the lives of cell populations are not dependent on their capacity to replicate — though this was not altogether Hayflick's argument. But they go on to re-examine mortality statistics and discover a trend for the survival curve to 'de-rectangularize' at 85 and above. Grundy (1984) also suggests that Fries's 'optimistic' prediction may be based on faulty interpretation of the data. In the early part of the century, inflation of age at a census was a serious problem in England and Wales, for example; investigators who have taken into account this and other similar sources of error, writes Grundy, have concluded that there has been a real and significant fall in morbidity among those aged over 85, with no indication that mortality rates among the very old are reaching a ceiling.

The 'rectangularization' model is of course the more appealing to a clinician

— who must therefore be doubly wary of it — but it is, on the other hand, difficult to believe in the infinitely extensible human life-span and to accept that such factors as, for instance, the widespread attrition of connective tissue and loss of immune capacity that has occurred by the tenth decade even in healthy individuals can be argued away by means of statistical projections.

The debate is an intriguing one, but the question is not altogether one of whether a doctor dealing with the elderly has simply to prevent his patient foundering in Fries's Bermuda Triangle of morbidity or to care for an ever-elongating 'tail' of the very old and enfeebled; the question being addressed here, in particular, is whether the quality of mental life can be maintained in either case — this more than anything else by the prevention or more effective management of dementia. Or, as an elderly patient of mine put it, 'I just want to keep all my wits until the Almighty finally taps me on the shoulder'.

SUMMARY AND CONCLUSIONS

Dementia is defined as acquired brain disease which is both diffuse and chronic; the most common morphological type in adults of all ages is that originally described by Alzheimer, at present known variously as 'senile dementia', 'senile dementia of Alzheimer's type (SDAT)' or 'Alzheimer's disease (AD). The last term is likely in time to replace the others. The present book is concerned mainly with dementia of this type.

Only a minority of elderly people suffer from dementia of any type. Most people, even the very old, retain an adequate degree of mental capacity; only one octogenarian in five, for example, is significantly demented, and the expectation of dementia appears to fall off slightly in extreme old age. A disease model is therefore more appropriate for dementia than one in which severe mental impairment is seen as an inevitable part of the ageing process.

Alzheimer's disease accounts predominantly for about 55 per cent of all dementias, and in part for a further 20–25 per cent; damage is selective to higher brain functioning, with the result that the condition creates severe handicap in sufferers without a drastic reduction in life expectancy, making for heavy and long-term care commitments.

The cause of AD is still unknown; there may, however, be genetic vulnerability in three-quarters or more of all cases, the possible mechanism being a mendelian dominant with age-dependent penetrance, but there is no clear evidence to implicate factors that may either influence gene expression or act as independent causes of the disease. There are some similarities between the morphological features of AD and certain transmissible brain disorders, but these changes are non-specific, occurring across a wide range of brain disease, and they do not in themselves indicate an infective origin for AD. In addition, AD has not, as far as is known, been passed from one host to another by way of the known mechanisms of disease transmission. The search for other possible causes of AD has proved equally unrewarding and, in the medium term, investigation of the biochemical abnormalities that underlie the *symptoms* of the disease is more likely to lead to some means of managing it effectively.

The prevalence of all forms of dementia in populations aged 65 and over is in the range 5–7 per cent; age-related prevalence thereafter rises steeply until age 85–90 and then levels out or falls off slightly. The lifetime expectancy of dementia is about 1.8 per cent for males and 2.1 per cent for females.

The age-specific rates for AD in males and females do not appear to differ substantially. Females are, however, at greater lifetime risk due to relative female longevity; females with the disease also survive longer. Social class, environment and culture do not appear to be risk factors for AD.

Less than one-fifth of patients with AD are in institutional care; patients in an institution are not necessarily more demented than those being cared for at home. Social and family factors strongly determine patterns both of admission and of discharge.

The proportion of people at maximum risk for AD (i.e. those aged 75 and over) will increase until about the year 2000. There will, for example, be a 34 per cent increase in those aged 85 and over during this period, and the life expectancy of demented patients in this age-group is also expected to increase.

If AD remains resistant to treatment, it can be calculated that overall provision for the demented elderly will need to be expanded by some 20 per cent over the course of the next 25 years simply to maintain current levels of care. There is, however, decreasing utilization of mental hospital beds for the demented, and the number of such beds in the UK is being reduced. There will therefore be an acute need for more and better nursing homes and other residential provision for the demented, and even more for an expansion of domiciliary care.

CHAPTER 2

Alzheimer's disease: the biochemical lesion

Investigation of the biochemical changes that underlie Alzheimer's disease is, for the clinician, an examination of the seductive possibility that there is at some point in the chain of causation leading to cell death an abnormality which could be rectified. Lack of knowledge of the primary cause of the disease would not necessarily be an obstacle; medicine abounds in instances of diseases whose cause is either unknown or impossible to eradicate, but which can be treated with partial or even complete success. Examples are:

(a) Correction of a neurotransmitter imbalance (models: Parkinson's disease, myasthenia gravis).
(b) Replacement of a deficient hormone (diabetes, hypothyroidism).
(c) Damage limitation by nutritional or dietary means (phenylketonuria, alcoholism).
(d) Prevention by vaccination (measles encephalitis, rabies).
(e) Slowing down of an irreversible process (steroids in brain tumour).
(f) Genetic counselling (Down's syndrome, Huntingdon's chorea).
(g) Alleviation of some symptoms (Huntingdon's chorea, idiopathic epilepsy).
(h) Surgery (brain tumour, hydrocephalus).
(i) Avoidance of a toxin (alcoholism, lead and aluminium encephalopathies).

Most of the above conditions represent or cause severe brain disease, but all can be medically controlled. By contrast, the 'treatments' for AD remain in general primitive and haphazard — either largely untried 'cerebral enhancers' or a range of tranquillizers that are as likely to make the patient's confusion worse as to bring about any benefit. Interest has in recent years been focused on the possibility of correcting neurotransmitter abnormalities which may underlie the condition, but a problem is that in established AD there has already been massive and widespread brain damage (and probably cell death) on a scale far exceeding that in, say, Parkinson's disease, so very little could be expected from interventions in brain biochemistry; given the unique vulnerability of brain cells, the effectiveness of therapy will have to depend on early diagnosis to perhaps a greater degree than in any other condition. At the stage when dementia is commonly diagnosed at present, the most that can be hoped for is that the process of destruction may be halted or at least slowed down. Even this hope requires many assumptions, one being that neurotransmitters are trophic to brain cells. Many treatments being evaluated at present are directed towards neurotransmitter replenishment, and it is not yet clear whether these are simply messenger substances or whether they contribute to brain cell metabolism. Even if they do not, however, such trials can rationally proceed on the theoretical basis that, even in the presence of established or progressive brain damage, correction of certain known neurotransmitter abnormalities will bring about clinical improvement. In the medium term, most clinicians would happily settle for such an objective, and it may — in the medium term — be attainable.

It would be convenient to view AD as a 'clean' disorder —that is, one associated with a specific chemical defect — but it is now evident that there is more than one abnormality, and probably an array of abnormalities, each in ascending neuronal clusters which are largely distinct from one another. To complicate matters further, there may be at least two subtypes of AD distinguished by different degrees of degeneration in neurotransmitter systems and a difference in clinical course and prognosis. There is nevertheless extensive common ground among neurochemists; it is generally agreed that in AD there are widespread abnormalities in the cholinergic transmitter system and, to a lesser extent, in the noradrenergic system.

THE CHOLINERGIC SYSTEM

Acetylcholine metabolism

Acetylcholine was the first neurotransmitter to be identified; it is the neuro-transmitter for voluntary movement, and it is released by the end-plate termination for axons from the anterior horn cells of the spinal cord on to striated muscle. Its activity at the neuromuscular junction has been intensively studied; to this work we owe a great deal of our understanding of the mechanism of synaptic transmission generally. Within the past decade or so, mainly because of the apparent association between acetylcholine and AD, considerable attention has been given to the mapping out of cholinergic neurone systems within the brain.

Acetylcholine is synthesized mainly in cholinergic nerve terminals by the action of the enzyme choline acetyltransferase on choline and acetyl coenzyme A (Figure 3). Choline is present in a variety of foods (e.g. egg yolk, soya beans and liver) and is taken up from the blood either as free choline or in its lipid-bound form phosphatidylcholine (lecithin). Choline acetyltransferase (CAT) is probably metabolized in the nerve-cell body and transferred to the nerve ending by means of axonal transport; the source of acetyl coenzyme A is

Choline   Phospholipid choline (lecithin)

Choline

+   Glucose

Acetyl coenzyme A

Choline acetyltransferase

Acetylcholine

Choline   Acetate

Receptor
(nicotinic or muscarinic)

Acetylcholinesterase

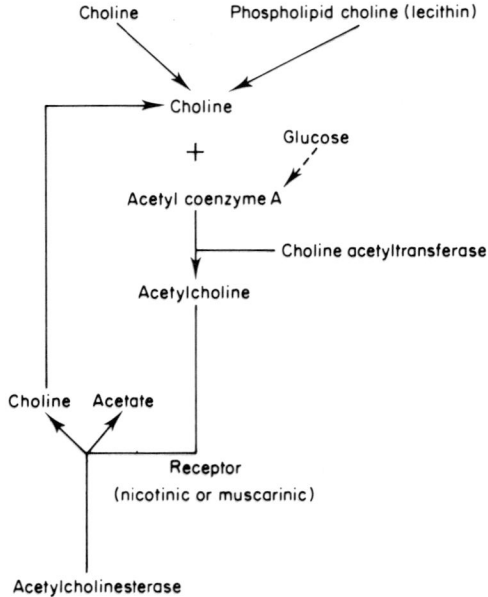

Figure 3   Choline metabolism.

not altogether clear, but it is at least partly derived from brain glucose (Tucek, 1978). The catalytic action of CAT combines the acetyl portion of the coenzyme with the choline to form the acetylcholine molecule.

Acetylcholine has generally been visualized as stored in the synaptic vesicles of neurones which are purely cholinergic, although it is possible that some is stored in cytoplasm (Dunant and Israel, 1985), and also that Dale's principle (that a neurone releases only one neurotransmitter from all its terminals) cannot be rigidly applied, since additional messenger substances may coexist in the same neurones with acetylcholine (for a review, see Iversen, 1979). It can be said, however, that there are distinct cell populations whose mode of synaptic transmission is predominantly cholinergic. Acetylcholine (ACh) is released into the synaptic cleft on the arrival of the electrical impulse at the nerve terminal and binds to the ACh receptor; these receptors are huge protein molecules partly embedded in the postsynaptic membrane, protruding slightly above the surface, iceberg-fashion. They are of two kinds, nicotinic and muscarinic, and the action of ACh on both is excitatatory. ('Nicotinic' and 'muscarinic' mean that ACh action on each type of receptor mimics the action of nicotine and muscarine respectively.) By binding to the receptors, the ACh molecules change the receptors' configuration and open a chemical 'gate' that allows ion passage, with consequent excitation of the postsynaptic neurone. The ACh is subsequently inactivated by acetylcholinesterase, contained mainly in the postsynaptic membrane but also found in the presynaptic terminal, its purpose there probably being to destroy ACh which is produced in excess of vesical storage capacity (Shaw et al., 1982). The ACh is split into choline and acetate, and the choline is reabsorbed into the presynaptic terminal.

Distribution of cholinergic neurones

Cholinergic nerve terminals are widely distributed in the cerebral cortex and in the basal forebrain, especially the hippocampus, but their origin seems to be essentially subcortical. The ascending cholinergic fibres appear to arise in a relatively small cluster of nuclei in the septal region and the structures adjacent to it. The septum, a vertical sheet of grey matter traversed by many fibres, is located in the medial wall of the anterior horn of the lateral ventricle, mainly in front of the anterior commissure. It contains the *septal nuclei*, the main source of cholinergic afferents to the hippocampus. The cell–body complex incorporating the septal nuclei extends posteriorly and ventrally to form the *nucleus of the diagonal band* and the *nucleus basalis of Meynert*; the two latter appear to be the principal sources of the cholinergic projections to the cerebral cortex (Figure 4). These are the major cholinergic pathways; others, especially within the limbic system, have been identified and mapped in detail (Brodal, 1981), although our understanding of the system is still incomplete due to the lack of a consistent and reliable method of localizing cholinergic neurones. Acetylcholine itself cannot be directly identified, and it therefore has to be located by means of identification of 'markers'; the enzyme choline acetyltransferase (CAT) is, for example, a reliable marker for ACh, and in one method acetyl coenzyme A is trapped with lead as it is released from CAT. Or a reaction may be stimulated by the preparation of an antibody to CAT (Kuhar and Atweh, 1978).

Much of our present knowledge about the cholinergic system comes from work on mammalian brains; means of mapping out neurotransmitter pathways in the human are still in a state of evolution. Techniques for neurotransmitter assay in preserved human post-mortem tissue need to be perfected — a problem being, for example, that ACh is rapidly hydrolysed after death (Richter et al., 1980) — and safe, non-invasion techniques that can be applied to the living brain are even further away, although NMR spectroscopy (p. 141) may provide some indirect information. As indicated earlier, however, almost all of the work now proceeding in the area has been stimulated by the group of observations which have associated abnormalities in the cholinergic system with the symptoms of AD and which are usually referred to collectively, though not very accurately, as the 'choline hypothesis'. Does this lead to the much sought after 'specific defect'?

The cholinergic system and Alzheimer's disease

The evidence which links AD with cholinergic system defects falls generally into two categories. First, there is now an immense literature describing cell damage or biochemical change which is relatively restricted to the cholinergic

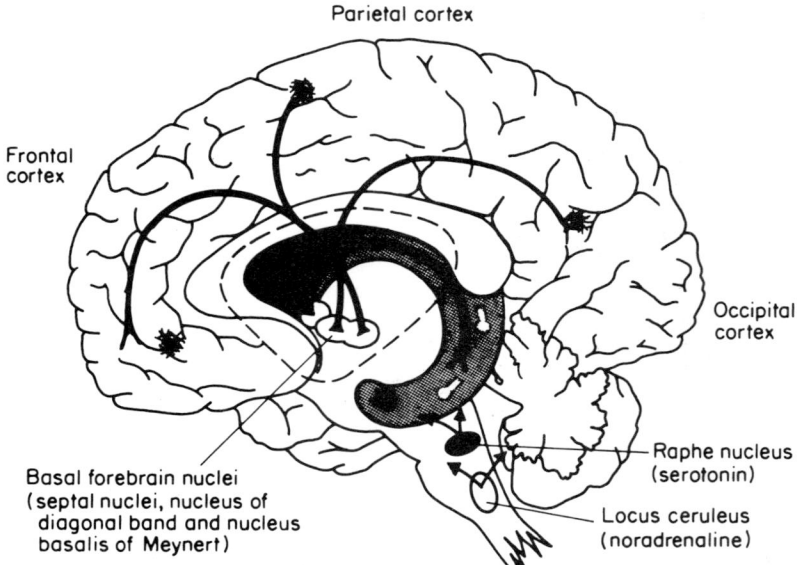

Figure 4 The central cholinergic pathways. (Reproduced from Davison, 1985, by permission of the author and the Medical Tribune Group.)

system, at least in the early stages of AD. These alterations have been shown to correspond closely with the clinical features of the disease, both in terms of the sites of damage and its degree. A good deal of this work depends (as did the initial identification of the cholinergic pathways) on assay of key enzymatic markets, such as choline acetyltransferase and acetylcholinesterase.

Second, evidence has come from 'challenge tests' which examine the effects of substances that act as agonists or antagonists within the cholinergic system. A study within this category might, for example, test the hypothesis that an acetylcholine antagonist will induce a 'model dementia'.

Selective damage

Bowen and Davison (1977) estimated cell loss in AD. They measured levels of chemical markers for nerve cells (there being no direct means of estimating atrophy under the microscope) and concluded that in AD about half of the cells were lost, as compared with numbers in normal (biopsy) controls. They estimated numbers of CAT-containing and GABA-containing neurones and concluded that the former were selectively vulnerable. Davies (1977) also evaluated the status of neurotransmitter systems in autopsied AD brains. As compared with controls, there were reductions to less than 25 per cent of normal values in the activity of CAT and acetylcholinesterase (ACE) in the hippocampal, frontal and parietal cortices. Perry and Perry (1977) examined the activity of various enzymes in post-mortem brains of patients with AD, multi-infarct dementia, depression and schizophrenia, and found significant

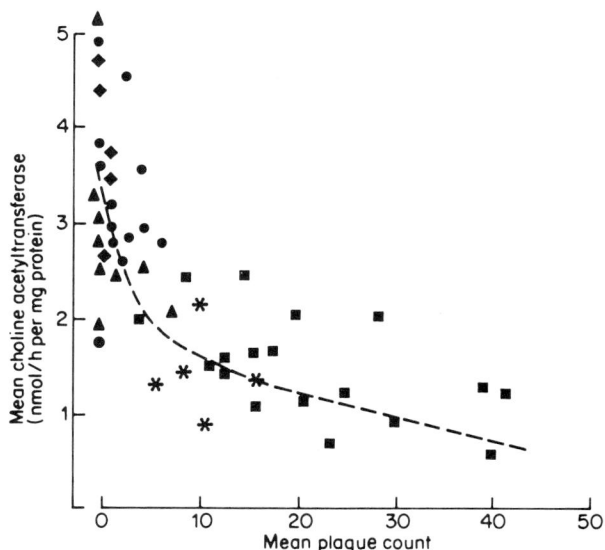

Figure 5 Choline acetyltransferase (CAT) activity and plaque formation in the neocortex. Individual plaque counts plotted against mean cortical enzyme activities in 51 cases. ●, normal; ▲, depression; ♦, multi-infarct dementia; ■, Alzheimer's disease. The correlation between CAT and plaque is significant for the entire series and for the 23 cases of Alzheimer's disease. (Reproduced from Perry and Perry (1980) by permission of the publishers. © John Wiley & Sons Limited.)

reductions in CAT levels almost solely in the AD brains. The loss was greatest in the hippocampal area. In the only major study of biopsies from living brain AD tissue, Bowen *et al.* (1982) examined surplus tissue from a number of cortical biopsies and compared several indices of ACh synthesis in samples showing AD changes (21) with those in the remainder (15). These were frontal and temporal biopsies, and in both areas there was significant reduction of ACh synthesis in the AD group.

CAT activity is selectively decreased in areas already known to be selectively affected in AD — mainly the frontal and temporal cortices and, more particularly, the hippocampus. Perry and Perry (1980) showed that CAT activity falls to about half as the plaque count rises above the normal range, and falls steeply as the plaque count rises further (Figure 5). Compared with changes in other cholinergic activities, CAT deficiency appears to be an early change, if plaque count is to be taken as a time-base for the disease (Perry *et al.*, 1978). CAT loss was also shown to correlate positively with intellectual impairment, in the same way as does plaque count (Roth *et al.*, 1967). Measuring levels of the other main marker enzyme ACE in the hippocampus, Perry *et al.* (1980) found a general reduction in ACE staining, but positive ACE staining in the processes of senile plaques, suggesting that these were derived from damaged cholinergic nerve-endings. There were also abundant neurofibrillary tangles in the hippocampus, which almost invariably shows severe damage in AD (Ball *et al.*, 1985; Collerton and Fairbairn, 1985).

The ACh defect is more likely to be one of synthesis in the cell body than one of axonal transport; there is no evidence of ACh accumulation in the axon (Perry and Perry, 1980). Also, ligand binding studies have indicated that the ACh receptors remain intact (Bowen, 1980). By contrast, there are marked changes in the cell bodies from which the cholinergic fibres originate. Clark *et al.* (1983) found severe neurone depopulation in the nucleus basalis of Meynert (nbM), and Mann and Yates (1982) also found neuronal loss in the nbM. Mann and Yates measured CAT levels in the nuclei of the septal region (which group includes the nbM), together with other indices of cell population in necropsy specimens from AD patients, multi-infarct dementia and controls; significant changes were found only in the AD brains, again indicating reduced levels of functioning in these key cholinergic cell bodies.

'Challenge' tests

It has been known for some time that hyoscine (scopolamine) premedication may impair recall of events immediately preceding anaesthesia (Hardy and Wakely, 1962; Pandit and Dundee, 1970). Experimental studies later confirmed that hyoscine, which blocks muscarinic ACh receptors, causes memory defects in young normal subjects similar to those found in (normal) elderly subjects (Drachman and Leavitt, 1974). Comparison of its effect with that of hyoscine methobromide (methscopolamine), which does not enter the central nervous system, showed impairment of memory storage and cognitive non-memory tasks only on admistration of hyoscine; there was no effect on immediate memory.

The effect of hyoscine on memory function was examined by Crow *et al.* (1982); the group confirmed an effect on delayed recall as opposed to immediate recall; further tests showed that this specific effect on delayed recall did not occur with amylobarbitone, diazepam or chlorpromazine; the effect of these drugs on delayed recall was either insignificant (diazepam) or was associated with more widespread cognitive impairment (amylobarbitone and chlorpromazine).

Conversely, physostigmine, an ACE inhibitor, and arecoline, a choline agonist at muscarinic sites, have been shown to enhance memory in normal young subjects (Davies *et al.*, 1976; Sitaram *et al.*, 1978). The effect is again specifically on ability to assimilate new information into long-term memory; the drugs do not enhance short-term memory.

Inability to transfer information from short-term to long-term storage is highly characteristic of AD (Baddeley and Warrington, 1970). Short-term memory, a matter only of seconds, is often tested by measuring a subject's 'digit span'; that is, asking him to repeat a series of unrelated numbers immediately after the examiner — usually eight to ten numbers in all. An AD patient might well have no difficulty on a digit span test, but might have much more difficulty in dialling the same numbers on a telephone (because of the inevitable slight delay between each digit). This test, using a circular telephone dial, is used in some test batteries which have been assembled to elicit evidence of dementia. This and other tests of 'delayed recall' are described in more detail on p. 111.

A similar defect has been observed in patients with hippocampal lesions (Milner, 1970).

There is therefore wide agreement that reduced cholinergic activity is seen to occur in close parallel with the clinical changes characteristic of AD. There are other neurotransmitter abnormalities (to be described later), but those in the cholinergic system have been the most consistently associated with both the clinical symptoms and the known anatomical changes of the disease. Since the primary site of damage within the cholinergic system appears to be the cell bodies of the septal area, it has been suggested that AD could be considered as essentially a disease of subcortical origin — akin, for example, to Parkinson's disease and the dementia sometimes associated with it (Rossor *et al.*, 1981). In the present state of our knowledge this requires too many assumptions about cause and effect; neurotransmitter abnormalities can so far only be regarded as productive of the clinical symptoms of the AD, rather than of the underlying disease itself.

Can any of these symptoms be relieved by interventions within the cho-linergic system?

Treatment possibilities

There are three kinds of possibility. First, excess substrate (choline or lecithin) might be given in order to increase end-product (acetylcholine) synthesis; this is the strategy known as 'precursor loading'. Second, attempts might be made to enhance the effect of ACh on its muscarinic receptors, using choline agonists such as arecoline. Third, anticholinesterases such as physostigmine might be used in order to inhibit ACh breakdown. All of these possibilities have been tested by means of clinical trials, and some are still being tested.

Precursor loading

Neurotransmitter synthesis is not necessarily subject to precursor control. Excess precursor will stimulate increased production of ACh, for example, only if the enzyme system is not already fully saturated. Wurtman and Fernstrom (1976) were able to establish a positive relationship between choline dosage and the rate of cholinergic nerve firing (the means by which the neurone varies stimulus intensity) in experimental animals, suggesting that the precursor is indeed 'rate limiting' in that it will enhance ACh synthesis if given in excess. Labelled ACh is, in fact, found in the brains of experimental animals within minutes of the intravenous injection of labelled choline (Schuberth and

Jenden, 1975). Choline is also rapidly taken up from the gut, and in healthy human subjects levels of choline in the blood and central nervous system rise after oral administration by a degree that would be sufficient to increase the neuronal firing rate in experimental animals (Wurtman and Fernstrom, 1976).

In 1978 Smith *et al.* studied the effect of choline on ten patients with AD; this was a double-blind cross-over trial in which each patient received two weeks' treatment with oral choline and two with a matched placebo. The results were disappointing in that there were unwanted side-effects with choline treatment (gastric discomfort and exacerbation of existing incontinence), and no significant improvement on a battery of tests of cognitive function. The authors comment, however, that three patients seemed less confused after two weeks of choline treatment, but it seems exceedingly optimistic to have expected patients with established AD to improve over such a short period.

Later in 1978, Signoret *et al.* reported a trial of choline in patients with early AD — that is, patients who showed memory disturbance but little intellectual deterioration. There was slight improvement on some recall tests, with reporting of improvement in everyday memory by patients and their relatives; the effect on learning was greatest in patients under 65 with the least severe memory loss. The trial did not include a placebo group.

Other trials have evaluated choline therapy over slightly longer periods (reviewed by Chaqui and Levy, 1982), but none has shown clear benefit to AD patients and the experimental designs of most have been adversely criticized (Perry and Perry, 1980; Chaqui and Levy, 1982). One problem, for example, is that free choline in the blood apparently needs to be maintained at several times its normal level in order to increase ACh synthesis significantly (Levy, 1978), and it is probable that these levels were not maintained in clinical trials.

Choline is no longer, in any case, the precursor of choice for clinical trials. It is partly wasted in the gut by bacteria with the formation of trimethylamine derivatives (Marks *et al.*, 1978), which have an unfortunate fish-like odour (although this effect has not been apparent in all studies (Yates *et al.*, 1980)). Lecithin is more fully absorbed from the gut (Wurtman *et al.*, 1977); it may also be the case that neurones require at least some choline in the phosphatidyl form, since the latter is a constituent of cell membranes (Ceder and Schuberth, 1977; Wurtman, 1983).

Yates *et al.* (1980) studied the effects of choline and lecithin in 12 patients with a clinical diagnosis of AD with onset before the age of 65. This was a cross-over trial in which the patients were given choline or lecithin or no medication for periods of up to ten days. There were mild side-effects with both choline and lecithin (transient diarrhoea and faecal incontinence in one patient, but no urinary incontinence). Neither treatment showed a 'dramatic' effect — although again one wonders slightly at the degree of optimism required to expect such an effect in so short a time — but there was some suggestion of a positive response to lecithin in three patients with mild to moderate dementia; there were improved ratings for speech, orientation and praxis. There were improvements in nurses' overall ratings for both the choline and lecithin patients, although these were all inpatients doubtless becoming accustomed to the ward environment and getting to know the staff; there was no control group. The trial was not double-blind; neither was the trial of lecithin by Etienne *et al.* (1978), in which three out of seven patients showed improved new learning ability.

Little *et al.* (1984) and Levy (1985) have reported preliminary results from a double-blind placebo-controlled trial of lecithin with assessments at six months and a year; this investigation clearly does not have the serious methodological defects of earlier studies; it is also the first study to use a 90% pure lecithin preparation. The investigators have thus far found continuing behavioural improvement in 8 out of the 24 AD patients treated. The average age of the responders was 79, whereas the average age of the non-responders was 69. It is possible that there may be two subtypes of AD (see also p. 54): 'old' AD patients with relatively isolated cholinergic deficiency, and younger patients with additional neurotransmitter defects (in the noradrenergic system, for example). It is also possible — which complicates matters further — that there may be a 'therapeutic window' effect, where there is little benefit to patients who receive either too little or too much lecithin.

These aspects still have to be properly examined; the results of trials of choline and lecithin thus far are summarized in Table 8. A few trials show some promise, but a continuing obstacle is the difficulty and expense of preparing lecithin in a sufficiently purified form. There are, incidentally, some misunderstandings about lecithin; to biochemists it is a specific chemical compound, phosphatidylcholine, while to the food industry the term refers to a wide variety of substances, the phosphatides. There is understandable lay interest in nutrients that might be prophylactic for AD, but 'lecithin' preparations sold in health-food shops are probably much too impure to be of any value in this regard (Wurtman, 1983).

Choline agonists

Studies have measured the effect of *arecoline* (which enhances the effect of ACh at muscarinic receptors) on elderly humans and on young and aged primates. This might in theory be an effective therapy, since the receptors are intact — although it has been pointed out that such substances might have a paradoxical effect as a result of receptor flooding (Davis *et al.*, 1982). There has, however, been evidence of memory improvement in some studies. Bartus (1979), for example, compared the effects of choline, physostigmine and arecoline in aged monkeys and found significant improvement in the performance of delayed recall tasks with arecoline and a similar result (though with more individual variation) with physostigmine. Arecoline has also been shown to improve performance in serial learning in both young and elderly normal human subjects (Davis *et al.*, 1982).

Christie (1982), in a randomized double-blind trial, compared the effects of physostigmine and arecoline in 11 AD patients with onset of the condition

48

Table 8. Clinical trials of choline and lecithin

Study	Patients	Treatment	Response
Boyd *et al.* (1977)	7 advanced cases aged over 70	Choline chloride 5 g per day for 2 wk, 10 g per day for 2 wk	No change in psychological tests; some patients more manageable
Etienne *et al.* (1978)	3 advanced cases aged 76–86	Choline bitartrate 8 g per day for 8 wk	One patient slightly better on nurses' rating
Smith *et al.* (1978)	10 cases, mean age 77	Choline bitartrate 9 g per day for 2 wk, double-blind placebo	No improvement on psychological tests; three patients less confused
Signoret *et al.* (1978)	8 mixed cases, aged 59–78	Choline citrate 9 g per day for 3 wk	Three younger patients had improved short-term recall
Etienne *et al.* (1979)	7 cases, onset within 3 years, aged 42–81	Lecithin granules 25–100 g per day for 4 wk	Three patients had improved new learning
Yates *et al.* (1980)	12 cases aged 53–76, mean time since onset 3.8 years	Cross-over with choline chloride and lecithin granules	Improved behavioural scores in all groups; improved cognition in 3 lecithin patients
Little *et al.* (1984)	24 patients	90% pure lecithin double-blind placebo	Behavioural improvement in 8 patients, mainly younger group

(Partly based on Yates *et al.* (1980) and reproduced by permission of the publishers. © 1980 John Wiley & Sons Limited.)

before age 65. Both improved performance on picture recognition tests as compared with a placebo; the difference was statistically significant in patients receiving arecoline. The improvement was not great, however, and the memory of all patients remained grossly impaired as compared with normal subjects. Arecoline also has the disadvantage of a short half-life, and has to be given by infusion. It has been suggested that oxotremorine, a longer-acting muscarinic agonist, is more likely to prove clinically useful, but it has not yet been evaluated (Davis *et al.*, 1982).

Piracetam, a derivative of GABA, can be classified with the choline agonists although its mode of action is uncertain; it is said to increase synthesis of ATP and to augment the release of ACh in the hippocampus (Wurtman, 1982). Animal studies have shown that piracetam improves performance on memory tasks as compared with a placebo; its effect is greatly enhanced if it is combined with choline (Bartus and Lambert, 1978). Curiously, however, the drug appears to be effective only in 'naïve' laboratory animals (those newly arrived at the laboratory), as compared with those that are 'acclimatized'. Studies in humans have in general been disappointing, showing only some weak, stimulant-like effects on attention, on some performance measures and on memory retrieval; one double-blind cross-over trial found no improvement in an extensive battery of cognitive and behavioural tests (Ferris *et al.*, 1982). In a smaller open study of choline and piracetam combined, by the same investigators, there was, however, clinical improvement in 4 out of 15 patients, with marked improvement in memory storage and retrieval; this difference was greater than any that had been observed with either substance alone. The authors plan a larger double-blind trial.

Cholinesterase inhibitors

Physostigmine inhibits hydrolysis of ACh throughout the body although its peripheral action can be partially blocked by administration of hyoscine methobromide (methscopolamine), which does not cross the blood–brain barrier. It appears to potentiate ACh action in the cerebral cortex to a greater extent than does choline (Krnjević *et al.*, 1980), and in young normal subjects it has been shown, like hyoscine, to improve ability to store information in long-term memory (p. 110) without affecting either short-term memory or retrieval (Mohs *et al.*, 1982).

Smith *et al.* (1982) studied the effect of physostigmine in three patients with AD in a placebo-controlled double-blind trial but the results were disappointing, the only effect being suppression of incorrect responses in memory tests (in which the subjects were required to learn lists of words). A similar effect was noted by Peters and Levin (1979), who observed a reduction in the number of 'intrusion errors', but disadvantages were significantly increased ratings for depressed mood and, in one patient, worsening of parkinsonian features.

Davis *et al.* (1982) treated ten AD patients aged between 50 and 68 with intravenous physostigmine under double-blind conditions using three different dosage regimes, randomly administered. They found significantly improved performance on recognition memory tasks (involving long-term memory: p. 110) in all patients. In a partial replication, patients were given either a placebo or the dose of physostigmine previously associated with a good response; the latter again enhanced performance on a recognition memory task. The effect was transient, persisting only for the 30 minutes during which the drug was being administered, and test performance, though improved, was still impaired in comparison with that of non-demented subjects. The authors conclude that their results thus far are of theoretical rather than practical interest; the hypothesis that memory in AD patients might be improved by substances active in the cholinergic system could only be tested by the use of agents which elevate cholinergic activity over extended periods.

Physostigmine has been combined with choline and with lecithin (Peters and Levin, 1979), achieving some improvement in long-term memory with the second combination, but the problem of the short half-life of physostigmine (30 minutes) has not been surmounted and, even if the drug's peripheral side-effects are blocked with hyoscine methobromide (methscopolamine), there may still be a number of centrally mediated effects; Janowsky *et al.* (1985) observed 'profound' changes in adrenaline level, pulse rate and blood pressure in younger patients infused with physostigmine after administration of meth-scopolamine. Clearly such effects in the elderly would be highly undesirable.

To sum up, trials of cholinergic agents in the treatments of AD have been almost uniformly unrewarding thus far in terms of yielding treatment that might be clinically useful, although it has been suggested that such agents might be more effectively given in combination — for example, a choline precursor together with an anticholinesterase (Wurtman, 1982). But there is now a good deal of evidence that the biochemical defect in AD is not restricted to the cholinergic transmission system, so any benefits from treatments aimed purely at rectifying an ACh defect would probably be very small and might be outweighed by factors such as cost, difficulty in administration and toxicity. Effective drug treatments for AD will most likely have to take into account not one but a number of neurotransmitter defects. Evidence for the existence of these additional defects is set out in the following paragraphs.

THE NORADRENERGIC SYSTEM

Noradrenaline (NA) is synthesized from the amino acid tyrosine, a constituent of dietary protein. Tyrosine loading does not appear to have any effect on NA synthesis; hydroxylation appears to be the rate-limiting step (Green and Costain, 1981). In noradrenergic nerve-endings, NA is inactivated by a number of metabolic steps (monoamine oxidase is involved in the initial metabolism) to the end-product vanillylmandelic acid (VMA).

Noradrenergic cell bodies in the CNS are concentrated in the locus ceruleus (Figure 4), a nucleus in the mid-pontine region so called because of the cells' melanin content. Ascending noradrenergic fibres project widely to the cerebral cortex, hippocampus and cerebellum.

Crow *et al.* (1982) have reviewed work which suggests that this system functions as part of a reward mechanism and could be partly instrumental, as is the cholinergic system, in converting short-term changes in intracortical synapses into the longer-term changes assumed to underlie permanent memory. For example, inhibition of a NA-synthetic enzyme in turn inhibits the acquisition of a passive avoidance response in rats; this is reversed by intramuscular administration of NA, provided that administration immediately follows learning — which suggests a specific role for the system in short-term to long-term memory conversion. Lesioning studies have been less conclusive, but Crow *et al.* conclude from the evidence as a whole that the cerulocortical NA system is likely to play at least some part in the reward element in learning.

Defects in the NA system have been demonstrated in AD. In some patients with AD there were lowered levels of homovanillic acid (HVA) in the cerebrospinal fluid as compared to controls (Gottfries and Roos, 1973), though these results have not been confirmed in other studies (Parkes *et al.*, 1974; Fischer, 1975). However, Adolfsson *et al.* (1979) measured brain monoamine concentration *post mortem* in 19 patients with autopsy-proven AD and found significantly lowered levels of HVA (as compared with age-matched controls) in the basal ganglia. There was also some decrease in NA levels, with significant differences from normals in the putamen and frontal cortex. There was a positive correlation between reduction of NA level in the hypothalamus and the degree of cognitive impairment, which is noteworthy in view of the well-established role of the hypothalamus in learning.

Mann *et al.* (1980) found severe loss of cells from the locus ceruleus in AD patients, as did Tomonaga (1984). The second study established a correlation with senile plaque numbers. A similar correlation was suggested by the findings of Berger *et al* (1976), who demonstrated loss of the fluorescent varicosities associated with plaques together with loss of noradrenergic fibre fluorescence in the cerebral cortex. Winblad *et al.* (1982) found consistent reduction in NA levels in the hypothalamus, caudate nucleus, hippocampus and gyrus cinguli of AD patients; they also found that HVA levels in the caudate nucleus correlated negatively with intellectual impairment, and that patients with an early onset and early death showed lower concentrations of NA and HVA than did older demented patients. Since other monoamines and their metabolites were reduced in patients with early-onset AD, the authors suggest that these might represent a biochemically distinct group.

Noradrenergic receptors appear to be intact in AD (Perry, 1984). Some investigators (Sharma *et al.*, 1979) have found increased noradrenergic receptor binding, which may be compensatory, following lesions of the locus ceruleus.

Forms of therapy based on the presumed NA defect have not yet been considered; problems are that the system is resistant both to precursor loading and to monoamine oxidase inhibition.

THE DOPAMINERGIC SYSTEM

The cell bodies of dopaminergic neurones are clustered in two small regions of the mid-brain. These neurones project on to the corpus striatum (this is the system affected in Parkinson's disease) and on to the limbic system and the hypothalamus. Dopamine is synthesized as in Figure 6; it is subsequently degraded to homovanillic acid (HVA). As is the case with NA, the rate-limiting factors in synthesis are not clear; concentrations are not increased either by precursor loading or by monoamine oxidase inhibition (Wurtman and Fernstrom, 1976; Green and Costain, 1981).

Some of the investigators who measured other neurotransmitter activity have indicated that there may also be a dopaminergic defect in AD. Adolfsson *et al.* (1979) found significantly reduced levels of dopamine (DA) in the thalamus and pons, and reduced levels of HVA in the caudate nucleus and the

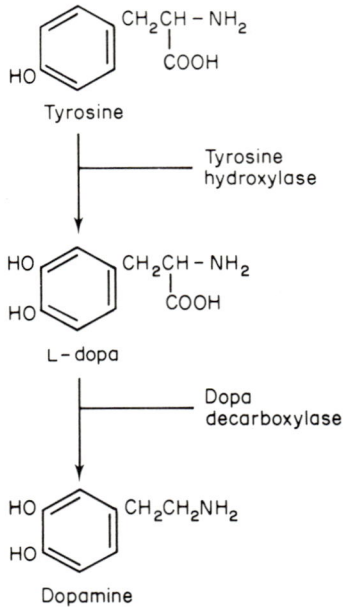

Figure 6   Synthesis of dopamine.

putamen; concentrations of HVA were lowest in the patients who were most severely intellectually impaired. Gottfries and Ross (1973) found a lowered level of HVA in the cerebrospinal fluid, and Fischer (1975) found that the urinary excretion of HVA was decreased in a group of demented patients as compared with controls. But Parkes *et al.* (1974) found no differences in cerebrospinal fluid HVA concentrations in AD patients as compared with age-matched normals. Diagnostic criteria in the two latter studies are not altogether clear.

Mann *et al.* (1980) found DA concentration in the frontal cortex, caudate nucleus and putamen to be reduced by an average of 26 per cent in three patients with AD as compared with age-matched controls, but there was no clear evidence of loss of dopaminergic cells. The authors suggest that this reduction in dopamine synthesis may be secondary to cholinergic damage, since there is some cholinergic innervation of the corpus striatum. (AD therefore contrasts with Parkinson's disease, in which there is relative over-activity of the cholinergic system; the reason that AD patients do not all develop parkinsonian symptoms is probably that they are 'protected' by the reduced cholinergic activity.)

The role of dopamine in cognition is not clear. However, on the basis of work such as that described above, suggesting a correlation between intellectual impairment and dopamine deficiency, there have been some small studies of the effects of L-dopa in patients with AD.

A double-blind study by Lewis *et al.* (1978) found that AD patients rated significantly better for 'communication' and 'continence' when treated with L-dopa. Other groups of AD patients treated with L-dopa showed no benefit either in cognitive functioning or in other areas (Parkes *et al.*, 1974; Kristensen *et al.*, 1977). In an open trial by Adolfsson *et al.* (1978) AD patients were treated with L-dopa and also with bromocriptine, a dopamine agonist. The L-dopa treatment yielded significantly higher HVA concentrations in the CSF and significantly improved overall psychomotor and motor functions. There was also some improvement on some psychological measures, but no memory improvement. Bromocriptine treatment did not bring about any positive results, and some patients became more confused.

Subsequently Adolfsson *et al.* (1982) undertook a double-blind trial of L-dopa in patients with AD, diagnosed on Roth's 1955 criteria. Results were again generally negative, with no evidence of benefit either in terms of cognition or in overall behaviour.

The activity of the other 'classic' neurotransmitters in AD have been investigated, and most of the studies have been summarized by Perry and Perry (1980). There have been few consistent results, but it does appear that the GABA system is usually unaffected, at least in older patients. Some postmortem reductions in the marker enzyme glutamate decarboxylase have been reported, but these have not been confirmed in biopsy studies and are discounted on the grounds that the GABA system is particularly vulnerable to post-mortem damage. There has been one report of decreased GABA receptor binding in AD; this did not correlate with decreased CAT levels (Reisine *et al.*, 1978).

Adolfsson *et al.* (1979) found a slight reduction in 5-hydroxytryptamine (5-HT) levels in the hippocampus, mid-brain and gyrus cinguli in patients with AD, but these differences did not reach statistical significance. Winblad *et al.* (1982), however, found marked diminution of 5-HT levels (to 22–49 per cent of normal control values) in the hypothalamus, caudate nucleus, gyrus cinguli and hippocampus. In some brain regions there was a negative correlation between the levels of 5-hydroxyindoleacetic acid (5-HIAA, the 5-HT end-product) and intellectual performance, but this did not reach statistical significance. The activity of monoamine oxidase A (MAO-A), a marker enzyme for 5-HT, was unchanged; normally it rises with age. The level of monoamine oxidase B is increased in AD; since MAO-B is localized to the glial cells and MAO-A to the neurones, Gottfries (1980) suggests that the increased level of the latter may reflect glial proliferation. But, as with the changes in dopamine levels, neuronal loss from the corresponding subcortical nuclei has not been established — in this case, in the somewhat scattered formation of cell bodies in the brain-stem raphe region that supply serotonergic fibres to the cortex.

Perry (1984), reviewing the various neurotransmitter studies, reaches a general conclusion that in AD not all neurotransmitter systems projecting to the cortex from underlying nuclei are equally involved — so the condition cannot be regarded as general 'brain failure'. Winblad *et al.* (1982) arrived at

Table 9. Subtypes of Alzheimer's disease

	AD-1	AD-2
Onset	Late: 9th or 10th decade	Early: 7th or 8th decade
Course	Insidious	Rapid
Cognitive change	memory loss is main defect	Widespread cognitive change
Cell loss	Moderate loss in nbM	Massive loss in nbM and locus ceruleus
Sites of plaques and tangles	Mainly temporal lobe; frontal lobe largely spared	Plaques and tangles widespread

much the same conclusion, having observed a poor correlation between the various neurotransmitter abnormalities in individuals; they make what can only be the tenative suggestion that there may be subgroups of AD patients in whom different systems or types of transmitter are insufficient and for whom, possibly, different kinds of replacement therapy would be effective.

A number of investigators now believe that there are in fact two major AD subtypes. Rossor *et al.* (1981) focused attention on the 'isodendritic core', the dense group of cell bodies and intermingling dendrites containing the nuclei from which the ascending cholinergic, noradrenergic and dopaminergic fibres originate, and proposed that both AD and Parkinson's disease are primarily disorders of this area. Other morphological features of the disease such as plaques and tangles are, it is suggested, secondary and non-specific responses to loss of neurotransmitter input. Rossor *et al.* (1984) subsequently examined the post-mortem brains of 49 AD patients and demonstrated that the older patients had a relatively pure cholinergic deficit confined to the temporal lobe and hippocampus, while the younger patients had a widespread and severe cholinergic deficit together with abnormalities of noradrenaline, GABA and somatostatin. The biochemical losses in young subjects did not resemble those seen in normal elderly subjects. In the latter group there were only modest losses of ACh and GABA, and none of AD or somatostatin; thus no support was given to the concept of AD as 'accelerated ageing'.

Bondareff (1983) suggested the characterizations AD-1 and AD-2. In AD-1 damage is relatively confined to the cholinergic system and onset is relatively late and insidious with slow progression and with cognitive damage relatively limited to effects on memory. In AD-2 there is massive loss of neurones from the locus ceruleus and the nucleus basalis of Meynert, and early onset with widespread cognitive damage and rapid progression. There is greater density of plaques and tangles than in AD-1.

The features of these two subtypes are listed in Table 9. The concept is not altogether new; clinical terminology has for a long time acknowledged the fact that dementia may be of early onset and relatively severe in its effects (i.e. 'Alzheimer's disease' as used exclusively when onset is before age 65) or of late onset and comparatively benign ('senile dementia' or 'benign senescent forget-fulness'). The two types cannot, however, be regarded as distinct disease entities because the morphological changes are essentially similar, differing only in degree. The biochemical distinctions are by no means absolute, either; Iversen *et al.* (1983), for example, observed loss of cells from the locus ceruleus in a small group of elderly patients with AD. Mann *et al.* (1984) plotted morphological change and cell loss from the nucleus basalis of Meynert and locus ceruleus in 26 patients with AD ranging from 50 to 92 against age and found an inverse linear relationship. There was a similar relationship between age and plaque and tangle formation in the temporal cortex. In short, the younger the patient, the greater were the changes, with no discontinuity.

The indications are therefore that AD is a single entity which occurs in a continuum of severity in which the disease at its most 'malignant' declares itself, as one might perhaps expect, at a relatively early age (see Figure 1).

PEPTIDES

These are chains of amino-acids (ranging in length from 2 amino-acids to 39) produced by the diffuse endocrine system and widely distributed throughout endocrine and non-endocrine cells; they are active both in the CNS and in other organs, and the same peptide may have different actions in quite separate areas. Substance P, for example, is an 11-amine compound which stimulates smooth muscle in the gut and which is also present in nerve-endings in the CNS.

Table 10. Some neuropeptides in Alzheimer's disease

Neuropeptide	Reported findings
Vasoactive intestinal polypeptide	Consistently normal
Cholecystokinin	Normal, although may be reduced in advanced cases
Substance P	Inconsistent: normal, reduced, or possibly increased in advanced cases
Met-enkephalin	Normal; also normal opiate-receptor binding
Vasopressin	Normal (one report)
Somatostatin	Reductions variously reported for many cortical areas, temporal cortex only or advanced cases only. Immunohistochemical reductions also seen
Thyrotropin-releasing hormone	Normal (one report)
Neurotensin	Normal (one report). May be reduced in advanced cases
Angiotensin	Reductions in angiotensin-converting enzyme reported in some areas
Insulin	Normal

(Reproduced from Perry (1984) by permission of Blackwell Scientific Publications Limited.)

where it may possibly influence both dopamine and 5-HT activity. Detailed accounts of the identification of the peptides and their actions within the CNS can be found in Iversen (1979) and Green and Costain (1981). Green and Costain point out that this use of the same compounds in different ways is not unique to the peptides, and draw a parallel with the role of 5-HT in the platelets as a vasoconstrictor substance, in the gut as a factor involved in motility and in the brain as a transmitter probably concerned with sleep and mood.

It is now considered that at least 24 peptides act as CNS transmitters; they appear to coexist in nerve terminals with the 'classic' neurotransmitters and to act as modulators, regulating their action in various ways. Enkephalin, for example, is stored in noradrenergic terminals. Substance P and β-endorphin have been identified in cholinergic terminals and appear to influence the turnover of ACh in certain brain areas, including the cortex and hippocampus (Cheney et al., 1978). It is likely, however, that no one peptide is associated with a single neurotransmitter, and that there are complex subgroupings.

Endorphins are extremely potent; minute amounts of substance P, for example, have been shown to stimulate intense dopamine-mediated behaviour (Kelley et al., 1979); another fascinating finding was that that stimulation of certain areas produced analgesia, which was blocked by the morphine antagonist naloxone (Pert and Snyder, 1973); this in turn led to the identification of the 'endogenous opiates', or the endorphins. It has been suggested that acupuncture may act by eliciting the release of specific peptides, such as endorphins, in the brain and spinal cord.

Are there peptide disturbances in AD? Information thus far comes only from post-mortem assay and has been reviewed in detail by Perry (1984); some of the abnormalities that have been reported are summarized in Table 10. Results are clearly inconclusive; however, ACTH, analogues of ACTH and vasopressin have been strongly implicated in the control of learning and memory in work both with animals and with humans. The first indications came from study of the changes which follow hypophysectomy; the pioneer work in this area is reviewed by Rigter (1982). In a succession of studies, De Wied (e.g. 1969, 1977) showed that learned avoidance responses (to electric shock) were impaired in hypophysectomized rats, but that learning ability could be restored by treatment with ACTH or with a fragment of its 39-peptide chain, $ACTH_{4-10}$. This latter substance is apparently devoid of peripheral endocrine activity. Some other ACTH fragments have not shown a similar effect on learning and memory, but Rigter, analysing subsequent work with ACTH-like peptides, suggests that at least some substances in this category enhance arousal in response to motivation-relevant cues (i.e. those related to pain-avoidance or reward-seeking) or, putting it slightly differently, that they enhance selective attention.

A number of other peptides, closely related to ACTH, have been tested in animal learning tasks; one is a synthetic peptide produced by means of three substitutions within the $ACTH_{4-9}$ peptide chain which has been named Org 2766. The substance appears to be considerably more potent than other ACTH peptides in enhancing long-term memory storage in animal studies (Pigache and Rigter, 1981). There have been only a few studies of ACTH peptides in man; these are reviewed by Pigache (1982). In short, no positive effects on memory have been demonstrated; however, there has been improvement of selective attention, vigilance and mood in elderly and younger normal subjects treated with $ACTH_{4-10}$ and Org 2766. Thus far there have been no trials in AD patients; present indications are that ACTH peptides would be, at best, adjuncts to therapy in the condition.

There have been some apparent benefits from trials with vasopressin, a peptide released by the posterior pituitary gland, which shows effects similar to those of ACTH in enhancing learning in both normal and hypophysectomized animals (Chase et al., 1982). Some studies have also demonstrated memory improvement in young and elderly normal volunteers; for example, Legros et al. (1978) found significant improvement both in short-term and long-term memory in a placebo-controlled study in which vasopressin was given to 23 subjects aged over 50. But Chase et al. found no improvement in a group of 17 patients with AD treated with vasopressin, although the duration of the trial (ten days) was fairly brief. Tinklenberg et al. (1982) found general improvement in overall function in trials with demented patients given two vasopressin analogues, but these changes were non-specific, relating only to nurses' impressions of a general increase in activity and alertness, and they also appear to have correlated positively with improvement on a depression rating scale.

The studies with peptides, therefore, share a problem common to many other drug trials in dementia, in that effects on learning have not been convincingly disentangled from what may be effects primarily on mood and alertness. It is noteworthy that in the other study cited above (Legros et al., 1978), where they appeared to be improvements in learning, the subjects, though not demented, were hospitalized with 'minor pulmonary or gastroenterological diseases'. This group would probably be highly sensitive to a drug with non-specific positive effects on mood and alertness. Kaye et al. (1982) found that demented patients responded to a vasopressin analogue with increased alertness and talkativeness but that memory did not improve.

It is likely that, in further trials of drug therapy in dementia, peptides will be combined with other agents, such as substances active in the cholinergic system. There are also likely to be trials of drugs thought to be active in the intracellular 'second messenger' system. This system conceives of the classic neurotransmitter as the 'first messenger'; on binding to its receptor, it mediates the conversion of the energy-carrying substance adenosine triphosphate (ATP) into cyclic adenosine monophosphate (cyclic AMP), and this chemical initiates cellular response to the transmitter. Drugs which enhance the synthesis or block the inactivation of cyclic AMP would theoretically improve target-cell responsiveness and might therefore be of clinical benefit. Ergot alkaloids (p. 155) are possible candidates in this respect.

It would be a mistake, however, to think of the neurotransmitter systems as completely distinct, separate or independent. In the same way, none of the degenerative brain diseases appears to be altogether 'clean', with damage confined to a single area or ascending system. One system is likely to be affected predominantly, and specific intervention may well lead to improvement. But evidence presented largely in this and the two following chapters suggests that there is, in almost all such conditions, some degree of 'overspill' of the disease into adjacent systems, this for reasons which are far from clear.

SUMMARY AND CONCLUSIONS

For almost all medical disorders of which the cause is unknown, there exist treatments that will at least alleviate some symptoms. The search for a treatment for AD can continue only in the hope that this disorder is no exception. The brain is, on the other hand, an exceptionally vulnerable organ, and a treatment capable of correcting biochemical abnormalities is unlikely to be of value if widespread tissue destruction has already taken place. Unfortunately, the diagnosis of AD is almost invariably made only when the disease is well established; effective treatment will require greatly improved diagnostic methods.

The cholinergic transmitter system in the brain appears to fall victim to the disease at a fairly early stage; there is selective loss of cholinergic cells and of marker enzymes for acetylcholine before there is appreciable damage in other systems. A number of treatments designed to intervene in the cholinergic system are at present under trial; 'precursor loading' with purified lecithin looks like a promising strategy, but it might be effective only where AD is of the late-onset and relatively mild type.

There are also defects in the noradrenergic and dopaminergic systems; as their nerve fibres, like the cholinergic fibres, appear to originate almost exclusively in nuclei extrinsic to the cerebral cortex, it has been suggested that AD could be categorized as a 'subcortical' dementia, in which brain-stem disease is the primary lesion leading to a cascade of ascending changes and ultimately to target-cell atrophy in the cortex. This view can be only tentative. It is not established that cortical cells require neurotransmitter input in order to survive; if they do, the link with the neurotransmitter is likely to be complex, perhaps mediated by changes in the microcirculation. But even the apparently simple question of whether or not there is significant cortical cell loss in AD remains open.

It is believed that there are two AD subtypes: a late-onset and relatively mild type in which there is a fairly pure cholinergic defect, and an early-onset and more 'malignant' type in which there is widespread neurotransmitter change, involving, for example, the noradrenergic system. These two types probably represent two ends of a continuum of severity within what is essentially the same disease.

There are a number of peptide abnormalities in AD; peptides coexist with the 'classic' neurotransmitters in nerve terminals and affect signalling; whether or not they can themselves be regarded as neurotransmitters is largely a matter of terminology. They may have some role in the treatment of AD; the peptides secreted by the pituitary gland have been shown to enhance memory in experimental animals, although studies with normal human subjects and AD patients have established positive effects only on mood and vigilance. These substances would thus probably be no more than adjuncts to therapy — but any drug treatment which will improve AD patients, given what we now known about the condition, is likely to be of the 'cocktail' variety. There is a surprising lack of studies evaluating combined therapy with substances active in different biochemical systems.

CHAPTER 3

The morphology of Alzheimer's disease

The morphological changes typical of AD were described some 80 years ago, but there is still uncertainty about the precise origin of these changes and about how specific they are to the disease; opinions have therefore varied about which conditions can be placed in the AD category, and unfortunately they still do. In younger patients degenerative brain disease is rare, and there is little difficulty in distinguishing between normal and diseased tissue and in identifying the relatively few types of dementia; the main difficulty arises in the elderly, in whom the changes characteristic of the various dementias tend to merge both with one another and with the features of normal ageing. An accurate diagnosis can still be made (and, for several reasons, should be made), but the obstacles, including the problem of terminology, are of very long standing.

Torak (1978), in the course of a brief history of AD as a diagnostic entity, has described the way in which early work on AD, Pick's disease and similar conditions proceeded against the strongly countervailing current of the new gospel, psychoanalysis, and of the pressing need of 'organic' psychiatry virtually to find a *raison d'être* in the face of the conversion of Charcot and others from microscopy to mesmerism, and the astonishing rise of Freud in Europe and his disciple Brill in the USA.

But, for the organic psychiatrists, the ground had been well prepared. In 1875 the Italian anatomist Camillo Golgi had come upon a form of silver impregnation which stained only one neurone in a hundred (for reasons still not fully understood), providing for the first time a clear microscopic view of individual cells and their interconnections; using the Golgi stain, Ramon y Cajal identified and named the main CNS structures and many of their connecting pathways, and in 1904 published his textbook of human and vertebrate histology. It was only following this work that the description and siting of the changes underlying AD were possible.

Alois Alzheimer had already, in 1894, described the features of arteriosclerotic brain disease (Mahendra, 1984); these were observed in patients in the fifth and sixth decades of life who developed pareses, fits, labile effect, failure of reasoning and loss of memory. He found arteriosclerosis, associated with areas of softening, in the brain and also in other organs (e.g. the heart and the kidneys). In the same year, Emil Kraepelin set out, in his *Lehrbuch*, a clear differentiation between dementia arising from vascular disease and non-vascular, or 'senile', dementia. Kraepelin had already drawn the boundaries of the organic dementias, defining them as those due to structural disease of the CNS; he later (1893) introduced the term 'dementia praecox' to describe what we now call schizophrenia, and which was presumed to be functional — that is, there was no underlying CNS disease. Unfortunately the title itself blurred this distinction, and Kraepelin acknowledged that it was not ideal (Scharfetter, 1975); it was superseded by Bleuler's 'schizophrenia' in 1908 (Bleuler, 1911).

Meanwhile, Alzheimer (1899) had turned his attention to 'non-vascular' dementia; he suggested that this was after all due to blood vessel disease, but to disease of the arterioles rather than of the arteries; the result was ischaemia of a degree sufficient to kill nerve cells but not to create an infarct. Kraepelin, however, doubted that dementia in old age was invariably the result of vascular disease; change in the blood vessels was, he suggested, 'an accompaniment of only secondary importance in a disease process which is highly destructive of nerve tissue' (1912).

Alzheimer was not the first to describe the 'senile plaques' which are so closely associated with AD. Blocq and Marinesco (1892), using a modified version of the Golgi stain, identified these structures in the brain of an elderly epileptic; Redlich (1898) described miliary plaques in two cases of senility and brain atrophy, and Alzheimer described them in patients with 'senile dementia'. Torak (1978) comments that Alzheimer seemed oddly uninterested in senile plaques — oddly because they did not bear any notable relationship to vascular disease.

In 1903 Bielschowsky completed his own studies of metal impregnation and found that he could stain thread-like structures in neurones which he called neurofilbrils; in 1906 Alzheimer used the technique to examine the brain of a 51-year-old woman who had died following a rapidly progressive dementia with memory loss, delusions and personality deterioration (Alzheimer, 1907). He found senile plaques in abnormal numbers, but also saw clusters of thickened argentophilic fibres within the cells, mainly those of the upper layers of the cerebral cortex. He termed these 'neurofibrillary tangles', and considered them to be the main features of a specific disease process.

During the next four years, 13 similar cases were described; some writers already referred to the condition as 'Alzheimer's disease'. All descriptions were of patients with dementia of onset before the age of 65 (average age 59), with rapid progression (average duration 5.6 years) and with severe memory loss together with agnosia, apraxia and aphasia. In all cases there were neurofibrillary tangles, and senile plaques were present in all cases but one; four of the patients had suffered from *grand mal* fits.

Kraepelin referred briefly to Alzheimer's disease in the eighth edition of *Psychiatrie* (1910), but questioned whether the anatomical changes were unique to the condition, which could possibly be 'an especially severe form of

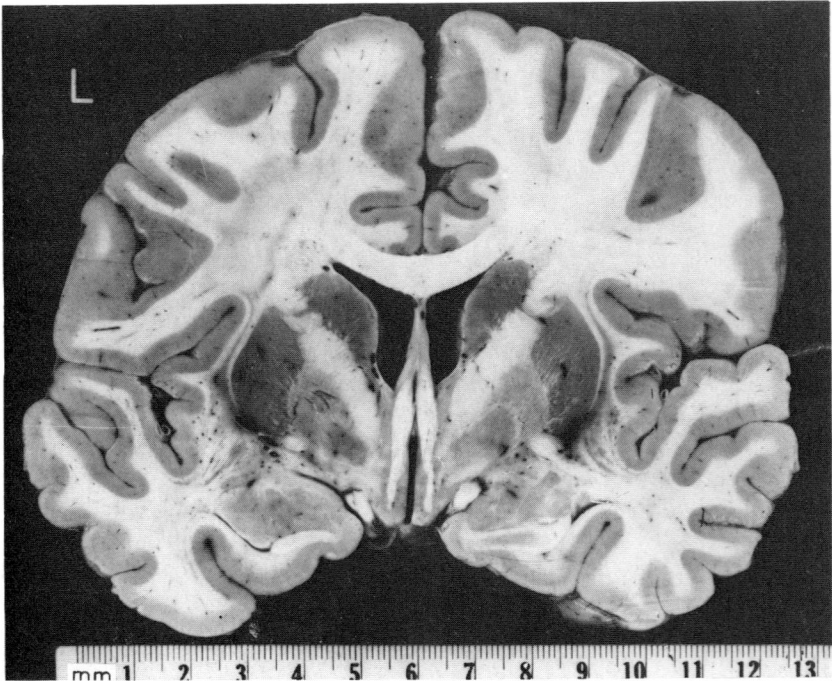

Figure 7   Coronal section of normal brain.

senile dementia'. He suggested, however, that there might be grounds for distinguishing AD from 'senile dementia' by the presence of aphasia, agnosia and apraxia.

It is now well recognized that these clinical features are not unique to presenile forms of dementia (e.g. Sourander and Sjörgen, 1970), and, even within a few years of Alzheimer's 1906 paper, plaques and tangles had been demonstrated in the brains of patients with dementia of late onset (Torak, 1978). But by 1912 the identity of 'Alzheimer's disease' had been firmly wedded to dementia with onset before the age of 65, and presenile dementia had been diagnosed as AD (Lafora, 1911; Schnitzler, 1911) even in the absence of the typical morphological features.

Alzheimer was appointed to the Chair of Psychiatry at the University of Breslau in 1912, but died of rheumatic heart disease in 1915, aged only 51. His death marked the end of a 'golden age' of organic psychiatry, a brief span of some thirty years during which the main types of dementia had been identified and described (including Huntingdon's chorea, Pick's disease and neurosyphilis), and there has scarcely been widespread interest in dementia until fairly recent years. The reputation of organic psychiatry suffered an eclipse partly because work was interrupted by the First World War but also because Kraepelin, Alzheimer and their colleagues could offer little more than morphological and clinical descriptions, in contrast to the glittering promises of

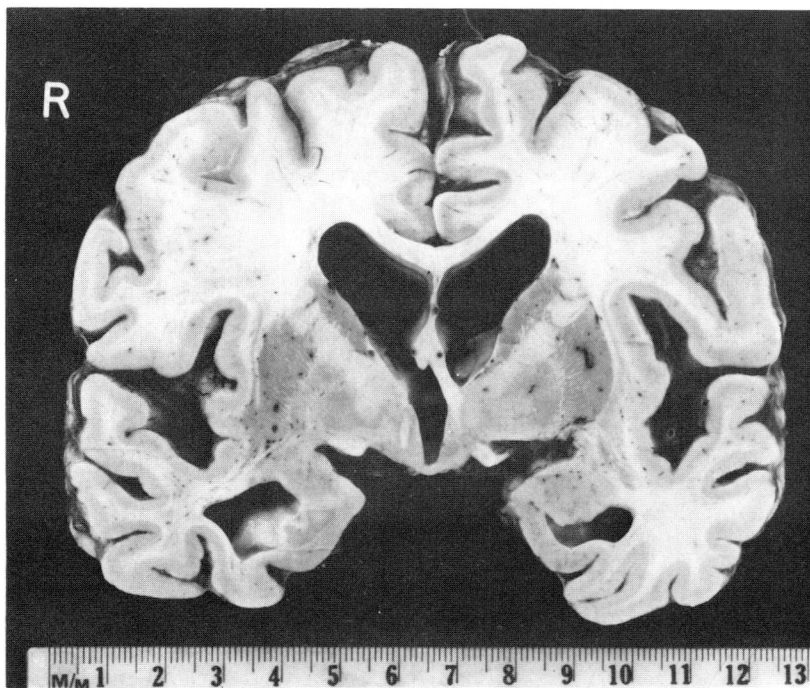

Figure 8   Severe cerebral atrophy and ventricular enlargement in Alzheimer's disease.

psychoanalysis; furthermore, organic psychiatry benefited hardly at all from the advances which revolutionized psychiatry from 1940 to 1960: the introduction of ECT, the phenothiazine tranquillizers and the antidepressants; dementia (with the exception of only a few types such as neurosyphilis) remained as intractable as ever, and advances were confined to more precise classification and description (esp. Roth, 1955; Corsellis, 1962). Even this work is incomplete; it is a chastening thought that recent work has served more than anything to reopen fundamental questions raised nearly 80 years ago (e.g. the specificity of the changes in presenile Alzheimer-type dementia, their origin and the contribution of circulatory disorder of the condition) and has gone only a little way towards answering any of them.

MACROSCOPIC CHANGES

Fairly widespread atrophy is the predominant macroscopic change in AD (Figures 7 and 8); in younger patients there may be dramatic weight and volume loss as compared with normal brains, but in older subjects there is greater overlap between changes due to ageing and those of normal ageing. *Brain weight*, in particular, is an unreliable index of severity of the disease. Brain weight declines from about 45 years, falling steeply after age 60, and even in 50 per cent of normal brains there is clear gyral narrowing with sulcal widening mainly in the frontal and temporal areas (Tomlinson *et al.*, 1968; Tomlinson, 1980). In 1970 Tomlinson *et al.*, who had previously studied the brains of 28 non-demented old people in detail, described the changes found in the brains of 50 patients who showed the clinical features of dementia; in 25 patients there were microscopic changes typical of AD. The ages of the group ranged from 62 to 92. Surprisingly, brain weights of AD patients (and also of those with other forms of dementia) did not differ significantly from that of age-matched controls. *Convolutional atrophy* of moderate or severe degree was, however, limited to the demented group; it was present to a severe degree in 32 per cent of the group. Atrophy was more widespread in AD than in ischaemic-type dementia; in the former type, atrophy involved both grey and white matter and was particularly severe in the temporal convolutions and in the hippocampal and adjacent gyri. The most striking difference between the normal and demented brain was in *ventricular dilatation*; in the demented series, the ventricles of 70 per cent of brains were described as moderately or severely dilated; the mean ventricular capacity in these averaged more than twice the mean for the non-demented series. Moderate dilation was present in 39 per cent of the normals, but none showed severe dilatation.

Corsellis, who in 1962 provided the major endorsement of Kraepelin's distinction between vascular and non-vascular dementia, measured atrophy by combining measurement of gyral shrinkage and ventricular enlargement. There was a clear difference in terms of atrophy between the brains of elderly patients who had died of Alzheimer-type dementia and those who had died of functional disorder; there was again only a small amount of overlap (Table 11).

Table 11. Cerebral atrophy in elderly patients with Alzheimer's disease and functional disorder
(Percentage of patients with atrophy at post-mortem)

	SDAT	Functional disorder
None	6	36
Slight	23	48
Moderate	60	14
Severe	11	2

(Reproduced from Corsellis (1962) by permission of the author and Oxford University Press)

MICROSCOPIC CHANGES

General

The most prominent general feature is disorganization of the cortical architecture with neurone loss and some glial proliferation, but there is a surprisingly poor degree of concurrence about the amounts and sites of these changes. Tomlinson (1980), from whom most of the following is drawn, reviews some of the studies which reported major cell loss throughout the neocortex and concludes that there is little evidence of a *general* fall in nerve-cell density in Alzheimer-type dementia by comparison with age-matched controls; nerve cell loss is largely confined to the hippocampus and anterior temporal lobes. Terry *et al.*, (1977) found that counts of cortical cells outside these areas in AD patients were not significantly different from similar counts in age-matched controls, although variance was greater in the former group. The issue has therefore been at times confused by failure to control, since there is in any case substantial cell loss in old age (Tomlinson and Henderson, 1976). Furthermore, as Tomlinson points out, questions of tissue volume have been neglected in nerve cell counts. Unchanged cell density in the presence of reduced volume would, of course, represent an absolute loss of cells.

Perry (1984) suggests that a distinction in terms of cell loss can be drawn between AD of presenile and senile onset. In the former there is almost certainly loss both in archicortical regions such as the hippocampus, and also in the neocortical lobes. In senile AD the amount of neuronal loss is not as pronounced, but there may be losses of up to 40 per cent in the large pyramidal neurones in the deeper cortical layers in certain regions of the frontal and temporal cortex.

All that can be stated with any confidence at present is that there are clear regional differences where most cases of AD are concerned; the hippocampal formation and temporal lobe, and to a lesser degree the frontal lobe, are most vulnerable to atrophy and cell loss. The almost invariable involvement of the hippocampus has led to the suggestion that AD could be primarily a disorder of the hippocampus or, perhaps, of the 'isodendritic core' (p. 45), with neurone loss in defined neocortical areas occurring secondarily to loss of subcortical inputs. These views will probably have to remain tentative until more sophisticated diagnostic methods provide means of 'staging' AD in life.

Other general changes are a substantial reduction in dendritic arborization as compared with the normal loss of old age, and a similar reduction in nucleolar volume and RNA production (Scheibel and Scheibel, 1976; Mann and Sinclair, 1978; Bowen, 1981); unexpectedly, some of these changes have been found in areas generally thought to be spared in AD — for example, the cerebellum.

Glial proliferation is not widespread, and it is apparent to only a slight degree even in areas where there is substantial cell loss or plaque formation. The blood vessels in general resemble those seen in age-matched normals; in some cases there is infiltration of intracerebral and pial arterioles with amyloid, but this may also occur in elderly subjects without the typical features of AD.

The specific features of AD are usually divided into two categories — the 'major' features (senile plaques, neurofibrillary tangles) and the 'minor' changes (granulovacuolar degeneration, Hirano bodies, congophilic angiopathy).

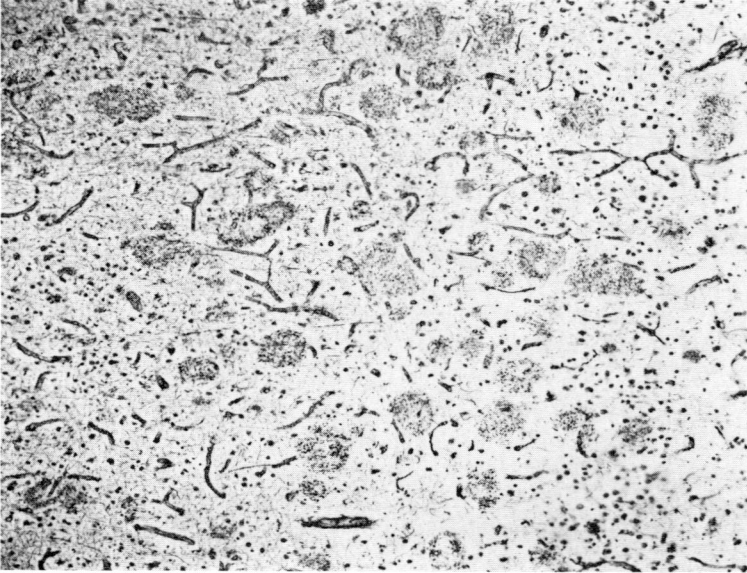

Figure 9   Heavy plaque formation in Alzheimer's disease.

Senile plaques

Senile plaques are by no means unique to AD, but they are an invariable feature of the condition (Figure 9). They were first described in the brain of an elderly epileptic by Blocq and Marinesco in 1892 and in two cases of senility with brain atrophy by Redlich in 1898; they were specifically associated with senile dementia by Alzheimer in 1904 and were also described in his 1906 case of presenile dementia. Alzheimer considered plaques to be glial in origin and of no great significance; during his lifetime the presence of plaques was also demonstrated in cerebrovascular disease and in normal ageing. The importance of plaques was not fully appreciated until the work by Tomlinson *et al.* (1970) showed both that they existed in abnormal abundance in Alzheimer-type dementia and that their numbers and siting could be related to the clinical severity of the disease.

A senile plaque is seen in silver-impregnated preparations by light microscopy; it is roughly spheroidal, made up of a central amyloid core surrounded by an unstained halo and an outer zone made up of densely packed and mainly radiating fibres resembling neuronal processes, dense bodies and microglia (Figure 10). Plaques vary somewhat in form — a core is not always present — and they range in size from 10 to 200 nm in diameter. (for comparison, the large Betz cell bodies in the cortex range from 7 to 10 nm in diameter.)

Electron microscopy has shown that the plaque core, commonly presenting a 'paper flower' or 'sea sponge' appearance (Nikaido *et al.*, 1971), is made up of dense amyloid filamentous material (Terry, 1978); the composition of the core

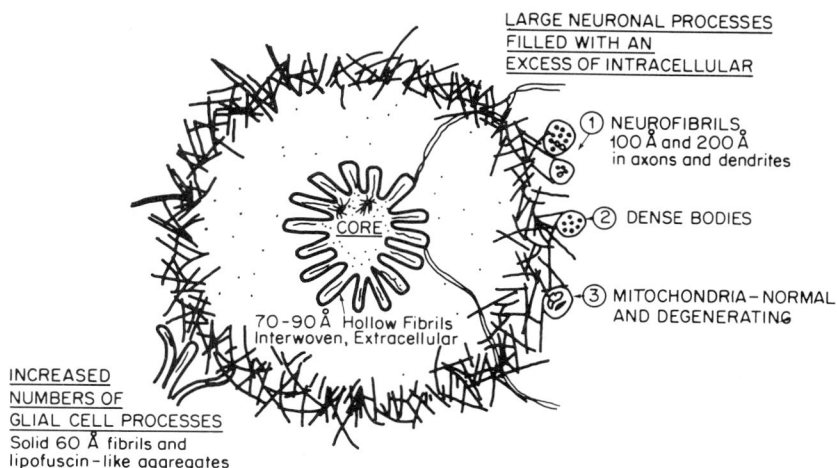

Figure 10   Schematic representation of a senile plaque. The rim of the plaque is made up of large neuronal processes filled with an excess of intracellular neorofibrils, dense bodies and mitochondria. The rim also contains increased numbers of glial cell processes containing fibrils and lipofuscin aggregates. In contrast, the central core lies extracellulary. It is composed of hollow fibrils which are interwoven like those of conventional amyloid. (Reproduced from Nikaido *et al.* (1971) by permission of the authors and the publishers. © 1971 American Medical Association.)

appears identical to that of systemic amyloid. The outer ring is made up of dendrites and small axons swollen by masses of filaments, dense bodies containing fibrillary material, and mitochondria. The glial component is made up of microglial cells, which may produce the amyloid, and of fibrous astrocytes.

Plaques are seen mainly in the cerebral cortex and hippocampus; they are present in non-demented individuals, increasing in number with age; they are not seen in the white matter. Present knowledge about plaque distribution, based largely on studies by himself and his co-workers, is summarized by Tomlinson (1980). Some plaques are present as early as the third decade, and by the eighth decade about 80 per cent of non-demented brains will show some plaque formation. Corsellis (1962) showed, however, that plaques may be absent in normal subjects aged even 90 and over. In normal elderly brains plaque density is usually below $10/mm^2$, whereas in elderly patients with AD plaque density can range from 15 to $40/mm^2$, and in cases of clinically severe dementia, particularly in presenile AD, it may reach densities of $50{-}60/mm^2$. In such instances plaques may appear to occupy almost half of the cerebral cortex, in places separated only by fibrillary or glial tissue. In established dementia no area of the neocortex is free of plaques, and the hippocampus, amygdaloid and hippocampal gyrus are usually heavily affected; plaques may also be found around the third ventricle, in the mammillary bodies and in the upper brain stem, but in relatively small numbers.

The origin of plaques is uncertain. They are seen in numerous brain diseases, including head injury (Corsellis, 1962), and, as far as is known, plaque structure is the same both in AD and in normal ageing (Roth *et al.*, 1966). In experimental scrapie in some animals, plaques are often seen in the white matter, suggesting that nerve-cell bodies or terminals are not necessarily involved in plaque formation and that deposition of amyloid fibrils may be the primary event (Bruce and Frazer, 1981), although the scrapie plaque does not appear to have a neuritic component and therefore has limitations as a model. Plaques in man owe at least some of their origin to nerve cell degeneration; unmyelinated neuronal processes, including synaptic boutons, have been identified in plaques (Terry and Wisniewski, 1970), but nerve cell death alone is considered unlikely to account for the amyloid deposition (Torak, 1978). Equally, although the outer ring of a plaque is partly glial, the astrocytes which collect round the margin are believed simply to be reactive; the microglia may be the source of the amyloid, but some substrate protein would be required for its production (Glenner *et al.*, 1973). It has been suggested (Walford, 1970) that with ageing there is gradual erosion of the blood–brain barrier; as plasma begins to leak into the brain tissue, circulating antibodies meet molecular configurations with which they have not been in contact before. These are interpreted as 'foreign' antigens and are 'neutralized' through formation of antigen–antibody complexes. The result is the destruction of neurones and the deposition of amyloid. Plaque formation would therefore be an autoimmune phenomenon secondary to almost any form of cerebral insult; it has in fact been experimentally induced in animal brains by trauma (Wisniewski, 1975). This view is therefore consistent with the fact that plaque formation does not appear to be restricted to specific types of brain disease and with the relative uniformity of plaque structure throughout a wide range of pathological contexts.

Plaque counts

Senile plaques relate *quantitatively* to AD. As part of his study of 300 patients who had died in Runwell Hospital between 1953 and 1957, Corsellis (1962) assessed the density of plaque formation on a four-point scale from 'none' to 'severe'. He found that plaque density discriminated strongly between organic and functional disorder in the elderly and, within the range of organic disorder, between vascular and senile dementia. Ninety-one per cent of functional patients showed no more than a slight degree of plaque formation, as distinct from 64 per cent of organic patients (Table 12). Four-fifths of the senile dementia group showed moderate or severe plaque formation, while in the other organic groups about the same proportion showed only slight plaque formation or none. Table 13 shows figures for patients with senile and vascular dementia.

Tomlinson *et al.* (1970) measured plaque density in the brains of demented subjects aged 64–92 and found significantly greater density than in age-matched controls. In 52 per cent of the demented patients there were 14 plaques or more per microscopic field, as compared with none of the controls.

Table 12. Plaque formation in elderly patients
(Percentages at post-mortem)

	Organic disorder	Functional disorder
None	55	66
Slight	9	25
Moderate	22	7
Severe	14	2

(Reproduced from Corsellis (1962) by permission of the author and Oxford University Press.)

Table 13. Plaque formation in elderly patients with dementia
(Percentages at post-mortem)

	Vascular dementia	Senile dementia
None	63	12
Slight	10	8
Moderate	17	42
Severe	10	38

(Reproduced from Corsellis (1962) by permission of the author and Oxford University Press.)

In severely affected patients plaques were present throughout the cortex and in all neuronal layers.

Sixteen cases were classified as Alzheimer-type dementia, both because heavy and uniform plaque formation distinguished them from the controls and because other AD-type changes (neurofibrillary tangles and granulovacuolar degeneration) were present to a degree greater than in any control. In six cases of arteriosclerotic dementia associated with extensive cerebral softening there was either no plaque formation or very small numbers of plaques. Patients with mixed senile and arteriosclerotic dementia occupied an intermediate position both in terms of cerebral softening and plaque formation. There appeared to be a threshold of cerebral degeneration beyond which some degree of intellectual deterioration was inevitable; a mean plaque count of 15–18 per field separated demented patients from normals. Within the general range of 10–50 plaques per field there was subsequently shown to be a clear positive correlation between plaque density and severity of dementia as measured by psychological and behavioural scales and a negative correlation with an orientation, concentration and memory score (Roth et al., 1966; Blessed et al., 1968). These correlations ceased to exist where dementia was severe.

Perry et al. (1978), using the same mental tests, established positive correlations between impairment, plaque density and diminished choline acetyltransferase content in the cerebral cortex. This applied to a group of patients suffering from depression, multi-infarct dementia, 'mixed' dementia and non-neurological diseases. Only in patients with AD, however, were there plaque counts of 17 or more per field.

70

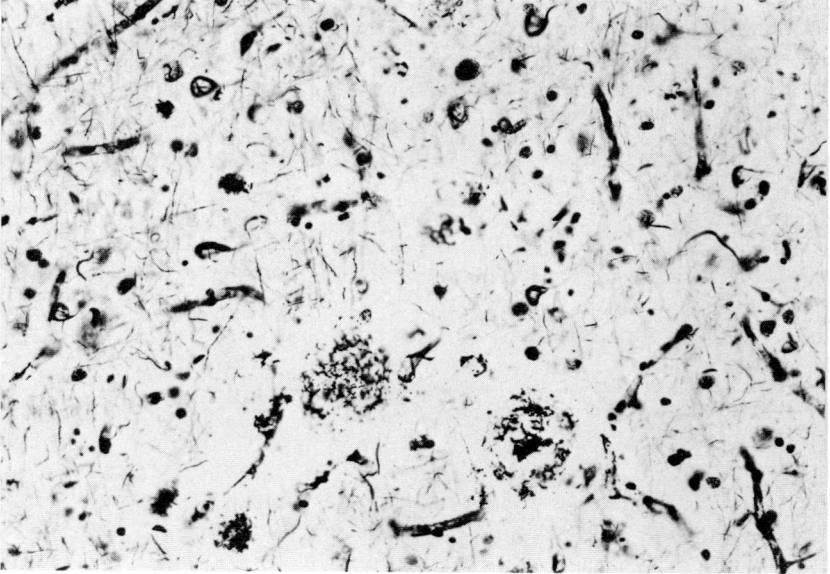

Figure 11   Heavy tangle formation in Alzheimer's disease.

High plaque concentration, therefore, virtually sets AD apart from other conditions, including normal old age. Around the age of 90 the density of plaque formation in normals approximates to that seen in patients with AD who have died at this age (Mann *et al.*, 1984). Presumably these patients are suffering from less severe disease; the same study indicated that the lower the age of death of an AD patient, the greater is the concentration of plaques (and tangles). Measurement of plaque and tangle frequency in the temporal lobes of patients who had died of AD aged from 50 to 92 established a high negative correlation between age of death and (a) plaque frequency, (b) tangle frequency and (c) cell loss and reduction of nucleolar volume in the locus ceruleus and the nucleus basalis. The correlations were linear, and there was no discontinuity between 'presenile' and 'senile' AD brains.

Neurofibrils

Neurofibrillary changes (Figure 11) have always been considered a necessary element in the AD entity. In sections prepared with the Bielschowsky silver method, remarkable changes in the neurofibrils within cell bodies were seen. In cells that otherwise appeared normal, one or several fibrils stood out due to their unusual thickness and impregnability. In more severely diseased cases many fibrils appeared, situated side by side and altered in the same way; at a later stage they merged into dense bundles and reached the surface of the cell. Finally, the nucleus and the cell disintegrated, and only a dense bundle of fibrils

Table 14. Tangle formation in elderly patients with dementia
(Percentages at post-mortem)

	Vascular dementia	Senile dementia
None or slight	87	54
Moderate	10	29
Severe	3	16

(Reproduced from Corsellis (1982) by permission of the author and Oxford University Press.)

indicated the site where the cell had been (Alzheimer, 1907; Wilkins and Brody, 1969).

These intracellular structures have usually been referred to as 'neurofibrillary tangles'; electron microscopy has, however, shown that each 'tangle' is a proliferation of paired filaments, each filament twisted helically round the other at fairly regular intervals (Terry, 1963). In the cortex they are seen mainly in the cytoplasm of the large pyramidal cells; they displace other extranuclear structures to a greater or lesser extent, and sometimes extend into the axon; they may also occasionally be seen in the outer rim of senile plaques.

Tangles (as they will be called for convenience) are present in normal old age, but in small numbers (Tomlinson et al., 1968). They are seen almost invariably only in the archicortex; from his studies of the brains of intellectually well-preserved elderly people — amounting to more than 100 subjects — Tomlinson found tangle formation to be most prominent in the hippocampus, but also to be frequent in other anteriomedian structures of the temporal lobe (e.g. the amygdaloid nucleus and the subiculum). Tangles appear in about 50 per cent of normal individuals in the fifth decade, and by the tenth decade virtually all brains show some tangles. Tangles are, by contrast, rare in the *neocortex* of normals, this often in the presence of considerable plaque density. Tangle count and distribution, in fact, sharply separate AD brains from those of age-matched brains of patients with functional disorder, and also from those in which change is primarily vascular. Corsellis (1962) found that 90 per cent of all patients with functional mental disease showed no tangle formation, whereas none showed severe tangle formation. Corresponding figures for organic brain disease were 69 per cent and 8 per cent. Table 14 compares tangle formation in senile and cerebrovascular dementia.

In one-third of senile dementia patients there was, however, no tangle formation in the areas examined — the frontal and occipital lobes, the diencephalon and the pons.

Tomlinson et al. (1970) found hippocampal tangle formation in both demented and normal elderly brains, but in 38 per cent of the demented brains the change was 'severe'; this applied to none of the normals. In the neocortex, tangle formation was present in 62 per cent of the dements as compared with only 11 per cent of the non-dements. In all 16 cases in which there was heavy plaque formation (p. 69) and which were classified as AD, there was also tangle formation greater than in any control. In the cases where the dementia was predominantly vascular, and in cases where vascular disease appeared to have contributed in some degree to the dementia, tangle formation was not seen in the neocortex.

Fibrillary change correlates with the clinical severity of dementia in the same way as does plaque density. The more severely demented the patient, the more dense is tangle formation (Tomlinson *et al.*, 1970). The presence of tangles in large numbers has also been shown to coexist with the characteristic features of AD; Constantinidis (1978) found that 91 per cent of cases with a high tangle density showed aphasia, apraxia and agnosia, regardless of age. High tangle concentration also correlates negatively with age of death from AD (Mann *et al.*, 1984). Individuals with late-onset AD have a tangle density in the temporal cortex only slightly greater than that of age-matched controls, but with a rather greater separation between the two groups than in the case of plaque count. High tangle density in the neocortex therefore appears to be an even more distinct index of AD in both younger and older groups.

In areas other than the neocortex there may be more overlap between dements and normals; from an examination of tangle formation in the hippocampus, Anderson and Hubbard (1985) suggested that the presence of tangles in more than 2.5 per cent of hippocampal neurones defined AD; there was, however, dense tangle formation in 2 out of 20 apparently normal elderly subjects.

As with plaques, the difference in terms of tangle formation between AD patients and normals would appear only to be quantitative; AD tangles do not appear to be unique structurally. Do plaques and tangles have a common origin? The origin of neither is certain. The scrutiny of tangles in particular has taken researchers down many fascinating alleyways — for example, neurofibrils occur in experimentally induced aluminium encephalopathies (p. 19) but they occur as single strands rather than in pairs. Again, scrapie-associated fibrils have been identified, and they may be present as helical pairs although their structure and the amino-acid sequence of their (protein) composition differ from those of tangles in man (Somerville, 1985).

Broadly, what plaques and tangles have in common is their relation to amyloid. Amyloid — literally 'wax-like' material — is produced when normal host protein is degraded by disease, assembled into insoluble fibrils and then deposited in the affected tissue. Most amyloid is probably of immunoglobulin origin and the substance is frequently laid down following prolonged antigen challenge (Scheinberg and Cathcart, 1976); the mechanism is frequently but not invariably autoimmune. Under the electron microscope, amyloid is seen to consist of non-branching filaments, mostly helically wound in pairs (Robbins and Cotran, 1979); the amyloid of plaques is indistinguishable from other amyloids. As tangles are also made up of paired and helically wound protein filaments, the question of whether they can be classed together with plaques as amyloid structures is largely a matter of terminology. The fibrils are about the same diameter as amyloid fibrils (about 11 nm (Robbins and Cotran, 1979)), and they appear on X-ray crystallographic analysis to show the β-plated sheet which is characteristic of amyloid (Termine *et al.*, 1972; Somerville, 1985). The periodicity of the wound pairs and the amino-acid sequences may be different where plaques and tangles are concerned, but amyloids do vary in these infrastructural details. Tangles could, in short, quite reasonably be regarded as the intracellular equivalent of plaques — accumulations of amyloid resulting from non-specific cell injury. In supranuclear palsy and in brains damaged by trauma and other conditions, intracellular filaments are sometimes seen to be arranged in pairs similar to those of AD (Torak, 1978); although the work with aluminium- and scrapie-induced filaments is interesting in itself, the closest *experimental* model of paired helical filament formation is induced by axon section, which results in the formation of filamentous pairs in the cell body seemingly identical to AD pairs (Pannese, 1963). It has therefore been suggested (Torak, 1978) that the sequence of plaque and tangle formation could begin with the destruction of dendrites, axons and synapses as amyloid is laid down and disrupts axonal flow; it could then proceed with neurofibrillary reaction in the cell bodies.

Granulovacuolar degeneration

This change is virtually confined to the pyramidal cells of the hippocampus. It is a cytoplasmic abnormality; within affected cells there are vacuoles of about 5 nm in diameter, each containing a central haematoxyphilic and argyrophilic granule of about 1 nm in diameter. There may be up to 15 of these structures in a single cell (Tomlinson, 1980). Their significance is not known, but their density correlates with the clinical severity of the dementia.

Hirano bodies

These also occur almost exclusively in the hippocampus; they are seen adjacent to and sometimes within the perikaryon of the pyramidal cells, and are round, oval or rod-like eosinophilic bodies varying from 8 to 15 nm across and up to about 30 nm in length (Hirano, 1965). As with vacuoles, the number of Hirano bodies reflects the severity of dementia; both structures are seen, though in relatively small numbers, in normal elderly subjects (Tomlinson *et al.*, 1970; Gibson and Tomlinson, 1977). For the time being, both can be taken only to represent the byproducts of cell degeneration.

Congophilic angiopathy

In some AD brains there is infiltration of the walls of arterioles, pial arteries and, occasionally, venules, with amyloid (which takes up Congo red stain). This finding is inconsistent; congophilic angiopathy is present in only a small proportion of cases, and it may be seen in some elderly subjects in the absence of plaque formation (Tomlinson, 1980). On section, the blood vessels are seen to be greatly thickened by amyloid; small and roughly spherical amyloid deposits may also be seen in close proximity to the vessels. Torak (1978) has suggested that these deposits may represent the primary event in senile plaque formation, although the sequence of events in the human is at present probably impossible to establish with certainty. But in certain animal disease models (e.g. aluminium intoxication, cortical undercutting and experimental scrapie) there is also amyloid thickening of blood vessel walls and perivascular amyloid deposits (Wisniewski *et al.*, 1970; Wisniewski and Terry, 1973). Some of these deposits may be associated with neuritic change (which may be dendritic or axonal), and they may closely resemble senile plaques in man. Amyloid deposits with little or no associated neuritic change might therefore represent 'immature' senile plaques. It is not certain, however, whether this model is applicable to AD, since senile plaques in man do not appear to occur in especially close proximity to blood vessels.

These, then, are the main morphological changes of AD. None is specific to the disease, but in no other condition do these features appear together or in greater than certain defined densities. In particular, the presence of neurofibrillary tangles in the neocortex distinguishes the brains of AD subjects from those of the intellectually normal; numerous neurofibrillary tangles are never found throughout the neocortex in normal old age. Their presence in large numbers is confined to the demented population. It would therefore be incorrect to suppose that AD at any age represents nothing more than accelerated ageing, or that the ageing brain in due course becomes indistinguishable from the 'senile dementia' brain. AD can be defined as a pathological entity even in the very old. It is always abnormal.

Where the symptoms of AD are concerned, there is a broad correlation — as with the biochemical abnormalities — between sites of damage and clinical abnormality. The vulnerability of the hippocampal and adjacent structures to histological change is of particular interest in view of the known role of the hippocampus in memory processing (p. 110); the observation by Anderson and Hubbard (1985) of dense hippocampal tangle formation in mentally normal subjects in the absence of AD-type features of similar density elsewhere suggests a sequence of morphological change which accords with the typical clinical history of AD — the onset of a characteristic form of amnesia (p. 110) followed by signs of widespread damage in the neocortex.

There is little doubt that hippocampal damage underlies the amnesia of AD; studies have already been reviewed (p. 67) which indicate that in AD both morphological damage and biochemical change are maximal in the hippocampus, which appears to be affected at an early stage of the disease. Penfield and Mathieson (1974) have suggested that the 'keys of access' to the cortical memory bank are located in the hippocampal formation and that within it, during life, more and more 'lines of facilitation' are laid down. Hippocampal disease would reverse the process, with increasing restriction of access to the memory bank. It has been suggested, indeed, that AD could be defined as a 'hippocampal dementia'; Ball *et al.* (1985) examined the brains of 20 patients diagnosed as AD in life, and found that, while in all there was severe hippocampal damage, in one there were no plaques or tangles whatever in the hippocampus or neocortex but, instead, 'devastating' cell loss together with florid astrocytosis; in another, small numbers of plaques and tangles were seen (in addition to severe cell loss and astrocytosis) in the hippocampus only. The 'hippocampal dementia' theory begs two questions: the first is whether 'Alzheimer's disease' can be diagnosed in the absence of the classic histological changes, and the second is whether DSM III (the source of the diagnostic criteria used by the authors) is sufficiently rigorous in its definition of Alzheimer-type dementia. The answer to the first question is probably in the negative, and the second certainly is; the DSM III criteria could admit chronic brain diseases other than the now well-defined AD entity (p. 9). The findings of Ball *et al.* do not appear to represent a basis for the authors' discussion of possible sites for brain cell transplantation.

Perhaps the amnesia of AD can be more accurately seen as the outcome of hippocampal *isolation*. Hyman *et al.* (1984) examined the distribution of hippocampal and parahippocampal pathology in the brains of AD patients, and reported a specific pattern of cellular changes in the projection neurones of the hippocampal formation (see below) which isolated it from the association cortices, basal forebrain, thalamus and hypothalamus.

The hippocampus is a complex and multilayered structure which has been divided into a number of fields, each of which has its own cellular architecture and its separate interconnections (Brodal, 1981). The principal *input* is to the entorhinal cortex (which is continuous with the hippocampus proper) from the association and limbic cortices, and the principal *output* is from the subiculum (the upper portion of the parahippocampal gyrus) to the thalamus, hypothalamus, the association cortex and basal forebrain. Hyman *et al.* (1984) found consistent loss, in five AD brains, of the principal cells of the entorhinal cortex and also of the neurones of the subiculum and of the large pyramidal cells of the adjacent hippocampal region. In these areas there was also heavy tangle formation. By contrast, other hippocampal areas were unaffected, as were the brains of undemented controls (aged 50–83). Damage therefore was almost totally selective to the cells which constitute the main gateway of information to the hippocampus and to those which constitute its major gateway of information to the neocortex. Memory processing cannot be visualized in strictly anatomical terms, but there is undoubted consistency between these findings and the observation that AD amnesia represents mainly a failure to lay down information in the long-term memory store (p. 110); hippocampal isolation would appear to be equivalent to disconnection of the central memory processor.

In conclusion — the anatomical and biochemical changes in the AD cortex occur in parallel and influence one another. Which comes first? Do cortical cells degenerate because of failing input from subcortical nuclei, or do the subcortical nuclei degenerate as a result of damage to their ascending axons? There can be little doubt that, by the time AD is well established, both mechanisms have played a part. But present evidence (e.g. the relatively selective damage in the neocortex and the early involvement of the hippocampus) suggests that subcortical disease may be primary. One still cannot be sure. However, Anderson and Hubbard (1985) draw an analogy between AD and other chronic diseases of old age which are clinically silent yet which are regularly diagnosed at post-mortem; study of these early changes is of the greatest value in understanding how diseases originate and progress. In the same way, research into AD is likely to benefit from the examination of many more brains from the (apparently) undemented.

SUMMARY AND CONCLUSIONS

The principal features of AD were described some 80 years ago; subsequent investigations have confirmed the original separation of the disease from other forms of dementia, such as that caused by vascular disease, and from the changes of normal old age. Each of the changes characteristic of AD may be found in the ageing brain and in other conditions, but only in AD do they occur together and in greater than certain defined densities. In particular, the presence of large numbers of 'neurofibrillary tangles' in the neocortex strongly identifies AD.

The major gross changes of AD are ventricular dilatation and loss of tissue density, but in the very elderly differences from normal may be obscured by individual variation.

Microscopically there may be cell loss, but a great reduction in dendritic arborization is the most prominent general feature.

'Senile' plaques are invariably seen in the cortex of AD brains; they are spheroidal with a central amyloid core and an outer fibrillary ring which is probably of dendritic and glial origin.

Plaque density is significantly greater in AD than in functional disorder or in age-matched normals, and it correlates positively with the severity of cognitive impairment in AD. There appears to be a 'threshold effect'; at a level of plaque density which is fairly consistent from one individual to another, some degree of intellectual impairment is inevitable.

The cytoplasmic 'neurofibrillary tangles' of AD are made up of paired and helically wound filaments; they are present throughout the neocortex in most cases and they may initially appear in the hippocampus. Tangle density also correlates with the severity of AD symptoms.

The origin of plaques and tangles is obscure. The tangles of AD appear identical to those induced by axon section, so the likelihood is that amyloid (a product of protein degradation) is laid down as a result of a 'dying-back' process consequent on disrupted axonal flow. An acceptable hypothesis is that plaque formation also begins with the laying down of amyloid. As a result of damage to the blood–brain barrier by disease (not necessarily AD), circulating antibodies have encountered unfamiliar protein, with the result that antigen–antibody complexes have formed and amyloid has been deposited in a variety of sites, including blood vessel walls. Where neurone destruction has taken place, the remains of the dendrites and the glial reaction have surrounded the amyloid centre to form the 'mature' plaque.

A distinction can be drawn between 'senile' and 'presenile' AD only on the grounds of severity; the earlier the age of onset, the more profuse is plaque and tangle formation and the greater is cell damage.

The amnesia of AD, a prominent and early feature, is likely to reflect early involvement of the hippocampal formation — in particular, disruption of its main channels of output and input — resulting in isolation of the area and failure of access to information storage sites. This damage occurs in parallel with the decline of cholinergic and other subcortical innervation of the area, and is possibly part of a 'chain reaction' beginning in the corresponding subcortical nuclei. But this is not certain, and it is likely that more accurate staging of the AD process will result from more extensive post-mortem examination of the clinically unaffected.

CHAPTER 4

Other types of dementia

Dementia — to repeat the definition — is acquired, chronic and diffuse brain disease. Most forms are also primary to the brain and, in essence, dementia is diagnosed when there is evidence of widespread chronic impairment of brain function in the absence of affective or extracerebral disease which could be wholly responsible. Although Alzheimer's disease is the most common form of dementia it should, where possible, be distinguished from other types for the following reasons. First, some forms of dementia are treatable; normal pressure hydrocephalus and syphilis are the best-known examples. Second, there may be effective prophylactic measures; cigarette smoking and uncontrolled hypertension and diabetes favour the advance of vascular disease, and there are self-evident preventive measures in the case of alcoholic dementia (including the rectifying of nutritional defects). Third, genetic counselling may be indicated, as with Huntingdon's chorea. If neurosyphilis is diagnosed, members of the patient's family might require investigation. Fourth, the dementia might be one of the rare transmissible types, such as Creutzfeldt-Jakob disease, where certain precautions are necessary in order to prevent spread. Finally, some form of prognosis even for untreatable conditions is highly desirable. The patient and his relatives need to know what to expect, and both they and the doctor must make realistic plans for the future. Clearly a different prognosis would be given for an elderly patient with late-onset AD than for a younger patient with dementia that was probably due to vascular disease; there is a sharply contrasting course and life expectancy; management also would be different. The following is less a detailed account of the different types of dementia than it is a description of the clinical features that distinguish each type from AD, and about the essential differences in management which follow.

MULTI-INFARCT DEMENTIA

'Hardening of the arteries' is a quasi-technical term traditionally used in connection with dementia, usually by relatives, but sometimes by a doctor when explaining the illness. The concept of brain cells disadvantaged as a result of arterial thickening and occlusion is readily grasped and is, one suspects, readily accepted since it tends to transplant the patient's symptoms into the area of physical illness from that of 'mental disorder' or from whatever illimitable diagnostic realm is implied by such terms as 'brain failure'. But it is now fairly well established that dementia is the result of vascular disorder in only a minority of cases; even in these, the symptoms may not be the result of disease in the cerebral blood vessels.

Cerebral arteriosclerosis is common in old age, but studies of the brains of demented and non-demented elderly show no difference between the two groups in terms of either the degree or the extent of arteriosclerosis (Corsellis and Evans; 1965; Worm-Petersen and Pakkenberg, 1967). In brains of patients with AD the incidence of arteriosclerosis is actually lower than in age-matched controls (Jamada and Mehraein, 1968). On the basis of an extensive review of the pathological evidence, Hachinski *et al.* (1974) concluded that when vascular disease is responsible for the dementia of old age it is not as a result of cerebral arteriosclerosis, but as a result of multiple infarcts secondary to disease of the extracranial arteries and the heart (i.e. from embolism). Therefore the term 'multi-infarct dementia' is more accurate than 'arteriosclerotic dementia'.

In their 1970 study, Tomlinson *et al.* found that the brains of 6 out of 50 demented patients showed extensive cerebral softening indicative of ischaemia. In these brains there was little or no plaque formation. In 3 further cases there were moderate amounts of softening, and in a further 4 there was softening associated with Alzheimer-type changes. Tomlinson (1980), summing up the results of a number of studies, suggests that about 17 per cent of dementias are of vascular origin, and that a similar number are of mixed multi-infarct and Alzheimer type.

The quantity of cerebral softening has been shown to accord with the severity of dementia and, as with AD, a threshold effect is apparent, with 50 ml of softening differentiating to a high degree between the demented and the cognitively unimpaired (Roth, 1971). Also, measurement of softening allowed a high degree of discrimination between vascular dementia and AD. In the former group, 73 per cent of patients had more than 50 ml of softening, while in the latter 94 per cent had less than 50 ml of softening. The overlap between the two conditions therefore appears to be relatively small.

No clear inheritance pattern for vascular dementia is evident (Larsson *et al.*, 1963), although the fairly small numbers and the difficulty in diagnosis during life would make genetic studies even more difficult than in the case of AD.

Most studies have found the risk to males and females to be about equal (Corsellis, 1962; Larsson *et al.*, 1963; Tomlinson, 1972).

Clinical features

Multi-infarct dementia (MID) has been briskly described as 'a matter of strokes large and small' (Fisher, 1968). First then, as one might expect, the history is generally episodic, with what is usually described as 'step-wise' deterioration, though often with a slight degree of recovery after each ischaemic episode. The other main features are, next, that cognitive impairment tends to be selective and uneven (as distinct from the fairly consistent pattern of widespread impairment characteristic of AD) and that there is likely to be additional evidence of vascular disease both in the brain and elsewhere. Bucht *et al.* (1984) found that 65 per cent of patients with MID had a history of cardiovascular disease, as compared with only 11 per cent of AD patients.

The *history* may include headaches, tinnitus or dizziness; there may have been transient ischaemic episodes with falls or with short-lived episodes of hemiparesis, confusion, dysarthria or dysphasia. There may be symptoms indicative of vascular disease in other organs; for example, angina pectoris or leg cramp. All of these should be enquired about specifically in a patient with an apparent diagnosis of dementia. Specific points of enquiry in relation to past medical history are diabetes, hypertension and, in relation to habits, diet and smoking.

On *physical examination* particular attention should again be paid to the cardiovascular system; evidence of extracerebral disease may include hypertension, loss of peripheral pulses or fundal arteriopathy. Where the CNS is concerned, there may be minor focal signs even in early cases (Birkett, 1972); for example, asymmetrical reflexes, extensor plantar responses or impaired pupillary reactions. In more advanced cases there are likely to be upper motor neurone signs, 'primitive' reflexes (p. 109) or pseudobulbar palsy.

Mental state examination is likely to show deficiencies in some areas with relative sparing of others; there is no typical pattern. There could be severe memory loss with well-preserved verbal ability, or, perhaps, dysphasia and memory loss with well-preserved insight, judgement and emotional control. Emotional lability is often said to be a feature of MID although in my own experience depression is much more common. A patient with AD tends to lose insight into his disorder at a fairly early stage in the disease; in MID, in some ways an even less merciful condition from the patient's point of view, an acute awareness of cognitive loss (and motor disability if any) is often retained, and such patients, often younger than AD patients, can be resentful, angry and difficult to manage. Depression may indeed have preceded the onset of the dementia; Bucht *et al.* (1984) found that one-third of their subjects with brain infarcts had been depressed before the dementing illness started, whereas depression was rare before the onset of AD. Therefore a careful mental state examination for evidence of clinical depression is necessary, and there may be an excellent response to antidepressants. Lipsey *et al.* (1984) found that 57 per cent of 103 post-stroke patients showed some degree of depression, which tended to be persistent. Treatment with nortriptyline brought about a significant improvement in a double-blind trial.

While some investigations (see below) are particularly helpful in the diagnosis of MID, the selective nature of the damage may be apparent from the outset, whether or not 'hard' neurological signs are present.

Case No. 1

Mr A was 78, and was referred because of a recent onset of 'confusion'. All had been well until 12 weeks before referral, when he took to getting out of bed at night to make tea, insisting it was morning. According to his wife he became 'normal' again for a time, then began to speak 'gibberish'; this again varied from day to day. On some days he was said to be like his old self; on others he was completely incoherent.

He was a pleasant man who did his best to be co-operative; there was no localizing signs on CNS examination; he was right-handed. There were no abnormalities on general physical examination and, on the evidence of his behaviour, he was not disorientated in place or time; he behaved as if he knew the time of day: he came for meals at the proper times, he went shopping with his wife, and went out and came back alone.

He could obey simple instructions readily, and he gave the appearance of understanding questions, but his replies bore no relation to what he had been asked. For example, when asked his age, he said, 'Place', and when asked his address he said, 'Ocasionally'. Twice he said spontaneously, 'I don't speak the truth'.

In essence, therefore, he showed a relatively isolated expressive dysphasia, probably with a considerable degree of insight; presumptive diagnosis was of a left hemisphere lesion, and this was confirmed by a CT scan, which showed a wedge-shaped loss of density in the left temporoparietal region area indicative of an infarction (Plate 10); it will be noted, however, that there are other areas of loss of density together with ventricular enlargement. When he was last seen, two months after the first examination, Mr A had made an immense improvement and his speech was almost fully intelligible, but he will have to remain under medical supervision and his wife may expect to have to cope with future similar episodes.

Multi-infarct dementia can often be distinguished from AD by calculating the patient's 'ischaemia score' (Hachinski et al., 1975). Regional cerebral blood flow (indicating infarcted tissue) was reduced in patients with MID but not in those with AD, and an ischaemia score of 7 or more correlated with the presence of reduced blood flow and favours the former diagnosis (Table 15). A score of less than 4 favours a diagnosis of AD.

Investigations in any patient with signs of dementia will include estimation of blood sugar and cholesterol, but these, together with an EEG, will be of particular value in the diagnosis of MID. In the latter, three-quarters of patients show frequent arrhythmias and electrocardiographic changes of cardiac hypertrophy or coronary artery disease, whereas in AD the ECG is likely to be normal (Harrison et al., 1979). Computerized tomography (p. 132) may also be most helpful in demonstrating the patchy nature of the damage, and also in distinguishing between a stroke and a tumour or abscess. Changes will be detectable about 24 hours after the onset of a stroke, and appear as irregular or wedge-shaped low-density areas. Figures 23 and 24 show appearances in a

Table 15.   Ischaemia score

Abrupt onset	2
Stepwise deterioriation	1
Fluctuating course	2
Nocturnal confusion	1
Relative preservation of personality	1
Depression	1
Somatic complaints	1
Emotional incontinence	1
History of hypertension	1
History of stroke	2
Evidence of associated atherosclerosis	1
Focal neurological symptoms	2
Focal neurological signs	2

A score of 7 or more favours a diagnosis of multi-infarct dementia; a score of less than 4 favours a diagnosis of Alzheimer-type dementia.
(Reproduced from Hachinski *et al.* (1975) by permission of the author and the American Medical Association.)

severely demented patient, where there are multiple cystic areas; these are often referred to as 'lacunar infarcts'.

Management will follow the general principles set out in Chapters 6–8; in particular, blood pressure and blood sugar will be carefully monitored, and the patient will be strongly advised to abstain from smoking. The relation between cigarette smoking and the risk of stroke has been well established (Paffenbarger and Wing, 1971; Grainger and Mastaglia, 1976; Walker, 1976; Salonen *et al.*, 1982; Bell and Ambrose, 1982; Rogers *et al.*, 1983); indeed, a recent study suggested that cigarette smokers had a threefold increase in the risk of stroke compared with current non-smokers and that 37 per cent of stroke events could be attributed to cigarette smoking (Bonita *et al.*, 1986), so here is at least one piece of positive advice to be given to anyone who asks how he can lessen the chances of his becoming demented. And an elderly patient in particular is not to be allowed to get away with the usual, 'I've smoked all my life; it won't do me any harm now'. On the contrary, the older the patient, the more vulnerable is the cardiovascular system (Fisher, 1962).

Specific measures will naturally include attention to the primary disorder, bearing in mind that MID is usually the consequence of blood vessel disease elsewhere than in the brain. Patients in this diagnostic category will probably benefit more than any from the combinations of skills of a psychiatrist and a geriatrician, together with their associated staff; a patient with a combination of major and minor strokes may need a range of treatment and rehabilitative measures that cannot necessarily be provided within a single specialty — for example, physiotherapy, speech therapy and closely monitored dosage of antihypertensive and antidepressant drugs. Although the provision of joint geriatric/psychogeriatric 'assessment units' has rightly been recognized as a necessity for some time, the need to provide joint *management* of certain groups of elderly patients is rarely emphasized as it ought to be.

Survival is even less predictable than in AD, with greater variability. Comparative studies have found a slightly better two-year average survival than in senile dementia (Roth, 1955; Shah *et al.*, 1969), with slightly better prospects for females. Where females are concerned, Shah *et al.* found that 65 per cent of patients hospitalized with vascular dementia had survived for two years, as compared with 32 per cent of those with Alzheimer-type dementia. Death was most commonly attributable to ischaemic heart disease.

ALCOHOL AND DEMENTIA

Alcohol-related problems are common in older people; from a review of 1983, Wattis concludes that excessive drinking is a significant source of illness and disability, including cognitive deterioration, in older age-groups. There is a striking sex difference; Edwards *et al.* (1973) found that in 46.3 per cent of cases of alcoholism in women the patient was over 60, but that the corresponding figure for men was only 11.3 per cent. Glatt (1982) found that elderly female alcoholics outnumbered males in the ratio of 3:2 and that, while two-thirds of the total group studied were excessive drinkers of long standing, one-third had only started to abuse alcohol in old age.

Alcohol abuse must be considered as a possible diagnosis in any patient suffering from chronic confusion, especially if the confusion is episodic and associated with falls; in the latter case the diagnosis would be made at once in the case of a younger patient! But it is surprising how often the true nature of the problem in an older patient does not emerge until a fairly late stage; Wattis (1983) points out that there can be additional difficulties in diagnosis due to collusion by other alcohol-abusing members of the same family. But alcoholism is no respecter of age, sex or status; enquiry about drinking habits should always form part of the history and it can, without causing offence, follow naturally after questions about diet and smoking. It should be noted also that alcohol appears to be less rapidly metabolized in the elderly, who reach higher peak concentrations than younger subjects following an equivalent dose (Vestal *et al.*, 1977), so what would be a 'moderate' intake in middle age would represent 'heavy' drinking in an old person.

Alcohol-related confusion may amount to nothing more than episodes of intoxication, with total recovery following withdrawal. Otherwise, alcohol-induced brain disease is generally considered to fall into two categories. First, there is the relatively well-defined Wernicke–Korsakoff syndrome and, second, there is the fairly diffuse cerebral atrophy which has been described in chronic alcohol abusers and which approximates rather more closely to a 'true' dementia — although terminology is again a problem.

The Wernicke–Korsakoff syndrome has been described in detail elsewhere (Victor *et al.*, 1971; Lishman, 1978). In outline, its title represents two conditions, described at different times, but which are now generally taken to represent facets of the same disorder — that is, the cerebral response to thiamine deficiency which in turn is usually, but not invariably, the result of alcoholism. (This deficiency in alcoholics is considered to arise not through a single mechanism but from a combination of poor diet, poor absorption and liver disease.) Wernicke's encephalopathy, the acute reaction, usually presents as a confusional state associated with ataxia and eye signs (e.g. nystagmus or failure of conjugate gaze). Korsakoff's psychosis is the enduring defect resulting from damage to structures in the region of the third ventricle, mainly the thalamus and the mammillary bodies, but also the periaqueductal grey matter in the upper pons, other brain-stem nuclei and the anterior portion of the cerebellum (Victor and Banker, 1978); these changes are apparently identical to those responsible for Wernicke's encephalopahy (Malamud and Skillicorn, 1956), but where the syndrome becomes chronic, the recent memory loss becomes the central or only cognitive defect. It is often associated with confabulation; this combination, seen where other cognitive functions are relatively spared, strongly suggests Korsakoff's psychosis.

Case No. 2
Mrs B is 75 and has been an alcohol abuser for at least thirty years; she has a history both of hospitalization and imprisonment. She is grossly disorientated in both time and place; when asked her age she replies brightly, 'Twenty'. At the same time she can name simple and complex objects accurately and without hesitation, and there are no problems with fine motor or sensory co-ordination. By contrast, a patient with AD is likely to struggle painfully and unhappily with questions about, say, his age, and will finally do the best he can with an answer which is incorrect by no more than a decade or so; it is also much more likely that there will be some degree of nominal dysphasia together with signs of parietal lobe damage.

A condition that could more accurately be termed *alcoholic dementia* has been described in some fairly recent studies (Cutting, 1978; Bergman *et al.*, 1980; Ron *et al.*, 1983). Chronic alcohol abusers have been shown to have wider ventricles than age-matched controls, with widened sulci over the cortex and cerebellum; these changes may be apparent even in patients under the age of 30 and do not correlate with duration of drinking, although they do correlate with severity of cognitive impairment. This may be widespread, with memory, personality and visuospatial defects. It is not clear whether the abnormalities seen on CT scanning are invariably the result of alcohol abuse or whether they may in some way predispose to it, but there is some support for the former in that abstinence may lead to improvement in some cases, even with decrease in ventricular size (Lishman, 1981).

The microscopic changes that underlie the condition are also uncertain. Dreyfus (1974) has reviewed studies that describe cell loss, gliosis, spongiform degeneration and laminar sclerosis in alcohol abusers. These changes are mainly confined to the frontoparietal cortex and are seen in various combinations; there is, thus far, no real evidence that a characteristic pattern exists.

As regards management — in cases where there is some question of brain damage, total abstinence must be the rule and, as indicated above, there is some possibility of improvement. Parenteral vitamin B complex is necessary in the acute phase, and a tranquillizer such as chlormethiazole may be effective in controlling withdrawal symptoms. But it should be remembered that alcohol-related brain disease is rarely an isolated condition, especially in an old person. Other diseases and deficiencies are almost always present; in particular, peripheral neuropathy or gastrointestinal or liver disease. Mellstrom *et al.* (1981) demonstrated a high prevalence of physical morbidity in alcoholics aged over 70; there was a higher prevalence of diabetes and chronic bronchitis, among other conditions, than in age-matched controls; they needed more care and mortality was higher.

Finally, the possibility of recent trauma should be considered in any elderly alcoholic brought to medical attention; subdural haematoma is common (Selecki, 1965) and, occasionally, the appearance of healed rib fractures on X-ray may give the first hint of the underlying diagnosis.

TRAUMATIC DEMENTIA

The acute of subacute effects of head injury do not, strictly speaking, fall within the 'dementia' category; it should only be said that subdural haematoma must be considered a possibility in a patient, especially if elderly, with confusion of fairly recent onset, perhaps with a fluctuating level of consciousness. There is not always a history of trauma, and symptoms may appear weeks or even months after the injury. Unfortunately, there are no altogether typical signs (Bedford, 1958; Lishman, 1978) and diagnostic accuracy during life is low, especially as the elderly patient may already be confused in some degree. However, if a demented patient develops an abnormal state of drowsiness, continuous or episodic, or an 'acute-on-chronic' confusional state, subdural haematoma is one of the possibilities, and the possibility is strengthened if there are asymmetrical reflexes or unequal pupils. Localizing signs are not always present, but CT scanning can be helpful in diagnosing and locating the haematoma; although a haematoma is sometimes isodense with brain tissue, its presence may be detected by distortion of the ventricular system.

The form of dementia which occurs in professional boxers is encountered from time to time, although it is fortunately rare. The first detailed description of 'dementia pugilistica' was in a man of 38 with progressive confusion and parkinsonism; changes resembling those of AD were found at post-mortem (Bradenburg and Hallervorden, 1954). Corsellis *et al.* (1973) reviewed a number of subsequent descriptions of the syndrome; the salient clinical features were chronic confusion and ataxia, often with parkinsonism. Post-mortem examination showed change in the septal area, loss of pigment in the substantia nigra and an abundance of neurofibrillary tangles in the cerebral cortex, often without abnormal numbers of plaques. Corsellis *et al.* generally confirmed these findings in a detailed study of the brains of 15 ex-professional boxers. Loss of Purkinje cells in the cerebellum, septal cavum (i.e. separation of the two halves of the septum, seen on coronal section), substantia nigra degeneration and widely distributed tangles, sometimes with a total absence of plaques, were consistent findings. Clinical history was variable, but clumsiness of speech and movement and loss of memory were common; in severe cases there was gross ataxia, dysarthria and dementia.

All of these subjects boxed in the 1900–40 period, and were presumably a selected group. But Roberts in 1969, from a study of a large random sample of boxers (224) who had held licences between 1929 and 1955, found evidence of brain damage in 50 per cent. Boxing controls are now stricter, and Roberts found a trend towards a lower prevalence of neurological abnormality; however, it is indisputable that boxing can still cause brain damage; Corsellis, who ruled out other possible causes in his subjects, believes it to be unlikely that all risk has been eliminated. There is also some possibility that similar types of damage may follow the head-banging and shaking associated with some of the more agitated forms of teenage dancing (Wood, 1984).

NORMAL PRESSURE HYDROCEPHALUS (NPH)

In 1965 Adams *et al.* described the cases of three patients who presented with chronic symptomatic hydrocephalus and a normal CSF pressure; shunting procedures resulted in complete restoration of neurological function in all three 'helplessly demented' patients. They considered recognition of the condition to be important in 'rescuing from oblivion' at least some of the patients considered to be suffering from senile dementia, as indeed it is. The cardinal features of the condition were a gradual onset of confusion, gait ataxia and urinary incontinence; headache and papilloedema did not occur. One of the patients, a paediatrician, was able to return to active practice after insertion of a shunt into the lateral ventricle.

Lishman (1981) has discussed the mechanism of normal pressure hydrocephalus. It is a 'communicating' hydrocephalus in that CSF can pass freely from the ventricles into the subarachnoid space; it is, however, prevented from flowing over the surface of the hemispheres for absorption at the superior sagittal sinus. The primary cause of the condition is not always clear; in some cases there is a history of head injury or meningitis. In some, even when there is no history of trauma or infection, post-mortem examination may reveal obstruction of the basal cisterns with fibrous tissue, possibly indicating an undiagnosed infection or subarachnoid haemorrhage.

It has been suggested that the 'normal' in the title may be misleading, since the pressure may have been elevated at an earlier stage (Geschwind, 1968), but the dynamics of the condition are still uncertain.

Little has been added to the original description of the clinical features by Adams *et al.* (1965). A gradual onset of symptoms indicative of diffuse brain disease, incontinence and lower limb ataxia are the characteristic triad which mean that the condition should be considered. A form of ataxia in which the patient's feet seem glued to the floor is frequently seen (Knuttson and Lying-Tunnell, 1985). Ataxia is rarely a feature of early AD; it is believed to occur in NPH due to stretching of the long tract fibres in the region of the dilated ventricles (Yakovlev, 1947; Katzman, 1978). Signs and symptoms of raised intracranial pressure such as headache or papilloedema are, however, more likely to suggest a diagnosis of tumour or subdural haemorrhage.

Diagnosis is usually confirmed on CT scanning (Figure 26); the appearances are of fairly uniform ventricular dilatation, normally without the sulcal widening seen in cases of AD; there is often some degree of periventricular oedema (Hughes and Gado, 1984).

Treatment is by insertion of a one-way shunt, commonly between the lateral ventricle and the superior vena cava. (This, of course, reduces CSF pressure to *subnormal* levels. Unfortunately, although in AD there is also increased ventricular size in the presence of normal CSF pressure, measures that reduce pressure in AD brains do not bring about clinical improvement (Katzman, 1978)). In NPH where there are no significant AD changes, some improvement can be expected although recovery may not always be complete.

Case No. 3

Mr C, aged 73, was referred because of a two-year history of worsening confusion and frequent falls. He had in due course become unable to walk; his wife required assistance to lift him, so he spent most of his time in an armchair in front of the fire. His legs had become burned and oedematous. His wife also had to feed and dress him and he was incontinent of urine. There was a substantial degree of personality deterioration; he lived in a three-generation household, and the fact that he constantly manipulated his genitals caused particular difficulty.

On examination there was general spasticity, with bilateral grasp and pout reflexes and extensor plantar responses. There were no other focal signs in the CNS.

He was inattentive, euphoric and disorientated, with perseveration; there was gross nominal dysphasia and he was apraxic, with poor motor co-ordination of both upper and lower limbs. He scored nil on the Abbreviated Mental Test Score (p. 114).

CT scanning (Figure 26) showed some degree of ventricular enlargement with normal sulci but with marked periventricular oedema. A ventriculoperitoneal shunt was performed; now, two months later, he is walking with the aid of a frame, can do rather more for himself and appears much more mentally alert, although there is unfortunately only an increase of a point or two in his mental test score, and this is variable.

NEUROSYPHILIS

This is now rare, but syphilitic infection is one of the potentially reversible causes of dementia, and serological screening should be routine, especially where onset is in the presenium. The most common clinical presentation is of progressive global dementia (Wood, 1984); absence of the specific features associated in the literature with neurosyphilis does not exclude the diagnosis.

Subacute dementia due to neurosyphilis (general paresis of the insane) becomes evident usually within one to five years of the primary infection, although the organism may lie dormant for thirty years or more. The brain is atrophied, mainly in the frontal and parietal regions, and there is often evidence of chronic meningitis. The microscopic changes are perivascular infiltration by plasma cells and lymphocytes in the cortex, interstitial iron deposits, and loss of cells with neuroglial proliferation, in particular of microglial Hortega cells, which have become elongated into characteristic 'rod cells'; these are arranged in parallel rows at right angles to the surface of the cortex.

Clinically, personality change with grandiosity or confabulation may distinguish the pattern of onset from that of AD, but depression is rather more common (Dewhurst, 1969); there are, however, no altogether characteristic psychiatric symptoms, and a positive result on syphilis serology is now most commonly an unexpected finding on routine screening. But pupillary abnormalities do occur in about two-thirds of cases (usually the Argyll-Robertson pupil — small, irregular and reacting to accommodation but not to light), as do coarse limb tremors (Lishman, 1981). Dysarthria and hyper-reflexia in the lower limbs are also fairly common findings, and in about 20 per cent of cases tabes dorsalis is present.

Where blood tests are negative but there are clinical signs of neurosyphilis then the CSF should be examined, as there is approximately a 10 per cent incidence of false negatives in the former; CSF serology is invariably positive in untreated cases. Equally, a number of conditions (rheumatoid arthritis, for example) may yield false *positives* on blood tests. Positive blood tests, therefore, also need to be confirmed by means of CSF examination.

Treatment is normally with a ten-day course of procaine penicillin, given in hospital because of the possibility of a 'Herxheimer reaction' — an acute fever which may occur early in treatment. Clinical improvement, as one might expect, is inversely related to the length of the history, but some improvement may be seen even in chronically and severely affected patients (Hahn *et al.*, 1959).

CREUTZFELDT-JAKOB DISEASE (CJD)

This has already been referred to as one of the 'spongiform encephalopathies' and, though rare, it is of importance because of its transmissibility. The distribution of the pathological changes within the CNS is variable, but the usual clinical presentation is of a rapidly progressive dementia together with signs indicative of damage in subcortical areas — often the basal or brain-stem nuclei, the cerebellum and the spinal cord.

Intellectual deterioration tends to progress concurrently with the motor or extrapyramidal damage (May, 1968). At an earlier stage there may be incoordination, nystagmus or muscle fibrillation resulting from involvement of the anterior horn cells of the spinal cord. Severe speech or visual disorders, parkinsonian symptoms or fits may occur, and coarse myoclonic jerks are a highly characteristic feature. Attempts have been made to stage the condition rather more precisely, but the clinical pattern is highly variable, at least in the early stages of the disease. The ultimate state, however, is one of gross dementia, emaciation and 'decerebration', and death usually occurs within three to nine months of onset.

Diagnosis during life is usually based on the history and clinical findings. There may be slight elevation of protein and cell count in the CNS, but these abnormalities are present in only some cases; gross ventricular enlargement (as seen on the CT scan) is rarely a feature (Kirschbaum, 1968). Catecholamine metabolite levels in the CNS may, however, be sharply decreased (Brun *et al.*, 1971). The EEG also may be highly abnormal, though the typical pattern tends to develop late in the disease. It shows periodic, generalized and bilaterally synchronous waves of 1–2 c/s. These may be spontaneous or may be evoked by a sensory stimulus (Roberts, 1984).

Apparent genetic transmission of CJD has been described; in 10–15 per cent of cases two or more members of one family are affected and in some families the disease appears to follow an autosomal dominant pattern (Masters *et al.*, 1979; Baker *et al.*, 1985); there are also published examples of conjugal cases (Matthews, 1985). But the question of whether the disease ever has a true genetic origin is still debated. Masters *et al.*, suggest, for example, that disease which appears to be transmitted genetically may in fact result from an unusually virulent strain of agent transmitted between those in close contact. In either case, it is of particular clinical relevance that iatrogenic transmission (especially by corneal transplant and psychosurgery) has been well established, and certain precautions are necessary in order to prevent spread once the disease has been diagnosed; these are detailed by Masters and Gajdusek (1982) and relate mainly to non-routine procedures. There is no evidence of risk to staff engaged in the general medical and nursing care of an affected patient.

The condition is generally untreatable, but three incidences of response to amantadine have been reported (Braham, 1971; Sanders and Dunn, 1973).

PICK'S DISEASE

This was first described in 1892; its prevalence is only about one-hundredth of that of AD. Transmission appears to follow a mendelian dominant pattern (Sjörjen *et al.*, 1952); no instances of person-to-person transmission have been recorded. Onset is usually in middle age, and women are affected more frequently than men.

The gross appearance of the brain is of sharply circumscribed lobar atrophy confined to the frontal and temporal lobes (as students we were told that, in contrast to AD, the condition 'picks' out certain areas). The anterior portions of the frontal and temporal lobes are most affected; the narrowed gyri and deeply indented sulci give these areas a 'walnut' appearance; the left hemisphere is commonly more atrophied than the right. These changes are so characteristic that Sjörgen *et al.* were able as a rule to make an accurate naked-eye diagnosis on the post-mortem table.

Microscopically there is massive cell loss and gliosis in the cortex, mainly in the outer layers. This loss may be curiously patchy, made up of multiple small foci of severe damage adjacent to relatively normal cells (Seitelberger, 1983). The other unusual features, first described by Alzheimer in 1911, is the presence of 'balloon cells' — nerve cell bodies distended with argentophilic material, often to the extent that the nucleus is displaced and flattened against the cell wall. There may also be spongiform appearances resembling those of Creutzfeldt-Jakob disease. Senile plaques and neurofibrillary tangles are rare, and may be completely absent (Jervis, 1971).

Signs of frontal lobe damage often appear first, with personality deterioration and mood disorder as prominent features. The patient may present with emotional lability or apathy associated with deteriorating standards of self-care that suggest AD, but on formal mental state examination, memory and language functions may turn out to be surprisingly well preserved. Fits may occur, although they are less common than in AD.

At a later stage there is more general cognitive damage and the condition becomes indistinguishable from other severe dementias. The distinction between AD and Pick's disease is in fact rarely made during life, although the latter may be suggested by dilatation of the anterior portions of the anterior and inferior horns of the third ventricle as seen on CT scanning. The disease usually runs a five- to ten-year course.

HUNTINGDON'S CHOREA

This condition is described here only in outline; there are already many detailed accounts of the clinical aspects of the disease (e.g. Lishman, 1981; Office of Health Economics, 1980); the biochemistry of the disease is described by Green and Costain (1981).

Transmission in most cases follows an autosomal dominant pattern with complete penetration, although the symptoms may appear first in middle age or later. In terms of diagnosis, it is noteworthy that a family history is obtained in only about 20 per cent of cases. Some few of the remainder (perhaps 5 per cent) may represent mutations but, as noted by Mahendra (1984) in his historical outline of the disease, failure to obtain a family history is more often due to denial, unaccounted-for deaths or illegitimacy (since promiscuity or increased fertility is sometimes a feature in sufferers).

Onset is usually around the age of 30–40, but the disease may present in the seventh or eighth decade. The classic choreiform movements are distal, twisting and tic-like, and develop insidiously, together with progressive dementia. The disease may also present initially as a presenile dementia similar to Pick's disease or AD, or even as a severe affective disorder. Oliver (1970) found depression in 35 per cent of Huntingdon's chorea patients, and it is believed that 7 per cent of deaths in sufferers from the condition are due to suicide. Patients may also present with a schizophreniform illness or in a pecular state of chronic euphoria. The patient usually declines into a profound state of dementia and ataxia within five to ten years, although patients may survive in a grossly deteriorated condition for a surprisingly long period; on occasion a cruel irony is that the constant movements prevent the development of pressure sores, venous stasis or pneumonia, any of which may lead to an earlier death in patients with some other forms of dementia.

In the brain, damage is principally to the basal ganglia and the cerebral cortex. The caudate nucleus is extensively damaged in most cases and in some it is almost totally replaced by glial tissue (Tomlinson, 1980). In the cortex there is cell loss together with gliosis, mainly in the frontal lobe, and examination of the white matter usually shows diffuse loss of nerve fibres, with narrowing of the corpus callosum.

The predominant biochemical change is a substantial decrease in gamma-aminobutyric (GABA) levels; the greatest decreases, around 75 per cent, are in the GABA-rich caudate nucleus, putamen, globus pallidus, substantia nigra and occupital cortex. The disease has been described by Green and Costain (1981) as in some ways the reverse of Parkinson's disease. The former is a hypokinetic state resulting from dopamine deficiency; GABA is an inhibitory neurotransmitter within the dopaminergic system, so that with reduction of its influence there is a *hyper*kinetic state due to dopamine overactivity. Defects in acetylcholine and catecholamine levels have also been described, but results have been inconsistent.

The diagnosis is indicated by a positive family history and progressive dementia together with choreiform movements; CT scanning is likely to show ventricular dilatation, especially with widening of the lateral ventricles in the area of the caudate nucleus. The EEG characteristically shows disappearance of alpha activity with very low amplitude and sometimes with almost total loss of cerebral rhythmic potentials (Scott, 1972). In advanced cases the tracing is flattened and featureless apart from prominent bursts of muscle activity. But there may be no abnormalities in the early stages, and EEG studies in families of Huntingdon's chorea sufferers have failed to defect carriers of the disease (Patterson, *et al.*, 1948; Chandler, 1966).

Treatment can only be symptomatic. Rationally, GABA-mimetic drugs such as sodium valproate should be effective, but results have been disappointing (Bird and Iversen, 1977). Dopamine antagonists, such as tetrabenazine, phenothiazines or butyrophenones, may be effective in controlling the choreiform movements.

The diagnosis of Huntingdon's chorea is often made after the patient has already had children and, since the disease is inherited as a mendelian dominant, the children will have a 50 per cent chance of themselves becoming victims. It is likely that predictive tests to identify those at risk (by means of a polymorphic DNA marker) will soon become available, but the use of such tests raises a number of ethical problems recently discussed by Craufurd and Harris (1986). As matters stand, predictive tests have still only been used for research purposes and there are no generally available means of discovering which offspring of Huntingdon's chorea sufferers are gene carriers and which are not; for the present, then, none of these offspring should have children. Sometimes sterilization or therapeutic abortion may be indicated, but expert genetic counselling is imperative.

PARKINSON'S DISEASE AND DEMENTIA

It is generally estimated that one patient in three with a diagnosis of Parkinson's disease (PD) becomes intellectually impaired, but the nature of the impairment is not agreed, nor is the question of whether PD is responsible for a form of dementia which is distinct from other types.

Brown and Marsden (1984) re-examine the diagnostic criteria for dementia upon which the one-in-three estimate is based. Some of these are vague and show a high proportion of false positives; it is suggested that a more accurate prevalence figure would be in the range 15–20 per cent. The figure for the *additional* risk of dementia over and above that in the general population would probably be in the range 10–15 per cent.

The cognitive changes have at times been reported to resemble or be identical to the insidiously progressive and widespread losses of AD (Boller *et al.*, 1980), although other studies (reviewed by Huber and Paulson, 1985) suggest that there may be amnesia and personality deterioration in the absence of aphasia, apraxia and agnosia. McCarthy and Gresty (1985) detected impairment of abstract reasoning in 7 out of 30 patients with newly diagnosed PD.

Histological features in the cortex of PD patients with dementia appear identical with those of AD and, in the same way, the numbers of plaques and tangles correlate with the severity of the dementia (Hakim and Mathieson, 1979; Boller *et al.*, 1980); it has been suggested that these changes simply represent the presence of coexisting AD (Marsden, 1984). It has also been suggested that these patients represent one of two distinct subgroups of AD patients: one is made up of younger patients with an exclusively motor disorder and a good response to L-dopa therapy; the other is an older group with a motor disorder followed by a cognitive disorder, and with a poor response to L-dopa (Lieberman, 1983).

However, the increased risk of at least some PD patients to AD-type dementia does require explanation; Pearce (1974) suggested that the two may form part of a spectrum of degenerative disorder. The risk appears to apply in both directions; Pearce found that 62 per cent of patients admitted to hospital with dementia showed parkinsonian features, and proposed that a disorder of dopamine metabolism could be common to both conditions.

Agid *et al.* (1984) quote studies showing that, conversely, cortical choline acetyltransferase activity may be diminished in the brains of PD patients, as it is in those with AD; their suggestion is that this reflects the degeneration of the innominatocortical (cholinergic) pathway, which has been shown to be damaged in PD as well as the dopaminergic system.

As with the other 'subcortical' dementias, there is a logical difficulty in categorizing a condition as a distinct form of dementia when it does not produce changes in the neocortex peculiar to itself, but the notion of 'brady-phrenia' goes some way towards reconciling the differing concepts of dementia; it is generally taken to represent the overall slowing in intellectual responsiveness typical of PD, which is at least in part dopamine mediated, and which also commonly includes features identical to those of clinical depression (Mayeux *et al.*, 1981). But while L-dopa therapy may improve the performance of cognitively impaired PD patients (Beardsley and Puletti, 1971; Bernheimer *et al.*, 1973), the effect is modest and often transient (Halgin *et al.*, 1977). The value of L-dopa therapy in AD without parkinsonian symptoms has not been established (p. 54), and its use is not recommended as there is a high frequency of side-effects, such as toxic confusion, hallucinations and mania (Goodwin, 1971; Agid *et al.*, 1984).

SUMMARY

Clinical medicine can provide pitiably few therapeutic or preventive measures in the area of chronic brain disease, but some do exist, making it necessary to distinguish where possible between the different types of dementia. Accurate diagnosis even of an untreatable condition is of assistance to a patient and to those caring for him.

Multi-infarct dementia is the most common type next to AD, accounting for 15–20 per cent of all dementias. The primary disorder is not, as was previously thought, in the cerebral blood vessels, but in relatively remote areas of the cardiovascular system, with multiple infarctions in the brain due to embolism. The history is therefore likely to include an account of ischaemic episodes affecting both the brain and other organs, and evidence of vascular disease will probably be found on examination. Cognitive damage is likely to be more uneven than in AD, with areas of loss or preservation which vary from one individual to another. Effective management requires in particular control of blood pressure and blood sugar and avoidance of smoking.

Alcohol abuse is a possible cause of chronic or fluctuating confusion at any age. Acute symptoms may be seen as Wernicke's encephalopathy — confusion together with eye signs resulting from damage to structures in the region of the third ventricle — and there may be enduring damage to the same area presenting as Korsakoff's psychosis — a relatively isolated loss of recent memory often associated with confabulation. Both of these conditions result from thiamine deficiency. A true 'alcoholic dementia' has also been described — diffuse cerebral atrophy leading to global impairment. All forms of alcohol-related brain disease may respond to treatment, mainly with vitamin supplements in the acute phase, and withdrawal in all cases.

Alcohol abuse and *head injury* are not unrelated; subdural haematoma is a high risk in alcoholics, but is a possibility in anyone with a history of trauma or with otherwise unexplained alterations in level of consciousness. Repeated trauma to the head over a long period can result in 'boxer's dementia', where there is chronic confusion and ataxia. The risk is rather less than in the past, but it remains substantial.

Normal pressure hydrocephalus is caused by failure of CSF resorption, probably as a result of past infection or trauma. Confusion, incontinence and ataxia are the usual presenting features; there is no clinical evidence of increased intracranial pressure but there are characteristic appearances on the CT scan. Insertion of a shunt may lead to total recovery.

Neurosyphilis is still encountered at times, and serological tests should be routine in cases of chronic confusion. The classic neurological signs of GPI are usually present, but may be absent in 10 per cent of cases. In 20 per cent of cases tabes dorsalis may be present. Treatment with penicillin is of potential benefit even in advanced cases.

Creutzfeldt-Jakob disease is also a transmissible dementia; it has often been transmitted iatrogenically by way of surgical procedures. The condition presents as a rapidly progressive dementia associated with extrapyramidal and spinal cord signs, the latter usually motor; myoclonic jerking is a characteristic feature. The disease is untreatable, but certain precautions will reduce the risk of spread.

Pick's disease is probably transmitted as a mendelian dominant; there is severe atrophy of the frontal and temporal lobes, so personality change is an early feature, but the condition is often indistinguishable clinically from AD, especially in its later stages.

Huntingdon's chorea is also transmitted as a mendelian dominant, but may occur as a result of mutation; damage is to the basal ganglia and the cerebral cortex. The choreiform movements may appear early, or the condition may present as a presenile dementia similar to AD or as a severe affective or schizophreniform disorder. There are characteristic changes on the EEG and the CT scan. Symptomatic treatment only is possible. Genetic counselling is essential in order to minimize the risk of transmission.

About one-fifth of patients with *Parkinson's disease* become demented. There is no typical pattern. In patients with severe dementia the cortical changes appear identical to those of AD; in others the intellectual deterioration can be described as 'bradyphrenia' resulting from the dopamine underactivity. It is likely that no clear line of distinction can be drawn between PD and AD; both represent degeneration of more than one ascending system.

The above conditions together account for 30–40 per cent of all dementias. Nearly all, being in some degree preventable, are becoming less common, and there is little doubt that the present trend will continue, with some becoming almost unknown within the next few decades. Also, with improving diagnostic methods, some dementias now considered to be of AD type will turn out after all to be remediable conditions. Therefore AD will assume greater prominence and will account for an ever-larger proportion of the dementias. The painstaking research into diagnosis and treatment that has been applied to other forms of brain disease will be directed to this most intractable condition to an even greater degree than at present. Will the results be equally rewarding?

CHAPTER 5
Diagnosis

Dementia is not a mere diagnosis of exclusion. But it is unfortunately too often the flag of convenience under which a confused and otherwise undiagnosed patient sets out on his final passage to a mental hospital or a geriatric ward. The essential first stage in diagnosis is certainly to exclude any remediable causes of confusion that may mimic or complicate dementia, but the various types of dementia have their own clinical features that need next to be identified before a safe diagnosis can be made. The less common types of dementia have been described in the previous chapter; this section will deal mainly with the diagnosis of Alzheimer's disease, and in particular with its distinction from acute toxic and affective disorders.

Diagnosis in psychiatry is generally believed to be imprecise; it is asserted that psychiatrists lack even a definition of illness. We cannot decide, it is said, whether or not a person with symptoms of mild depression or anxiety is truly 'ill'. In the same way, patients with dementia may be as poorly tolerated in a psychiatric ward as in an acute medical ward; they are not ill, they are psychogeriatric. Quite probably they are also undiagnosed.

The definition of illness in psychiatry is, or should be, no different from that which applies in other areas of medicine. *Illness is loss of function*. In the case of depressive disorder, for example, a patient may show psychomotor retardation, sleep disturbance, constipation or weight loss. If he is anxious he may suffer from handicaps due to phobia, from tachycardia or tremor. There are objective ways in which an illness interferes with a full and normal life; outside the area of these measurable disabilities it is doubtful whether medicine or psychiatry can have any useful function. Indeed, harm can be done by the use of tranquillizers, or by the use of psychotherapies which make the patient even more discontented and self-obsessed. This applies to functional and to organic disorders, both of which have clear objective features that have to be sought. Furthermore, in neither area does a single symptom represent a diagnosis; in the simplest terms, a patient is not clinically depressed because he is tearful or depressed because he is forgetful. There is a tendency to overvalue such single symptoms, and this is how most of the difficulties in distinguishing between functional and organic disorder in the elderly arise, and how such non-diagnoses as 'pseudodementia' come into being. To arrive at an accurate diagnosis in psychiatry it is necessary, as in other areas, to identify a clinical syndrome — that is, the *group* of impairments of function which belong to a particular diagnostic category and which are fairly consistent from one patient to another. In the field of dementia in particular, it is upon such 'syndrome diagnosis' that most effective practice depends. A clinician who, for example, examines a patient systematically for the signs of AD will occasionally find symptoms that are unexpected, that don't fit in. The dementia may be associated with vivid auditory hallucinations, for example, leading to investigation of the patient for hypothyroidism. There may be ataxia, possibly indicating normal pressure hydrocephalus. Areas of preservation — for example, adequate memory functions in the presence of severe personality disorder or dysphasia — may suggest a tumour, and CT scanning is then indicated. Or other evidence (e.g. the presence of bowel or urinary symptoms) may suggest that the primary disease lies outside the brain altogether.

In instances where a patient appears to be confused, therefore, diagnosis is essentially a three-stage process. First, any remediable causes of confusion need to be sought — and this is necessary even if a diagnosis of dementia has been made previously. Second, symptoms of functional mental illness have to be distinguished from those of organic brain disease and, third, the nature of any organic brain disease has to be established.

ACUTE CONFUSIONAL STATES

Case No. 4

Mrs D was severely confused and incontinent; a place in a mental hospital was sought for her. On examination she was frail and could scarcely stand; when she was eventually helped to her feet a strong ammoniacal odour permeated the room. She was treated in a short-stay ward for a urinary tract infection and three weeks later returned home in a state of moderate mental alertness.

Case No. 5

Miss E was 60 and for many years had lived in a hostel for the homeless; during the year before referral she had shown signs of worsening confusion; it was episodic and heavy drinking was thought to be the cause. She was sent to a psychiatric clinic because she was 'much worse and peeing everywhere'. She was underweight and polyuric; her blood sugar turned out to be grossly elevated. Her diabetes was treated (under section 46 of the National Assistance Act in a general medical ward) and she made a substantial mental recovery and was placed in the hostel again, with a district nurse to give regular injections and test her urine.

Every severe illness leaves its mark and there is rarely a 'miracle cure' for any cause of acute confusion, but the detection of a treatable cause for what has been considered to be a hopeless case of dementia is an immensely rewarding experience for both patient and doctor, and by no means uncommon. It follows a systematic approach which depends on knowledge of which conditions are most likely to cause confusion in an elderly patient, and of the ways in which they usually present clinically.

The possibility of an acute confusional state will, in the first instance, be raised by the history. 'Take a full history' is standard and undoubtedly good advice, but the time that can be spent on history-taking is restricted and must be used to best advantage; the clinician must know what he is looking for. He will be concerned mainly with two aspects of the history of a confusional state: first, the pattern of onset and, second, the presence and nature of any associated features.

History: pattern of onset

An independent history from a relative, friend or other acquaintance is virtually essential. Alteration in a patient's everyday behaviour over a period of time is probably one of the most sensitive of all indicators of progressive brain disease and, not surprisingly, accounts given by a relative are much more reliable than those given by the patient himself and show a high degree of consistency (Kellett et al., 1975; Baddeley et al., 1982). It is also necessary to ask about any past medical history that the patient may have, although it is my experience that accounts in this area may be poor and omit important details; they need to be verified from medical sources.

Next, what are the patient's recent or present habits? Does he smoke or drink heavily? Is he receiving any medication? Sleeping tablets are often felt to be in a separate category from other tablets and need to be asked about specifically; the same applies to tranquillizers, which are a potent cause of confusion in old people. Learoyd (1972) found that, of 236 consecutive admissions to a psychogeriatric unit, 16 per cent were due to adverse reactions to psychotropic drugs; in a series of 50 patients referred to a clinic that had been established to diagnose memory problems in the elderly, we (Van der Cammen et al., 1987) found that the symptoms in two patients were entirely due to medically prescribed tranquillizers (flurazepam in one case, diazepam in another) and disappeared when the drugs were withdrawn. The drugs especially likely to cause confusion in the elderly are listed in Table 16.

Then, were the symptoms abrupt or insidious in their onset? Are there spells of severe confusion alternating with periods of relative lucidity? What were the first symptoms, how did they develop and what are the symptoms now? Were there problems with the patient's job or with housework? AD will tend to have become apparent over a period of months, and the changes most likely to have been noticed by other people are difficulties in a patient's employment — where applicable — or in the daily domestic routine (Simpson et al., 1984). A difficulty with people's names is also a common early symptom (names have no associative 'peg' on which they can be hung), and this may in due course progress to severe forgetfulness, repetitiousness, the loss of items in the house

Table 16.   Drugs liable to cause confusion in the elderly

Tranquillizers/hypnotics (esp. barbiturates and benzodiazepines)
Digoxin
Tricyclic antidepressants
Levodopa
Methyldopa
Beta blockers
Anticonvulsants
Anticholinergics
Steroids

---

or disorientation outdoors. Evidence of language disorder ('he sometimes mixes his words up') or personality deterioration (e.g. unaccountable bouts of depression, euphoria or rage) tend to follow at a somewhat later stage. There are also likely, at this stage, to be accounts of clumsiness (apraxia), with some inability to wash or dress. Incontinence is also a relatively late feature in AD, and is often due to the patient's losing his way about the house. Grand mal fits are also an occasional feature of AD.

Paranoid behaviour is extremely common in the earlier stages of AD; it may in fact be the presenting problem. Typically an elderly person misplaces items in the house and angrily accuses her relatives of having moved or hidden them. If she lives alone, she may insist that people enter her flat while she is absent and steal objects, break them or move them around. AD in a younger patient has more than once, in my experience, been diagnosed initially as paranoid schizophrenia.

Case No. 6
Miss F, aged 50, had lived alone for some years and was said to have become increasingly 'odd'. She locked her relatives and the doctor outside, insisting they were imposters, and took to hammering, both by day and by night, on the walls of the adjoining flats, accusing the occupants of interfering with her belongings; in the end she became so combative that she was compulsorily hospitalized. On examination there was evidence of severe memory loss, disorientation and dysphasia, and in due course AD was diagnosed. She was placed for a short time in a nursing home, but is now in a long-stay psychogeriatric ward with gross confusion, incontinence and a number of 'primitive' reflexes indicative of severe brain damage.

Case No. 7
Mr G, who was an author of some distinction, was admitted with an almost identical history; his CT scan (Figure 25) shows gross cerebral atrophy.

A fluctuating confusional state is rather more typical of cardiovascular disease than it is of AD; in particular, where there are brief episodes of confusion with near-total recovery after each, multi-infarct dementia is a strong possibility (p. 80). But any departure from the insidious and fairly typical history of AD as outlined above is noteworthy; it is highly improbable, for example, that confusion of abrupt or rapid onset is purely the result of AD. Again, one clinical feature may stand out in isolation. Early personality change might suggest a frontal tumour or Pick's disease; isolated memory loss, perhaps with confabulation, might suggest alcoholism or vitamin B_{12} deficiency. As in Case No. 1, an isolated expressive difficulty suggests a focal lesion, probably an infarct or tumour.

History: associated features

These are recent symptoms of disease both in the CNS and in other organs which may help to pinpoint the diagnosis, especially in the case of acute toxic confusion. First, has there been cough, sputum or fever? Then, have there been symptoms of cardiovascular disease? Heart failure or coronary thrombosis commonly cause confusion; there are also likely to be symptoms of extracerebral vascular disease if the patient is suffering from dementia of multi-infarct type. Has there been angina, or symptoms of intermittent claudication or of poor circulation in the extremities? Signs in the CNS suggestive of MID are headache, dizzy spells or falls. Also in the CNS, gait disorder or incontinence at an early stage may indicate normal pressure hydrocephalus; ataxia at an early stage, especially of the upper limbs, may indicate Huntingdon's chorea. Has there been any recent fall or head injury that may lead to a diagnosis of subdural haematoma?

Next, have there been any bladder or bowel problems? Dysuria will suggest infection and polyuria will suggest diabetes; changes of bowel habit or weight could indicate bowel carcinoma, which may be associated with confusion in an elderly patient.

Finally — although affective disorder scarcely fits into the 'acute confusion' category, this is a convenient time to ask whether the patient has shown recent evidence of anxiety or depression. Some 10–15 per cent of patients with apparent confusional states are in reality suffering from affective illness, most commonly depression (Fish and Williamson, 1964; Van der Cammen et al., 1987), and this possibility needs to be considered at an early stage. Has he been tearful? Has there been loss of sleep, appetite or weight? Has his conversation been depressive in content? Has there been slowing up or loss of interest in normal activities? True depressive illness will have a consistency over time which generally sets it apart from the emotional change characteristic of frontal lobe damage, where the patient is emotionally labile, easily swayed between one extreme and the other.

Physical examination

In the same way as when the history is taken, the principal causes of acute confusion are sought and excluded systematically; again, the salient points can generally be covered fairly quickly. The section that follows is not a detailed account of the acute confusional states, which are of course dealt with fully in textbooks of general psychiatry; it simply outlines the features that most usually differentiate the condition from dementia.

Chest infection

Respiratory disease is probably the most common single cause of acute confusional states in the elderly (Hodkinson, 1973); in particular, the pneumonias account for about one-quarter of all confusional states (Kay and Roth, 1955; Flint and Richards, 1956; Agate, 1960). Confusion may also result from acute exacerbations of chronic bronchitis. Where there are recurrent chest infections, malignancy should also be suspected, and the patient should be re-X-rayed after the acute infection has subsided, at which stage a bronchial carcinoma is more readily visualized.

Although not now common, tuberculosis is still from time to time encountered as a cause of resistant chest infections and a fluctuating confusional state.

Cardiovascular disease

Cardiac failure has been revealed as a causative factor in up to 22 per cent of groups of elderly people with confusion (Flint and Richards, 1956; Hodkinson, 1973). Confusion of relatively abrupt onset will suggest coronary thrombosis or stroke, both of which can be relatively 'silent' in terms of prominent physical signs. Patients with cardiac thrombosis may show arrhythmias or a fall in blood pressure or be diagnosed only by means of an ECG; in the case of stroke there may be 'soft' neurological signs such as mild apraxia, dysphasia or sensory inattention.

Urinary tract infection

This is the third of the triad of common causes of confusion in the elderly, and causes or contributes to perhaps 20 per cent of cases (Kay and Roth, 1955; Hodkinson, 1973). It may also be silent clinically, or there may be no symptoms other than incontinence; one should remember that a description of a patient as 'confused and incontinent' can be misleading; the urinary problem may well be primary. Incontinence is not an integral feature of dementia, and should always be investigated (p. 158).

Carcinoma

Carcinoma at virtually any site can present with confusion in an elderly patient; it was a significant factor in 5 per cent of Hodkinson's series of 144 patients aged 65 and over with confusion of recent onset. The bronchus or bowel is the most usual primary site; there may be localizing signs in the CNS indicative of cerebral secondaries, but this is uncommon. On physical examination, detection of liver deposits or a mass on per rectum examination tends to be more reliable than the palpation of masses in the large bowel, often due to constipation or impaction. Both the latter can, however, cause double incontinence and confusion in the elderly.

The presence of carcinoma is often first indicated by abnormal liver function tests.

Diabetes

Routine screening is essential, but the diagnosis may be indicated clinically by severe weight loss, peripheral neuropathy or polyuria (p. 97). Drug-induced hypoglycaemia may also cause confusion which, in the elderly, may not be associated with sweating or hypotension.

Hypothyroidism

This again needs to be screened for routinely, as it is not uncommon as a cause of confusion in old people; the classic physical signs of myxoedema are not necessarily present, but the confusion is often associated with fairly colourful delusions or hallucinations. These are of the type commonly encountered in patients with late paraphrenia — generally paranoid in type and often with a fairly overt sexual content. Hallucinations are probably more common and vivid than in 'functional' paraphrenia.

Case No. 8
Mrs H, aged 75, had been suffering from worsening memory loss and disorientation for more than a year; during the last few months, she had been complaining bitterly about the tenants who lived upstairs. These were two men whom she was convinced were homosexual, and she said that she could hear them making indecent propositions to one another; she was able to hear them through the ceiling, although they spoke only in whispers. However, she heard their voices only through one ear, while in the other (as if to redress the balance) she heard hymns. She did not know where these were coming from; the hymn was usually 'Abide with Me'. She could hear it while I was interviewing her and, by closing her eyes and concentrating, she was able to tell which verse was being sung.

On questioning, she said that she had been troubled by dry hair and skin in the recent past. Tests revealed gross hypothyroidism; she was treated with thyroxine replacement therapy and the hallucinations vanished within two weeks and did not recur. Her memory improved but there is some residual impairment, which is often the case in treated hypothyroid patients. The memory loss is, however, isolated and there is no dysphasia, dyspraxia or personality change.

An important point is that serum T4 is an unreliable test on which to base any view on thyroid function; especially where a patient is elderly or has had a number of infections, serum globulin levels may be sufficiently elevated to give a normal T4 level even in the presence of severe hypothyroidism. In another patient aged 73 at present under treatment, symptoms were severe isolated loss of recent memory together with confabulation and the belief that her bedroom was being entered and she was being raped almost nightly. In addition to other clinical features of hypothyroism, there were classic 'hung-up' reflexes. T4 level was within normal limits, but TSH was grossly elevated at 28 u./1. The latter is the more reliable index of thyroid deficiency and should always be included in screening. (This patient's normal CT scans are shown in Figures 17 and 18.)

Alcoholism

The diagnosis may be suggested by a number of features in the history and clinical presentation. In summary, these are a history of fluctuating confusion associated with falls or other injuries, social isolation, fits or hallucinations, a general appearance of self-neglect, peripheral neuropathy, tremor, gastric or liver disease. The types of alcoholic brain damage are dealt with on p. 83.

Drugs

The drugs that frequently cause confusion have already been listed (Table 16). The clinician will not be satisfied with the patient's or relatives' account of his current medication, but will want to see the tablets for himself; a full and rattling plastic bag of astonishing size is commonly produced — but questions of medication, alcohol intake and diet are often most quickly dealt with by means of a home visit.

Dunn and Arie (1973) reported a number of instances of improvement where medically prescribed drugs were withdrawn, and Van der Cammen *et al.* (1987) have described two in which apparent 'dementia' was entirely drug-induced (p. 98).

Electrolyte disturbances

Hypokalaemia is the electrolyte disturbance most commonly associated with confusion (Hodkinson, 1973), and usually results from vomiting, diarrhoea or the overuse of diuretics or laxatives. Hypocalcaemia may be a cause of confusion in patients with renal disease or with dietary calcium or vitamin D deficiencies.

Anaemia

This, like many of the other conditions listed here, often follows self-neglect, although the causes of anaemia in the elderly are of course legion, and its detection is only the starting-point in diagnosis. Vitamin B_{12} deficiency, with or without anaemia, is more likely to cause confusion in an elderly person than is iron deficiency.

Other conditions to be excluded at an early stage are liver and renal disease. Hypothermia is also a cause of confusion in the elderly; it is to some extent seasonal, and contributed to by poverty and poor housing conditions, but the majority of elderly people brought to hospital with the condition are suffering from 'secondary' hypothermia; the most common conditions that underlie hypothermia are infections, stroke, heart failure and hypothyroidism. The use of tranquillizing and antidepressant drugs also predisposes to hypothermia (Collins, 1983).

Defects of vision and hearing may also cause apparent confusion associated with hallucinations, illusions and paranoid symptoms (Herbst, 1982; Berrios and Brook, 1984; Christenson and Blazer, 1984). Finally, there is likely to be more than one cause of a severe confusional state; the 'acute-on-chronic' confusion caused by extracerebral illness in a demented person is fairly common, but it has also been said that a doctor who makes a single diagnosis in a confused elderly patient has missed at least two others!

The results of *investigations* usually add very little to what is already known about the patient. Kellett *et al.* (1975) found that an adequate initial interview of a patient and his next of kin was likely to achieve a correct diagnosis in 95 per cent of cases. Colgan and Philpot (1985), in a study of 167 patients admitted to a psychiatric ward for the elderly, found that only 4 per cent of investigations influenced future management. Victoratos *et al.* (1977) and Renvoise *et al.* (1985a,b) also found that about 5 per cent of apparent dementias were discovered to be reversible after full examination and investigation, but it is not clear in these studies how much the investigations contributed to diagnosis. In any case, when an elderly patient presents with confusion, the following should be carried out initially: full blood count and ESR or CRP, blood urea and electrolytes, liver function tests, serum glucose, vitamin B_{12} and folate, thyroid function tests, urine examination and culture, syphilis serology and chest X-ray. In a confusional state of acute onset, an ECG might be indicated. Other tests which might help to discriminate between various types of dementia (e.g. the EEG and CT scan) are dealt with from p. 127.

FUNCTIONAL OR ORGANIC?

This is the great watershed in psychiatric diagnosis; in the case of an elderly and uncommunicative person with memory loss, the difficulty is principally that of deciding whether the patient is suffering from dementia or depression. Severe depression can by itself cause memory loss, together with failure of grasp and apparent disorientation, and can impair performance on several formal tests of cognition (Nott and Fleminger, 1975; Ron *et al.*, 1979; Fraser and Glass, 1980);

depressed elderly patients as a result risk being misclassified (Post, 1975; Marsden and Harrison, 1972).

The difficulty in making the distinction is not, however, so great; as pointed out earlier, most errors in the area arise from confusing symptoms with syndromes. Generally speaking, diagnoses of both organic and functional disorders are unsafe unless the characteristic *group* of impairments that make up the syndrome in question is identified.

The diagnosis of depression is a good example and is, for the reasons given above, particularly relevant. The features of depressive illness should be sought even if the clinician is fairly sure that the patient is demented; depressive illness can still complicate and worsen the patient's overall condition. The depressive syndrome, like any other, is made up of a number of functional impairments; not only is there depression of mood, there is also 'depression' of sleep, appetite, weight, hydration, mobility, mental alertness and memory, and there is distorted and pathological thinking. Table 17 sets out the way in which these changes, seen together, translate into the clinical features of a depressive illness. In cases of doubt, one of the diagnostic scales which itemize the main symptoms of depression can be useful (p. 128) and will sensitize the clinician to the fairly consistent nature of the syndrome and its complications (Fraser, 1984).

With symptoms of affective disorder either identified or excluded, the next step is to attempt a *positive* diagnosis of AD, which is a psychiatric syndrome, with its typical set of impairments, like any other. There is an ample literature to show that the 'multidimensional', 'global' or 'cluster' diagnosis of AD is the only reliable one (Hare, 1978; Ballinger *et al.*, 1982; Gurland *et al.*, 1982; Rabins *et al.*, 1984). Isolated signs can be most misleading; Hare showed, for

Table 17.   Features of clinical depression in the elderly

'Depressed' function	Symptoms	Common complications
Mood	Sadness, tearfulness, guilt	Suicide, alcoholism, drug dependence
Appetite	Anorexia, weight loss	Dehydration, falls, fracture
Mobility } Speech }	Psychomotor retardation	Contractures, pressure sores, hypothermia, isolation and malnutrition, break-up of family or job
Sleep	Insomnia	Hypnotic dependence
Bowel function	Constipation	Single or double incontinence, impaction
Cognition	Impaired memory, concentration and attention	Misdiagnosis as dementia

example, that, of a group of patients with severe amnesia, 34 per cent had recovered within six months, and were depressed rather than demented. On the other hand, those with lesser memory defects but with temporoparietal signs had deteriorated cognitively.

The diagnosis of AD is therefore largely a clinical matter, requiring little more than orderly thinking; Rabins *et al.* (1984) were able, on the basis of standard clinical examination, to make diagnoses of depression and dementia that were stable at two-year follow-up, and they conclude that diagnosis in the area has nothing to do with mysterious disorders that only experts in the area can detect, but depends on the careful checking for signs and symptoms that would appear in any other area.

The key to accuracy is that *AD is a disorder consistently affecting certain areas of the brain, so that diagnosis depends on identifying symptoms and signs referrable to all or most of these areas.* It is true that one may encounter the late-onset and relatively benign form of AD (probably equivalent to 'AD-1', as described in Chapter 2), in which memory loss appears to be the most prominent defect, but careful testing even of these patients usually reveals deficits in other areas as well. It is questionable whether there exists a true *senium naturale* (Kral, 1962); the observations underlying Kral's view were confined to memory; there is no record of testing for other cognitive losses. These, like AD itself, are latent at earlier stages and are detectable only by challenge (Thompson, 1985). The following section, then, will describe the form of clinical examination recommended for accurate diagnosis and will deal with symptoms and signs in relation to the main sites of damage.

CLINICAL FEATURES OF ALZHEIMER'S DISEASE

The frontal lobe

Frontal lobe damage in AD brings about personality change, language disorder and, at a later stage, the emergence of neurological signs such as 'primitive' reflexes.

Personality change

There is no altogether typical pattern of change, but a state of *apathy* has generally been described (Sjörgen *et al.*, 1952; Miller, 1977). A common presentation is of a deeply anxious family together with a bland, slightly bewildered patient who has no idea what all the fuss is about. Memory defects or possibly wandering episodes are likely to be denied by the patient, perhaps with amusement, perhaps angrily. There may at an early stage be some insight into the memory loss and questions can be cleverly evaded (this, in my experience, depends largely on the previous intellectual endowment of the patient), but this is soon lost. The most sensitive account of personality change will of course come from the patient's relatives, but the clinician is likely to notice a certain blandness or detachment at interview. Bouts of irritability will often be described or be evident to the clinician, and the question will arise of whether there are significant depressive symptoms. The diagnosis of depression is described earlier — and a diagnosis of AD does not preclude the presence of coexisting depressive symptoms — but the emotions of uncomplicated AD, in contrast to those of true clinical depression, are shallow, fleeting and inconsistent. The well-recognized later state is one of *emotional incontinence*, where there is lability of mood to the extent that the patient is easily swayed by a few words (or for no apparent reason) either to laughter or to tears.

The patient's emotional disinhibition may also take the form of *restlessness* — probably the feature of dementia which causes most trouble to relatives and other carers. Sometimes this relates to earlier working habits — as where a former early-shift worker takes to rousing the household at 5 a.m. — but there is more usually an irrational restless pottering and wandering which cannot be related directly to any previous habits.

The personality change will also lead to a deterioration in self-care, with lack of attention to dress and hygiene, and to coarsening of behaviour and language. Excessive smoking and scattering of ash, untidy eating habits and indiscriminate urination may follow.

Paranoid behaviour is extremely common in patients with AD; some patterns have been described earlier (p. 99). Often, as with restlessness, it will appear almost as a natural consequence of the memory loss (misplacement of objects and angry accusations of theft or interference); however, elderly demented people living alone may develop quite vivid visual or auditory hallucinations on the basis of early AD, social deprivation and some form of sensory deficit. It is surprising how often, for example, patches of early cataract turn out to be at least the partial explanation for the sinister invaders in an old lady's flat. Unfortunately, eye and ear examination in the case of a hallucinated elderly patient is often omitted.

As the disease advances, there is a general flattening and impoverishment of emotion. To relatives this will represent a sad loss of contact with the person they have known — but it is often the case that a patient who has previously been restless and anguished (perhaps because of a degree of insight) will in due course enter a more tranquil and outwardly philosophical phase in his final years. It is reasonable to reassure anxious relatives (though it is only small comfort) that this is a likely progression.

Language disorder

Language disorder, or dysphasia, is well recognized as a reliable marker for the presence of AD and as an index of its severity. Language disorder is the result of damage in Broca's area (the posterior part of the inferior frontal gyrus) in the language-dominant hemisphere, usually the left. It is ironic that a difficulty with terminology arises here; the condition is also referred to as 'aphasia'; there is the same confusion over 'dyspraxia'. The prefixes 'a-' and 'dys-' tend to be used almost interchangeably to indicate disorder, and in the present work, although 'dys-' is preferred, the interchangeable use of the two cannot be avoided; the lack of any general convention is unfortunate.

Language disorder in relation to dementia has been a subject of close study only in fairly recent years; it is usually the case that dysphasia does not give rise to any noticeable difficulty in the patient's daily life in the early stages if AD, so it is missed if not tested for specifically (Rosen and Mohs, 1982). Skelton-Robinson and Jones (1984) have reviewed a number of studies which indicate that patients with various degrees of senile dementia show a significantly greater expressive difficulty (particularly delays in naming) than age-matched controls; there was a striking degree of correlation ($r=0.8$) between severity of dementia, as measured by a mental test score, and score on an object-naming test. Similarly, Kirshner (1984) found that scores on an aphasia test discriminated sharply between patients with early senile dementia and other elderly ill patients. Hare (1978) found that language disorder was a reliable predictor of progressive dementia, and Berg *et al.* (1984), from a study in which 53 subjects with mild senile dementia were compared with age-matched controls, found that aphasic disturbances as revealed on an aphasia test battery were predictive of progression to more severe dementia within 12 months. Similarly, Naguib and Levy (1982b) found decreased survival in patients with dysphasia, dysgraphia and dyspraxia — the 'instrumental dysfunctions' of AD.

Language disorder is a complex subject about which volumes have been written, but for the purpose of diagnosing AD it is sufficient to examine, broadly, for 'receptive' and 'expressive' dysphasia. Neither is especially difficult to elicit, and they should be sought routinely. There may be a history of language disorder, but this is unlikely in early AD; however, name-finding is extremely vulnerable in the condition, and problems can readily be elicited by clinical testing. Signs of receptive dysphasia are, by contrast, almost always of late onset.

The detection of a language problem needs to be approached with tact, especially in patients with only mild impairment. Often a naming test can be presented as one of vision. One might ask, 'How is your eyesight, Mrs Jones?', and then ask the patient to look out of the window (where convenient) and describe what she can see. Any lack of fluency will often be apparent at this stage. Then one can proceed to simple objects (a pen, a bunch of keys, a watch) and then to others that are progressively more complex — the point of the pen, the watch strap, the winder, the buckle. A patient with AD will almost invariably have difficulty at some stage. In early AD there will probably be hesitation, or evasions such as 'it's a thing' or 'it's a wassisname'; *circumlocution* is an extremely common response: a patient cannot name an object, but may be able to say what it is for, as 'It's for writing with' or 'You tell the time with it'. Patients with moderate degrees of preservation can use circumlocutory responses with great skill to conceal their handicap. Thus a retired authoress, tartly, when shown my pen and asked if she could see what it was: 'Of course I can. I didn't suppose that you wrote with your finger!' But the word 'pen' was never forthcoming. Other patients may show great irritation and impatience at being asked 'stupid questions'.

A dysphasic patient may show *paraphasia* — substitution or alteration of words; a pen may be a 'pill', for example. This tends to be a later phenomenon; also in more damaged patients there may be *perseveration*, where the answer to a former question is repeated. Or there may be *echolalia*, where the question itself is repeated. The change is in general in the direction of increasing poverty of language, and in severe AD there may be no useful words — simply a few syllables or a meaningless babble.

The above problems generally indicate *expressive* dysphasia. *Receptive* dysphasia is generally encountered in the later stages of AD. It can sometimes be presented as a test of hearing, as in asking a patient what a watch or a thermometer is. Or simple instructions may be given, though the ability to follow these may remain surprisingly well preserved. It is, indeed, a common and accurate observation that demented patients often understand more than they can express, and both relatives and doctors should be aware of this. When I had finished examining a man of 55 with AD who was totally disorientated and incoherent, his wife asked me how long he was likely to live. I said, unthinkingly, 'Perhaps only a few years', and saw, to my dismay, the patient's eyes suddenly fill with tears. It was a valuable object lesson.

'Primitive' reflexes

These are 'release' phenomena, found where the cortex fails to inhibit the subcortical centres that control motor activity; they are associated with immaturity and also with frontal lobe damage. They are almost invariably a late feature when they occur in AD.

The grasp reflex: the palm is stroked in an outward direction, usually with two or three fingers, resulting in a grasping response by the patient.

The palmomental reflex: the thenar eminence is stroked in an outward direction and the response is puckering of the contralateral lower lip.

The sucking reflex: the clinician's forefinger is brought towards the patient's mouth; the response is pouting of the lips.

The snout reflex: the lips are protruded in response to tapping of the upper or lower lip.

The extensor plantar or Babinski reflex: outward stroking of the inner aspect of the sole of the foot is followed by extension of one or all of the toes.

Some of these reflexes can be elicited in normal individuals, but they are usually indicative of severe frontal cortical damage. At an advanced stage of AD there may be widespread rigidity and a 'fetal' posture similar to that seen in other conditions where there is decerebration.

The temporal lobe

The temporal lobe, which includes the mesial limbic structures, is essentially the area that governs memory. The theories of memory, ever changing and much debated by psychologists, are not for dissection here; it is necessary, however, to have some understanding of what is at present known about memory in order to know what tests are clinically useful in the detection of disease. For a comprehensive and readable account of current professional views on memory, Baddeley (1983) is recommended. Much of what follows is drawn from this work, and also from Baddeley *et al.* (1982).

For clinical purposes, memory can be thought of as having two main constituents: short-term memory (STM) and long-term memory (LTM). STM has a duration measured only in seconds, and has a capacity for only about ten items; it is heavily reliant on phonemic coding. One thing that this means in practice is that remembering a list of unrelated numbers or words which the subject has heard only once depends largely on subvocal rehearsal. If this is prevented, for example by asking the patient to repeat some nonsense words, the memory is disrupted. If you look up a phone number and someone speaks to you as you are about to dial and you have to reply, then you will probably have to look up the number again.

As required, however, items are transferred into the main memory store (LTM). Coding here is quite different and is not altogether understood, but it certainly depends to a large degree on the association of new items with those that have been laid down previously. Names, as we have seen, are among the most difficult things of all to remember because of a lack of any easily found associative 'peg', and memory for names is thus especially vulnerable in AD; impairment is often one of the first symptoms.

It should be understood, then, that STM is *not* the same thing as 'recent memory', though the two are often confused. STM is very short-term indeed; memory for both remote and recent events are, after a matter of seconds, encoded into LTM.

The anatomical and biochemical substrates of this process have been examined briefly in earlier chapters. The hippocampal system has been experimentally linked with STM and the temporal cortex with LTM; writers in the area warn against 'boxology', and this is certainly an oversimplification, but the basic STM/LTM model does hold up well in practical terms when it comes to diagnosis and prediction in patients with dementia.

The principal memory defect in AD is inability to store new information. There is increasing difficulty in adding new information to LTM, and the record is also less durable — that is, the new information is more quickly forgotten. As in the case of other defects, an independent history relating to problems in the patient's everyday life may be much more informative than will standard clinical tests. Simpson *et al.* (1984) found that such 'behavioural' evidence of dementia was frequently described before clinical signs of dementia were apparent. The subject will not have remembered what has been said to him recently, items will need to be repeated to him, or he will repeat himself, often asking the same questions several times over. He will forget appointments unless reminded, and even then he may forget; he may leave the gas or electricity on or — very common — may put a saucepan or kettle on the stove and forget about it until it has boiled dry, and perhaps taken fire.

Certain standard tests of memory are not helpful in diagnosing early AD; for example, digit span (repeating back to the examiner seven or eight numbers) or serial 7s (repeatedly subtracting 7 from 100) are essentially tests of STM, which is generally well preserved in AD. The tests that are most sensitive at this stage are those which require information to be transferred to LTM. For example, the subject is given a simple name and address to remember. When he has repeated it correctly, he is then given a five-minute distractor task (serial 7s might serve at this stage) and then asked to repeat the name and address once more. He has not been told that this will be required, so as to preclude any subvocal rehearsal. An undemented person is likely to remember at least some part of the information but it is highly unlikely that a patient with AD, no matter how early, will remember any of it. This is known as a *delayed free recall* test ('free' because the elements can be repeated in any order). A group of five or six unrelated words can also be used.

Tests of *orientation* are standard, and they are useful in order to exclude severe memory loss; they do not, however, tell the examiner a great deal about the *pattern* of memory loss. If a patient is being interviewed at the house where he has lived for forty years, he is likely to know where he is even if moderately demented; he is less likely to know the name of the hospital into which he has been admitted an hour or so previously. So a statement that the patient is 'orientated in place' can be meaningless; the same can apply to tests of orientation for time and person.

It is better to test in an orderly sequence that depends on the recency of information. One might begin by testing delayed free recall, then go on to the most recent past, asking if the patient can remember the examiner's name and where they are, then asking the day, the month and the year. Where moderately recent events are concerned, I find that extremely useful assessments can be based on the patient's knowledge of current events. One might ask, 'Mrs Jones, do you watch TV/listen to the radio/read the papers?' and then ask what has been in the news in the past few days. Other questions might test the patient's memory of a slightly more remote period. At the time of writing, for example, both Mrs Thatcher and Ronald Reagan have been in office for some years, and there will be few problems of recall for mildly demented patients; by contrast, there may be great difficulty in recalling even major occurrences of the few days before the interview. Tests of memory for personal events can be related in the same way to recency; in these, also, a patient with AD will show a pattern in which recall becomes increasingly poor as the point of reference comes closer to the present.

As the condition worsens, increasingly remote memory is affected. Following on from what was said above — on a visit to a ward for the demented the British Prime Minister found herself completely unrecognized (by the patients), which was undoubtedly a novel experience for her. Furthermore, although it is often said that demented patients retain a good memory for events in the more distant past, this ability is often more apparent than real, since the accuracy of such memories is less easily checked; they have in fact

112

been shown to be seriously disrupted in almost all instances, with huge gaps and with faulty sequencing of events (Williams, 1968).

The parietal lobe

The parietal lobe processes and co-ordinates sensory information and also governs the perception of spatial relationships that is required in order to carry out fine or complex motor tasks. Defects in parietal lobe function are generally the result of right hemisphere damage.

It is usually possible to detect parietal lobe disorder by means of simple clinical tests. Where sensory defects are concerned, there may be failure of *two-point discrimination*: the patient (with eyes closed) is unable to tell whether the examiner is touching his palm with one finger or two. There may also be *astereognosis*: again with eyes closed, the patient is unable to identity an object placed in his hand (a pen or a coin, perhaps) because he lacks the ability to co-ordinate such tactile sensations as the shape, temperature or size of the object. Naturally this will be a simple object which the patient has earlier shown himself able to name on the tests of language ability. There may also be *agnosia* — that is, lack of ability to identify an object; a patient can be asked to explain (or demonstrate non-verbally) the use of a pencil or, say, a telephone. *Finger agnosia*, shown to be common in demented patients (Pearce, 1984), consists in an inability to name the patient's or examiner's fingers; if there is naming difficulty the patient may be asked to point to fingers named by the examiner.

A patient with severe agnosia may be uncertain how to respond when the doctor greets him initially by holding out a hand; there are many good reasons for shaking hands at the beginning of an interview!

There may also be *right–left disorientation*. The patient is asked to hold out his right or his left hand; if he can do this he is next asked to touch, say, his left ear, or to put his right hand on his left shoulder. These tests, of course, call upon both sensory and motor ability, but the two cannot always be completely separated.

Disorders of skilled motor movements (generally the result of parietal disease) are grouped together as *apraxia*. Mild apraxic disorders often appear early in the course of AD and may be one of the presenting features; a 'dressing apraxia' is, for example, very common. Other delicate movements (such as the use of a comb or scissors) may also have been difficult.

The presence of a degree of apraxia has been shown to correlate positively with overall severity of AD and also to predict a poor outcome. Naguib and Levy (1982a) demonstrated a strong correlation between scores on tests of parietal dysfunction (e.g. drawing a clock-face, finger recognition and digit copying) and survival in demented patients. The poorest-outcome patients also showed significantly lower radiological density (on CT scanning) in the parietal lobes. Previous studies by Hare (1978) and McDonald (1969) had also shown that impaired parietal lobe function indicated a poor prognosis. Moore and

Wyke (1984) found significant relationships between poor performance on simple drawing tests and overall degree of dementia. Drawings made spontaneously were impoverished, but copies of drawings showed faulty spatial positioning, indicating that a memory defect was not entirely responsible.

A good clinical test for apraxia consists in asking the patient to draw a clock-face (complete with numbers) or to copy simple diagrams. If these are completed without difficulty there is unlikely to be significant disorder, but one can go on to rather more exacting tasks, such as asking the patient to make squares or triangles with matches, or by giving him one of the formal block design tests, such as Kohs' blocks.

Apraxia of gait is a poorly recognized feature of AD; however, tests of gait and balance may reveal subclinical impairment even in apparently normally ambulant patients with dementia. In one study, patients were found to walk more slowly, to take shorter steps and to show greater body sway on both walking and standing than did age-matched controls (Visser, 1983). This, it is suggested, may explain the high frequency of falls in AD patients.

The above, then, represent the clinical tests of cognition that are most likely to be helpful in establishing a diagnosis of AD. Essentially the clinician is doing two things. First, he is further distinguishing between functional and organic disease. Functional disease is likely to show a pattern of cognitive impairment (if any) that is both inconsistent with the AD syndrome and inconsistent with time; there may, for example, be equal impairment of both recent and remote memory and an absence of dysphasia or dyspraxia. It will also show features that are *additional* to those of the AD syndrome — for example, depressive delusions and early waking or loss of appetite.

Second, he is distinguishing between diffuse and focal disease. There may, for example, be personality change in the absence of memory loss or there might be isolated language impairment. These would suggest that AD is most unlikely as an explanation and that stroke or tumour may be responsible. Or there may be isolated memory loss with relative impairment of other functions that could suggest toxic or deficiency states. 'Localizing signs' can be sought and identified on mental state examination just as they can on physical examination; a psychiatrist can probe with his questions just as a neurologist can with his pin or patella hammer. We will see from the work described in the 'formal testing' section that a careful clinical diagnosis of AD on the basis of a consistent set of impairments is almost never overturned by subsequent events or investigations.

FORMAL MENTAL TESTING

This is partly the province of psychologists, but a clinician may also carry out a formal test in order to confirm his diagnosis or, perhaps, to quantify for himself some aspect of the patient's illness — for example, the severity of his memory loss. A description of some tests in this 'bedside' category will follow, and after that a section on some tests that are usually administered by a psychologist. The second category will be dealt with only in outline; however, a doctor responsible for the diagnosis and management of demented patients needs to know which tests are in common use, how to interpret the results and, in general, what kind of help is to be expected from psychological testing.

It should first be appreciated that, no matter whether a test is carried out by a physician or a psychologist, it will only be of value in so far as it addresses a specific question. The clinician who asks, 'How can I test for dementia?' is lost at the outset. But some of the many and more specific questions he might ask, and which might be answered by tests, are:

(a) Is the patient significantly confused?
(b) Is the patient suffering from Alzheimer's disease?
(c) How severe is the disease?
(d) What outcome is to be expected?
(e) Where will the patient be best placed?

These are only a few examples of the questions that tests, innumerable tests, have been designed to answer. Many of these, often time consuming and difficult to administer, yield little more useful information than do some which are much simpler, and others, more complex, leave important areas untested; others still may not measure what the clinician thinks they measure. For example, a test of memory is a test of memory, not a test of the severity of dementia. Equally, a test showing that a patient is confused at some point in time shows simply this and no more; the patient might be suffering from dementia or he might equally well be suffering from an acute toxic disorder.

The tests described below have, generally speaking, all proved their value in resolving doubt within certain areas. They fall into the two categories outlined above: first, brief (or mostly brief) cognitive tests that are usually carried out by clinicians and, second, the more detailed psychological tests designed to map out the pattern of cognitive and behavioural impairment in a patient rather more fully and also, in many cases, to make clear predictions about outcome, helping the clinician towards the best plan for a patient's future care. There is some overlap between the two categories, but no one test is of great value in isolation. It is presumed, too, that the clinician has already taken an independent history relating to the patient's daily living pattern and has carried out a careful mental state examination. Both of these have in themselves considerable power of diagnosis and prediction; formal testing is an additional measure, not a substitute.

Brief cognitive tests

The abbreviated mental test score

This was developed from the 34-item Mental Test Score (Lloyd, 1970; Hodkinson, 1973). The MTS was a measure of mental impairment in the elderly; the test proved effective in separating the mentally normal from the confused, and

Table 18.   The abbreviated mental tests score (AMTS)

1. Age.
2. Time (to nearest hour)
3. Address to recall at end of test; this should be repeated by the patient to ensure that it has been heard correctly:
   42 West Street
4. Year
5. Name of hospital
6. Recognition of two persons (e.g. doctor, nurse)
7. Date of birth
8. Years of First World War
9. Name of present monarch
10. Count backwards from 20 to 1

Each question scores one mark for a correct answer.
(Reproduced from Hodkinson (1972) by permission of the author and Ballière Tindall.)

a score of 25 or more represented the acceptable range of normality. The test did not discriminate between demented patients and those with acute confusional states.

The Abbreviated Mental Test Score (Table 18) is a ten-item version of the MTS. It is equally effective in discriminating between the normal elderly and the demented (Hodkinson, 1972); it is therefore a useful screening instrument and is often used routinely in geriatric wards. It is less demanding than the longer test and patients tend to respond more co-operatively. Scores below 7 indicate a significant degree of confusion.

The AMTS is not designed to diagnose *dementia*. A high score is in fact diagnostically more helpful than a low score; the former excludes confusion but the latter simply indicates that a cause for the patient's confusion must be sought. Also, a low score does not necessarily exclude severe depressive illness; elderly patients with severe depression can score well within the 'confused' range of tests of memory and orientation (Fraser and Glass, 1980).

Following a firm diagnosis, however, serial use of the AMTS (or MTS) can be useful in detecting and quantifying change in the patient's condition, and can help with planning ahead. It should be remembered, incidentally, that both tests have been developed for use only in patients of 65 and over.

The mini-mental state examination

This (Figure 12) is really a 'mini-cognitive state' test. It was introduced as a simple screening instrument which would be acceptable to patients and which could be completed in about five minutes. It is designed to aid in the recognition and grading of cognitive impairment (Folstein *et al.*, 1975). The test has fairly high sensitivity for dementia and acute confusion; Anthony *et al.* (1982) found that 87 per cent of confused patients scored within the range

Orientation		Score	Points
1. What is the	Year?	....	1
	Season?	....	1
	Date?	....	1
	Day?	....	1
	Month?	....	1
2. Where are we?	State?	....	1
	County?	....	1
	Town or city?	....	1
	Hospital?	....	1
	Floor?	....	1

Registration

3. Name three objects, taking on second to say each. Then ask the patient all three after you have said them. Give one point for each correct answer. 3
Repeat the answers until the patient learns all three.

Attention and calculation

4. Serial sevens. Give one point for each correct answer. Stop after five answers. Alternative: Spell WORLD backwards. 5

Recall

5. Ask for names of three objects learned in Q3. Give one point for each correct answer. 3

Language

6. Point to a pencil and a watch. Have the patient name them as you point. 2
7. Have the patient repeat: 'No ifs, and or buts'.
8. Have the patient follow a three-stage command: 'Take a paper in your right hand. Fold the paper in half. Put the paper on the floor.' 3
9. Have the patient read and obey the following: 'CLOSE YOUR EYES'. (Write it in large letters). 1
10. Have the patient write a sentence of his or her choice. The sentence should contain a subject and an object, and should make sense. (Ignore spelling errors when scoring.)
11. Enlarge the design printed below to 1.5 cm per side, and have the patient copy it. (Give one point if all sides and angles are preserved and if the intersecting sides form a quadrangle.)

	....	1
Total	....	30

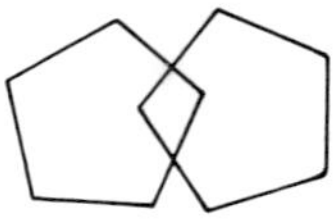

Figure 12   The mini-mental state examination. (Reproduced from Folstein *et al.* (1975) by permission of the publishers. © 1975 Pergamon Journals Ltd.)

indicating disturbance of cognition (i.e. 23 points or less). The test does, however, have serious limitations; there is a high false positive rate, mainly among patients whose educational level is poor or who are aged over 60. Studies have shown false positive rates of up to 39.4 per cent for subjects in

Age on testing.............................   Name ....
Age on admission ....   Notes ....

Mark a cross at the appropriate place to indicate failure

Memory

    What year are we in?   ....
    What month of the year is it? ....
    Who were we fighting in the Second World War?
        Germans   ....
        Japanese   ....
    What year were you born? ....

Error score ....

Aphasia

    Name a wrist watch ....
    Name the wrist strap or band ....
    Name the buckle or clasp ....
    What is a refrigerator for? ....
    What is a thermometer for? ....
    What is a barometer for? ....

Error score ....

Parietal

    Show me your left hand ....
    Touch your left ear with your right hand ....
    Name a coin in right hand ....
    No tactile sensory inattention present ....
    Normal two-point discrimination ....
    Construct a square with matches ....

Error score ....

Abstraction

    Subtract 27 from 65 (presented visually) ....
    Too many cooks spoil the broth ....
    A rolling stone gathers no moss ....

Error score ....

*Wiegl–Goldstein–Scheerer test**

    Able to sort by colour ....
    Able to sort by shape ....
    Able to sort when given an example ....

Error score ....

Figure 13　The Kew cognitive map. (Reproduced from McDonald (1969) by permission of *The British Journal of Psychiatry*.)

these groups (Anthony *et al.*, 1982; Dick *et al.*, 1984), and patients with depression or parkinsonism (Brown and Marsen, 1984) may also be incorrectly assigned to the 'confused' category. Furthermore, performances on widely

Mark each error with a cross

Memory

What year are we in?   ....
What month is it?   ....
Can you tell me two countries we fought in the Second World War   ....
What year were you born?   ....
What is the capital city of England?   ....

Error score   ....

Aphasia

What do you call this (a watch)?   ....
What do you call this (a wrist strap or band)?   ....
What do you call this (a buckle or clasp)?   ....
What is a refrigerator for?   ....
What is a thermometer for?   ....
What is a barometer for?   ....

Error score   ....

Parietal signs

Show me your left hand   ....
Touch your left ear with your right hand   ....
Name the coin in hand named (as 10p)   ....
No tactile inattention present   ....
Normal two-point discrimination   ....
Draw a square   ....

Error score   ....

Figure 14   Modified Kew cognitive test. (Reproduced from Hare (1978) by permission of the author and the Editor of the *British Medical Journal*.)

differing cognitive tasks are combined into a single score, with the result that substantial loss in a single area (in Korsakoff's psychosis, for example) might be obscured.

The test is therefore suitable only for patients under the age of 60 whose educational attainments are average or above. As with the AMTS in the case of older patients, it cannot in itself yield any diagnosis; it simply indicates the need for more intensive investigations.

The Kew Cognitive Map

This has the advantage that it not only samples a range of cognitive functions but also assigns each to a separate subscale (Figure 13). Therefore the tests will indicate the presence of confusion and may also take the clinician some way towards establishing its cause. In the same way as with the clinical examination, isolated losses will suggest a focal lesion, uneven change may suggest multi-infarct dementia, while global impairment will suggest Alzheimer-type dementia (McDonald, 1969). The tests of parietal lobe function would also appear to constitute a sensitive index of the severity of AD.

Hare (1978) tested 200 patients with a modification of the Kew Cognitive Map (Figure 14). She found that the 56 patients who in due course turned out to be suffering from progressive senile dementia had errors on all tests, and continued to show errors on all tests over the course of four to six weeks. By contrast, patients with other conditions, such as depressive illness or acute toxic confusion, showed a much less even pattern of impairment, which fluctuated with time. By the end of four to six weeks, most patients in the non-dementia categories were either error-free on testing or showed errors only on memory testing.

The CARE Tests

These are two scales requiring the use of a semi-structured interview — the Comprehensive Assessment and Referral Evaluation (Gurland et al., 1978). Their purpose is to discriminate between depression and dementia in patients of 65 and over. The principle is that multidimensional diagnosis is the most powerful means of distinguishing the two groups; in a study involving 841 patients there were highly satisfactory results in terms of separating the patients into two clear categories.

Depression is diagnosed if the score on the depression scale (Table 19) is greater than 2 and greater than the score on the dementia scale (Table 20). Dementia is diagnosed if the score on the dementia scale is greater than 5 and equal to or greater than the score on the depression scale. In essence, one diagnoses whichever of the two conditions is the more prominent.

The CARE tests take into account a good deal of information, and they are also suitable for use by non-psychiatrists. They are no longer used routinely in their original form, but are shown here as illustrative of the necessary multidimensional approach to diagnosis.

The Hachinski ischaemia score

This test, described on p. 82 (Table 15), is of proven validity in discriminating between multi-infarct and Alzheimer-type dementia. Scores of 7 or more favour the former diagnosis and scores below 4 favour the latter.

All of the above relatively brief cognitive tests simply represent abbreviations and formalizations of a good history and mental state examination; where the patient is in experienced hands, they will probably add very little to these, except that some tests may be useful as objective measures of severity or change. Brief cognitive tests are more useful for staff whose specialty is not psychiatry, or for those who are unaccustomed to dealing with the confused elderly; a poor performance on the AMTS will probably suggest, among other

Table 19.   The CARE tests: depression scale

---

1. Feels lonely
2. Is restless
3. Worries
4. Worries about everything
5. Sad or depressed
6. Has cried
7. Depression lasts several days
8. Time of day when depressed
9. Life isn't worth living
10. Worried about the future
11. Bleak future
12. Wished to be dead
13. Suicidal thoughts
14. Sleep disorder due to thoughts
15. Describes headaches
16. Lack of enjoyment
17. How happy subject is
18. Awakes early or tired

(Reproduced from Gurland *et al.* (1982) by permission of the Raven Press, New York.)

investigations, referral for psychogeriatric assessment. A formal check-list is not altogether to be despised even by the experienced practitioner; its routine use means that important items are not forgotten and, taken together with the results from a scale of severity, it can lead to a more precise diagnosis.

Severity scales

What does a clinician mean by 'mild' or 'severe' dementia? A number of groups have in recent years attempted to define the degrees of dementia more accurately and to provide simple scales that will fairly broadly quantify the severity of impairment. Reisberg *et al.* (1982) have, for example, published a seven-point scale from 1 (no cognitive decline) to 7 (very severe cognitive decline). The staging takes into account a good deal of information about the patient's abilities in his daily life, but there is no reference to clinical disorders of language and praxis, and defects in these areas require to be sought (and are usually apparent) virtually from the outset. On an investigation of 16 patients, the disagreement rate among five neurologists was 0.052, which is only just acceptable.

   Hughes *et al.* (1982) developed a five-point scale from 0 (healthy) to 3 (severe dementia). 'Questionable' is graded as 0.5. The grading is awkward and the measures are largely restricted to memory and social functioning, but inter-rater reliability was shown to be good and there was highly significant correlation with results on other dementia scales, such as that of Blessed *et al.* (1968), which is a 29-point behavioural check-list. The authors write that, while validation will require reassessments over a long period, followed ideally by

Table 20   The CARE tests: dementia scale

1. Doesn't know own age
2. Doesn't know birth year
3. Doesn't know years in area
4. Doesn't know address
5. Doesn't remember rater's name, first try
6. Forgets name of President or Prime Minister
7. Doesn't know month
8. Doesn't know year
9. Doesn't remember rater's name, second try
10. Knee–hand–ear test
11. Capacity to prepare own meals
12. Problem handling personal business
13. Difficulty dressing by self
14. Difficulty doing chores
15. Who does shopping?
16. Forgets television, conversations, etc.
17. Doesn't know phone number

(Reproduced from Gurland *et al.* (1982) by permission of the Raven Press, New York.)

autopsy, the original ratings have accurately predicted ratings after six to nine months.

In St Pancras Hospital we established a 'memory clinic' for the diagnosis of early dementia (Simpson *et al.*, 1984; Van der Cammen *et al.*, 1987); patients suffering from memory loss were examined independently by a geriatrician, a psychologist and a psychiatrist; I (the last of these) evolved a simple seven-point scale for the grading of AD-type dementia, based on clinical experience of the condition's natural history (Table 21). This proved useful in order to provide definitions of terms such as 'moderate' or 'severe', and most patients could without difficulty be fitted into one of the categories. As with similar scales, full validation will not be possible until two to three years have passed, but grading has shown a significant correlation with independent psychological testing. Correlation with scores on the Object Learning Test from the Modified Kendrick Battery (p. 123) was 0.77 ($N=52$, $p<0.001$). One advantage is that no additional time is required; a point on the scale can be assigned at the end of a normal clinical examination without further questioning or tests.

Psychological tests

The Wechsler Adult Intelligence Scale (WAIS)

This is a relatively blunt instrument; it may on occasion be helpful in distinguishing between the effects of dementia and those of normal ageing, but standardization is difficult, especially where the elderly are concerned. The theoretical difficulties have been reviewed elsewhere (Miller, 1977); the main problem is that 'normal ageing' is the yardstick in this as in several other psychological tests, and the process of cognitive change with ageing has been

122

Table 21.   Severity of Alzheimer type dementia: the St Pancras scale

0	Absent	No evidence of cognitive impairment
1	Equivocal	Slight memory impairment, definitely or possibly due to affective disorder
2	Minimal	Definite memory impairment or dubious or minimal memory impairment together with slight nominal dysphasia
3	Mild	Definite memory impairment together with definite nominal dysphasia
4	Moderate	Definite impairment of both recent and remote memory, possibly with confabulation. Moderate dysphasia (including difficulty in naming simple objects) and some failure of comprehension. Possibly some parietal features (e.g. dressing apraxia). Possibly some personality deterioration (e.g. emotional lability, paranoia)
5	Severe	As above, but all worse in degree and with definite personality deterioration
6	Profound	As above, but all worse in degree; totally dependent on others for self-care. Little coherent communication

(Reproduced from Van der Cammen *et al.* (1987) by permission of *The British Journal of Psychiatry*.)

generally mapped out by means of cross-sectional rather than longitudinal studies. The defects of the former have already been briefly pointed out (p. 25); results are distorted by factors such as changing educational opportunities, and there tends to be a false presumption that many cognitive abilities will decline with age. The few longitudinal studies, reviewed in detail by Torak (1978), yield results in striking contrast to those of the cross-sectional studies; far from showing the general decline recorded by the latter, performance on most subtests is actually shown to improve with age. This means that the standards for what is 'normal' are likely to be somewhat too low in many of the tests in common use at present, with the result that the changes of early dementia could be obscured.

The WAIS consists of six verbal subtests (information, arithmetic, similarities, comprehension, digit span, vocabulary) and five performance subtests (digit symbol, picture completion, block design, picture arrangement, object assembly). Where normal ageing is concerned, the consensus from longitudinal studies is that there is modest decline in certain aspects of performance in old age; for example, in the digit-symbol matching test. The performance tests are sometimes known as the 'don't hold' tests in contrast to the 'hold' verbal tests, and they are the more sensitive to organic brain disease. Therefore a marked verbal–performance discrepancy would suggest organic brain disease rather than normal ageing or functional disorder. Otherwise, measurement of performance on the various subtests has not proved helpful in distinguishing between different forms of brain disease (Lishman, 1978).

The WAIS, like many other tests of cognition, is most useful for serial testing of an individual rather than as a one-off measure; it can helpfully detect and measure change over a period of time.

The Wechsler Memory Scale (WMS)

This is made up of seven subtests: personal and current information, orientation, mental control (e.g. counting backwards), logical memory (repeating a short prose passage), digit span, visual reproduction and associate learning. The raw score is age-corrected, and a 'memory quotient' is derived. Norms for the elderly have been provided (Hulicka, 1966; Klonoff and Kennedy, 1965, 1966), and the test is available in two equivalent forms for serial use, although practice effect is in fact minimal (Stone *et al.*, 1946; Strömgren *et al.*, 1976). The WMS, however, has grave disadvantages. In essence, the idea of a single score which represents all memory functions would now be considered theoretically unsound; in practice, as with the Mini-Mental Test, isolated defects, in older patients at least, are obscured (Fraser and Glass, 1980). This last study showed that the WMS did not discriminate between depressed and demented elderly subjects; most of the former group showed significantly impaired performance on all subtests. Work by Kopelman (1986) indicated that the logical memory subtest discriminated satisfactorily between depressed and demented patients, but the mean age of the patients was fairly low (for the AD patients 65.6 and the depressed patients 60.6). The WMS tends to be used now only as a research instrument — for example, to detect memory impairment following ECT — but where the diagnosis of dementia is concerned it can achieve little more than the exclusion of severe impairment; tests which are simpler and much less time-consuming will serve this purpose equally well.

The Modified Kendrick Battery

Originally this consisted of a synonym learning test and a digit copying test (Kendrick, 1965, 1967). The synonym learning test was replaced by an object learning test (OLT), as the former was found to be too stressful for elderly subjects, many of whom refused to complete it (Irving *et al.*, 1970). In the OLT, the subject is simply shown a number of drawings of common objects on a card, and is required to remember as many as he can; a parallel form is available for retesting (Gibson and Kendrick, 1976). The digit copying test is a test of speed; performance on the latter is likely to be impaired in depressive illness (Cowan *et al.*, 1975), and the OLT is often used on its own. The two tests taken together have, nevertheless, shown a high degree of discrimination between dementia and depression (Gibson and Kendrick, 1979; Van der Cammen *et al.*, 1987), and a score below the cut-off point for dementia can satisfactorily predict organic mental deterioration over time (Cowan *et al.*, 1975; Gibson *et al.*, 1980). It should be noted, however, that the test has been designed to *detect* dementia rather than to measure its degree.

The Inglis Paired Associate Learning Test

Like the OLT, this is a measure of ability to establish new information in the long-term memory store, and it has also been shown to discriminate effectively between the normal and the demented elderly (Inglis, 1959; Caird *et al.*, 1962; Parsons, 1965). The test is extremely simple. There are two forms, in each of which the subject has to learn three pairs of unrelated words (e.g. pen — cabbage, sponge — trumpet, knife — chimney). The tester reads one of each pair and the subject has to provide the other; he is scored according to the number of repetitions necessary to learn all three pairs. Low scores have been shown, in the above studies, to identify patients with dementia in a mixed group of elderly patients and, as with the OLT, poor performance usually predicts fairly rapid cognitive deterioration (Cowan *et al.*, 1975; Whitehead, 1977, 1982).

The Clifton Assessment Procedures for the Elderly (CAPE)

These were developed by the Psychology Department at Clifton Hospital, York, the aim being to devise a 'reasonably brief' method for assessing the cognitive and behavioural competence of the elderly (Pattie and Gilleard, 1976, 1981). It has the great virtue of taking into account a patient's day-to-day behaviour as well as his test performance, and it is a worthwhile instrument for measuring the patient's overall degree of dependency, thus helping towards more realistic arrangements for future care.

There are two independent measures, the Cognitive Assessment Scale (CAS) and the Behavioural Rating Scale (BRS). The CAS consists of three sections, an information and orientation test, a mental ability test (which measures counting, reading and writing skills) and a spiral maze test (which measures fine motor co-ordination). These tests have been found to be brief and acceptable to the elderly, and require little training to administer.

The BRS is completed by an observer familiar with the subject's behaviour; this might be a relative or a hospital nurse, for example. There are 18 questions which provide measures of four principal areas of behavioural disability; that is, 'physical disability', 'apathy', 'communication difficulties' and 'social disturbance'. There are, for example, questions about continence, dressing ability, daytime or nocturnal restlessness.

The information obtained from the two scales is recorded on a CAPE report form and the patient's score is graded on a five-point scale from A to E, these grades representing progressive levels of impairment of function.

Grade A characterizes the independent elderly who make little or no demand on caring agencies

Grade B indicates mild impairment; these low-dependency individuals may be found in warden-supervised accommodation or living at home with one or more relatives.

Grade C represents moderate impairment and medium dependency. These people need considerable support in the community and are typically to be found in old people's homes.

Grade D represents marked impairment and high dependency. This group is usually institutionalized.

Grade E represents severe impairment and maximum dependency. These are usually psychogeriatric and geriatric patients, unable to look after their own needs.

The CAPE has shown satisfactory levels of discrimination between people in different types of provision, though there is inevitably some degree of overlap, often due to misplacement. More important, it has proved possible to discriminate between individuals with differing outcomes in groups of elderly psychiatric patients and to predict levels of adjustment among newly admitted residents in social services accommodation for the elderly (Pattie and Gilleard, 1978a), and also to predict death or survival in the elderly mentally infirm (Pattie and Gilleard, 1978b).

The CAPE tests have been thoroughly validated and are often used routinely in psychogeriatric units, where they can be of the greatest assistance in planning.

Automated psychological testing

A test battery is not of necessity the better for being automated, and it is not to be imagined that a computer can probe mysterious areas beyond the range of the perception of the averagely competent clinician or psychologist. But some automated test batteries do have value; several have been under evaluation for 10–15 years (Elithorn and Telford, 1969; Gedye and Miller, 1979), although the advent of less expensive and easy to use microprocessors has only recently provoked wide interest (Simpson and Linney, 1983).

Most tests in common use in the diagnosis of dementia, as we have seen, measure the subject's ability to establish items in long-term memory. One automated test, for example, consists of two parts. First, the subject's digit span is measured: he is shown sequences of numbers, displayed one by one on the monitor, and, on the instruction 'NOW DIAL', he dials the sequence on a dummy telephone (with a rotary dial); the maximum sequence of numbers that he can recall without errors is his digit span. He is then given a string of numbers *exceeding* his digit span, which will theoretically require utilization of LTM. The number of trials required to dial the sequence correctly is counted.

Another test is of recognition memory; the subject is shown a sequence of designs and, from a further sequence, he has to identify (by pressing a YES or a NO button) each of those he has seen before. This also is a test of LTM; dementing patients tend to show a high number of false positives.

Other tests are designed to measure capacity for abstraction; for example, the subject is shown a sequence of drawings and is required to press the YES or

NO button according to whether the object is man-made or not. He might be shown a pig, a ship, a plant or (this perhaps requiring a few milliseconds' additional thought) an overcoat. The measure here is time taken to respond, or 'latency'.

The tests are, all in all, less easy than they sound, and a certain amount of learning ability is necessary to do even the simplest of them; for example, one must remember to wait for the instruction 'NOW DIAL' before dialling. Some patients cannot remember the various test instructions, and the battery is not suitable for patients who are even moderately impaired; its value should lie primarily in the detection of *early* dementia.

The advantages and disadvantages of automated testing have been examined by Miller (1968) and by Simpson and Linney (1983) under four headings, discussed below.

Ease for subject and operator   In theory, less skilled staff can supervise the test sessions, though in practice the subject needs a good deal of guidance and instruction. Although the tests are not suitable for subjects with established dementia, experienced users of the tests may also be able to adjust them downwards in some degree to make them less challenging for those with slight impairment. In a classification test, for example, the subject may be asked whether the picture represents an animal or not. The program can also be made 'user-friendly'; the subject is 'addressed' by name and is also told 'GOOD' or 'WELL DONE' at the end of each task regardless of performance (as distinct from the stern admonitions delivered by earlier versions of the program, such as WRONG or TRY NOT TO MAKE AND MISTAKES NEXT TIME, following which elderly subjects sometimes made excuses and refused to finish the tests). Otherwise the tests tend to be enjoyed and to be treated as something of a game; they carry a great element of novelty for those not of the computer generation.

Speed of testing   Automation can save a great deal of time both by editing a test battery so that it conforms to the subject's ability and by recording results and performing analyses. Older people in particular will, quite naturally, require a certain amount of 'socializing' before and after the tests, but time is still used more economically.

Freedom of tester from routine tasks   The tester is free to observe and record behaviour during testing; there may, for example, be affective symptoms interfering with response.

Reliability   Test–retest reliability has thus far proved high where normal subjects are concerned, making standardization possible; however, slightly impaired subjects do show a small learning effect, so that results on serial testing (such as in a drug trial) might prove deceptive. Unfortunately, most trial populations have been quite small, so there are insufficient data to enable correction for this possible bias. It is likely that between-centre standardization of automated test batteries will be necessary in order to make them more useful; it is also likely that certain tests, such as those involving free verbal recall, will remain outside the area of automation for some time to come, and it may still be that a simple test such as recalling a fictitious name and address after a distractor task will turn out to be as good a predictor of pathology as more sophisticated measures (Simpson *et al.*, 1984). Indeed — to return to cognitive assessment generally — it has to be born in mind that many formal tests, especially the brief tests, have been validated only against clinical assessments made at the same time, so it is somewhat irrational to use such a test in order to 'confirm' a diagnosis arrived at after careful clinical examination. There is nevertheless something to be said for a test which will quantify disability at a given time or which can be used on different occasions to measure change, or for a test which, distilled from considerable clinical experience, constitutes an accurate screening instrument in the hands of a non-specialist. But the only diagnostic tests for AD that can properly be said to be valid are those which will identify those patients who will in due course develop a categorical global dementia; it is here that the more sophisticated tests are still in their infancy. As matters stand, an experienced psychologist will use not a single diagnostic test or even an off-the-shelf test battery, but a group of tests designed to answer specific questions about a number of areas of function and which will vary according both to the patient and to the tester's experience. For example, Whitehead (1982) was able to predict decline over a four-year period using the Parietal Scale (McDonald, 1969), the WAIS vocabulary and the Inglis tasks, and Berg *et al.* (1984) found that scores on two measures (the digit symbol subtest of the WAIS and an aphasia battery) correctly predicted deterioration over the course of a year in 95 per cent of subjects ($N=43$) with mild Alzheimer-type dementia.

Finally, Table 22 lists the questions which formal testing may help to answer and, against each question, indicates the test or tests which are likely to prove helpful. Each test is listed only once, but a single test can of course be informative in more than one area. For example, sensitive measures of clinical severity will naturally predict outcome and indicate what future provision is necessary.

THE EEG IN DEMENTIA

Electroencephalography is non-invasive, safe and widely available; it can be helpful in diagnosis within certain limits. It cannot be regarded as 'obsolete as a diagnostic test in dementia' (Pearce, 1984) with the advent of computerized tomography, since the latter is by no means universally available and is also much less sensitive to early disease (Harner, 1975; Soininen *et al.*, 1982) and probably also to the effects of relatively subtle change over time (Exton-Smith *et al.*, 1983).

There may be alterations both in spontaneous and in evoked EEG patterns.

128

Table 22.   Formal cognitive testing

Is there cognitive impairment?	
If patient is 65 or over:	Mental Test Score (Lloyd, 1970; p. 114) or: Abbreviated Mental Test Score (Hodkinson, 1972; Table 18; p. 115)
If patient is under 65:	Mini-Mental State (Folstein et al., 1975; Figure 12; p. 115)
Is the impairment due to depression?	Hamilton Rating Scale (Hamilton, 1960) or: CARE tests: Depression Scale (Gurland et al., 1982; Table 19; p. 120)
Is the diagnosis Alzheimer's disease?	Kew Cognitive Map (McDonald, 1969; Figure 13; p. 117) or: Modified Kew Cognitive Test (Hare, 1978; Figure 14; p. 118) or: OLT from Kendrick Test Battery (Kendrick, 1965; p. 123) and: PALT (Inglis, 1959; p. 124) and: 5-minute delayed free recall (p. 111)
Is the diagnosis multi-infarct dementia?	Hachinski Ischaemia Score (Hachinski et al., 1974; Table 15; p. 82)
If Alzheimer's disease, how severe is it?	Clinical Dementia Rating (Hughes et al., 1982; p. 120) or: St Pancras Scale (Van der Cammen et al., 1987; Table 21; p. 122)
What future provision will be required?	CAPE (Pattie and Gilleard, 1976; p. 124)

The spontaneous EEG

As is the case with other diagnostic procedures in dementia, changes from normal are less marked in older subjects, but the EEG in dementia regularly shows both quantitative and qualitative differences from that of age-matched controls. *Normal* subjects show an increasing frequency of EEG abnormalities as they age (Thompson, 1976); the principal changes associated with ageing are slowing of the alpha rhythm, the appearance of random delta and theta waves, and the development of localized temporal slow-wave activity (Busse et al., 1956). Conventional EEG recordings in patients with dementia show, generally speaking, an accentuation of all these changes; their frequency tends to correspond with the degree of intellectual impairment (Frey and Sjörgen, 1959; Roberts et al., 1978; and other studies cited by Soininen, 1983). In a group of 62 patients with AD, Soininen et al. (1982) found a highly significant difference from age-matched normal elderly subjects in respect of overall EEG disturbance, specifically accentuation of delta and theta waves and slowing of the dominant occipital rhythm. The last was the most effective discriminator between the two groups. Only three AD patients had a normal EEG; 82 per cent of the AD patients and 89 per cent of the controls were correctly classified on the basis of dominant occipital rhythm; slowing of the rhythm also correlated positively with clinical severity.

Patients with multi-infarct dementia showed changes similar to those of the AD group; the only difference was that asymmetrical findings were more than twice as common in MID.

There was a weak correlation ($r=0.35$) of the frequency of EEG abnormalites with third ventricle widening as seen on the CT scan, but not with cortical atrophy; this poor degree of correspondence between EEG changes and cerebral atrophy has been observed in other studies (Roberts et al., 1978; Stefoski et al., 1976). The EEG measures functional abnormality, and it is probable that EEG changes occur before the stage of permanent neuronal death and cerebral shrinkage.

Measurement of EEG coherence may provide a sensitive index of the presence and degree of a dementing process; analysis by computer of EEG synchronization between different brain areas can enable a 'coherence function' to be calculated. O'Connor et al. (1979) measured coherence in 24 elderly patients with a diagnosis of senile dementia, senile arteriosclerosis or depression, and found that coherence between the parietal and temporal areas, in particular, significantly discriminated between the two groups. The patients with senile dementia showed the greatest coherence between recording sites (doubtless reflecting the diffuse nature of the damage in AD) and those with arteriosclerotic disease the lowest, implying focal pathology. Patients with depression occupied an intermediate position. Coherence measures might therefore be of value in distinguishing between AD and MID in the earlier stages, though these measures have thus far been tested only against previous clinical diagnosis and there is no immediate likelihood of their becoming routine.

Evoked potentials

An evoked potential has two components — first, a stimulus-related component which is related to the physical characteristics of the stimulus and, second, an event-related component which is dependent on the information content of the stimulus. The event-related component appears only when the subject 'attends' to the stimulus and when it has meaning for him; it can therefore be regarded as the 'cognitive' element in the evoked complex (Goodin et al., 1980).

Two forms of event-related potential have received particular attention where the diagnosis of dementia is concerned: (a) The P300 component of the auditory evoked potential (AEV) and (b) the Contingent Negative Variation (CNV).

The P300

This is the most prominent of the event-related potentials, and is a positive

130

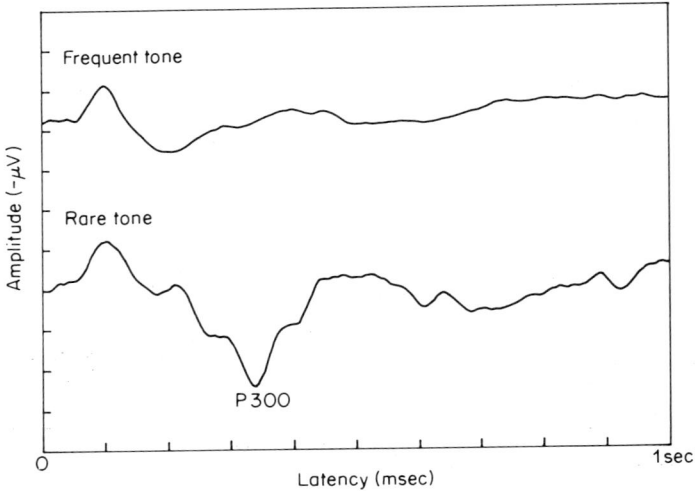

Figure 15 The auditory evoked potential. Response of a normal subject to frequent and rare tones.

wave occurring at a latency (i.e. time from stimulus) of 300–500 milliseconds (Figures 15 and 16). In tasks where discrimination is required, the latency of the P300 increases with age. The subject may, for example, hear two tones, one identified as 'rare' and the other as 'frequent'. He will then have the task of counting the rare tones in a sequence. The increase of P300 latency with age is linear, but the demented show a latency which exceeds the normal age-related value by about two standard deviations (Goodin *et al.*, 1980); it is likely that 80 per cent of patients with dementia have prolonged latencies (tentatively related by Slaets and Fortgens (1984) to slowing of 'memory updating'), though it should be noted that most of these figures have generally been derived from populations with *presenile* dementia. Where the elderly are concerned, the main interest lies in alterations in the P300 observed on serial testing and the fact that some forms of pharmacotherapy appear to reduce P300 latency. Exton-Smith *et al.* (1983) found in a small pilot study that five patients with AD showed prolonged P300 latencies on a task which involved counting rate tones, but that latencies were reduced in patients treated with the cerebral-activating drug dihydroergotoxine mesylate (p. 156) as compared with latencies in placebo-treated controls. There were no changes on clinical and psychological assessment, but trials are under way in which larger populations will be observed over a longer period, the question being whether this change in P300 latency heralds eventual clinical improvement.

Contingent Negative Variation (CNV)

This is a slow negative potential change which is recorded, mainly over the vertex, when a subject is preparing to respond to a stimulus (Walter *et al.*,

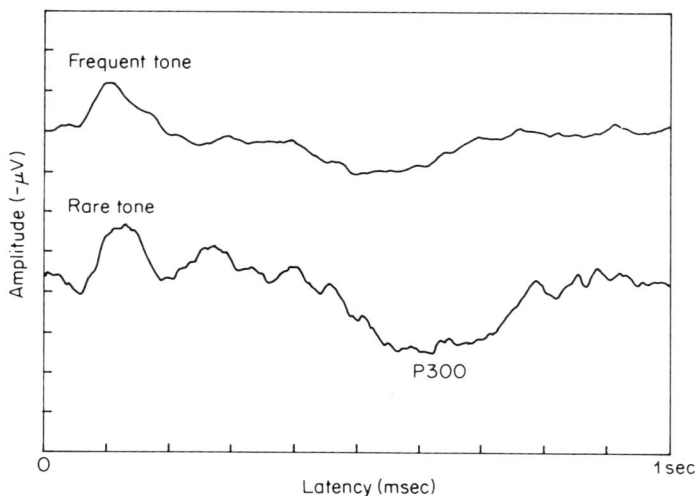

Figure 16   The auditory evoked potential. Response of a demented subject to frequent and rare tones.

1964). Classically the subject is given a warning signal followed by an imperative stimulus instructing the subject to respond. The CNV amplitude declines with age and it is also reduced in patients with AD, but *CNV rebound* is the usual measure. This is seen in divided attention tasks; if the warning tone is followed by some form of distraction (e.g. showing the subject letters that he has to repeat later), CNV amplitude is reduced. If the distraction is withdrawn then CNV is usually of supranormal value, this representing the 'rebound'. CNV rebound shows a stepwise decrement with age, and appears to be completely absent in many patients with AD although there is slight overlap with age-matched controls (Tecce *et al.*, 1983). This last study also showed, however, that where CNV rebound was absent in AD patients it could re-emerge on treatment with drugs in the 'cerebral activator' category; it is suggested that CNV rebound may represent a sensitive index of cognitive functioning and prove a useful objective means of evaluating pharmacotherapy in the demented.

These are all no more than straws in the wind, and there are obstacles to accepting changes in evoked potentials as valid diagnostic indices in dementia. First, as observed above, most of the results that show altered evoked potentials in dementia come from work with younger patients (e.g. Goodin *et al.*, 1980; Harding *et al.*, 1985; St Clair *et al.*, 1985). A test that discriminates between patients with presenile dementia and age-matched normals can be of little practical value, since clearly the dementing patients have already been identified and more precise diagnoses are not forthcoming. A study of Orwin *et al.* (1986) suggests that serial increase of response to flash stimulation (over the course of three years in the case described) may be specific for AD, but again the patient was aged 58 and AD had already been diagnosed. Curiously, one of the patients in the study of Goodin *et al.* (1980) was aged only 27 (scarcely a case of AD), but correspondence has failed to elicit details. The real difficulty continues to be in discrimination and prediction in the case of the older patient. Here there is wide variation, especially in P300 latency; Slaets and Fortgens (1984) were unable to distinguish between healthy and demented patients in the older age-groups and suggest that the value of the P300 might be limited to diagnosis of presenile dementia or to the serial measurement of change in individuals. A further difficulty is that evoked potentials might be altered by affective disorder; this question still has to be fully examined. Averaged evoked potentials to auditory stimuli show prolonged latency in elderly patients with depression (Hendrickson *et al.*, 1979). Depressed patients occupy an intermediate position in terms of latency between the demented and age-matched normals, though with some overlap. Prolonged P300 latency does not appear to be specific to dementia either; Brown *et al.* (1982) found normal P300 latencies in seven depressed patients, but Patterson *et al.* (1984) found that P300 latencies in depressed patients were prolonged; as in the study of averaged evoked potentials, the values occupied an intermediate position between those seen in normals and those in patients with dementia. In the study by Hendrickson *et al.* (1979), values of averaged evoked potential did not return to normal in depressives who recovered, and it is suggested that subtle organic changes, perhaps those of early dementia, may have underlain the depression, but this would require a longitudinal study. Unfortunately, there is no longer-term follow-up information on these patients (Levy, 1985, personal communication). The indications are, however, that this group of patients did *not* seem more likely to develop dementia. As with the P300, a measure that was vulnerable to affective change (as appears to be the case) would naturally be of little value in discriminating between depression and dementia, and there would also be problems with serial testing. Furthermore, changes in evoked potentials following treatment with 'cerebral activators' would not answer the possible assertion that such drugs are no more than mild euphoriants.

The EEG changes seen in AD are listed in Table 23. To sum up, the EEG is of value mainly in the diagnosis of presenile dementia; it may help to distinguish between organic and affective disorder, and may show characteristic changes both in AD and in some of the less common dementias (e.g. Huntingdon's chorea, p. 90); it may also indicate asymmetry or focal damage, in which case CT scanning is usually the next diagnostic step. The EEG is not as effective as the CT scan in the detection of small lesions, and it is not helpful in discriminating between types of lesion — for example, a tumour or an infarct.

Measurement of evoked potentials may also turn out to be of some value in diagnosing presenile dementia and in measuring response to drug therapy, but the indications at present are not especially promising.

CT SCANNING

The principles and the technique of computerized tomography are by now

Table 23.   The EEG in Alzheimer's disease

The spontaneous EEG
Slow alpha rhythm
Slow dominant occipital rhythm
Widespread random delta and theta activity
Abnormally high coherence between adjacent cortical areas

Evoked potentials
Reduced amplitude and latency of P300 component of auditory evoked potential
Reduced contingent negative variation (CNV) amplitude
Absence of CNV rebound

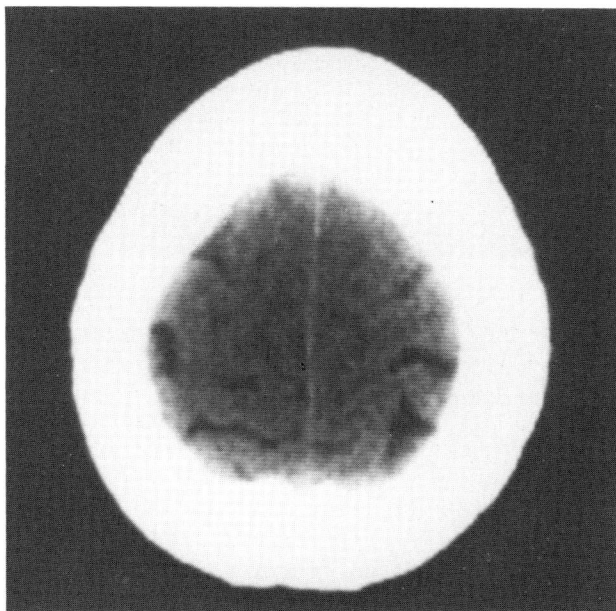

Figure 17   Normal CT scan (vertex).

fairly familiar. In brief, where head scanning is concerned, collimated X-rays (i.e. X-rays moving in parallel paths) are used to build up a picture of intracranial structures in eight to ten horizontal planes. Each of these 'slices' is constructed from about 250,000 density readings; the result looks something like a conventional X-ray but is, of course, a computerized artefact. Water is the standard for zero density, so the ventricles have very low density in relation to the grey and white matter; thus clear pictures are provided of the ventricular system and the brain surface. As the white matter is of lesser density than the grey matter, many of the brain structures can also be visualized.

CT scanning represents a huge advance in neurological diagnosis; it is safe, speedy, non-invasive and is not interfered with by drugs; its value in the diagnosis of dementia can be considered under the following three headings.

134

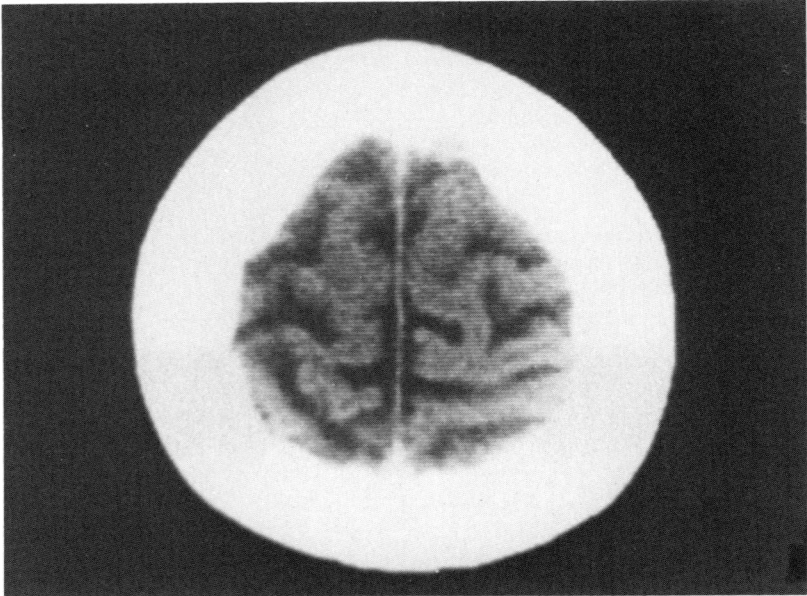

Figure 18   Severe atrophy at the vertex in Alzheimer's disease.

Detection of localized damage

This is probably where CT scanning has the greatest advantages over other techniques in general use. A scan can detect small lesions and can generally (though not always) indicate the nature of a lesion on the basis of shape and density. An example is Case No. 1 (p. 81), where the diagnosis of an isolated lesion was confirmed. Figures 23 and 24 show CT scanning results in a patient who presented with confusion and dizzy spells; the diagnosis of multi-infarct dementia was confirmed by the finding of multiple areas of low attenuation (reduced density), representing 'lacunar' infarcts. (The patient survived for only a matter of months following diagnosis.) CT scanning is usually indicated where an apparent dementia is in some way untypical: the patient may be young, the onset may be abnormally rapid, or the mental state examination may fail to show global impairment but, instead, an uneven pattern of impairment and sparing. Bradshaw *et al.* (1983) found that, of 500 demented patients referred for CT scanning, 10 per cent were discovered to have a treatable cause for their dementia. Of 327 patients who had no symptoms or signs other than of dementia, 5 per cent were found to have a treatable cause; the scan therefore provided new information in this group.

The mean age of all the patients was 68, but, as ventricular size and sulcal width increased with age, the boundary between changes related to ageing and to disease became indistinct. CT scanning was therefore of most value in

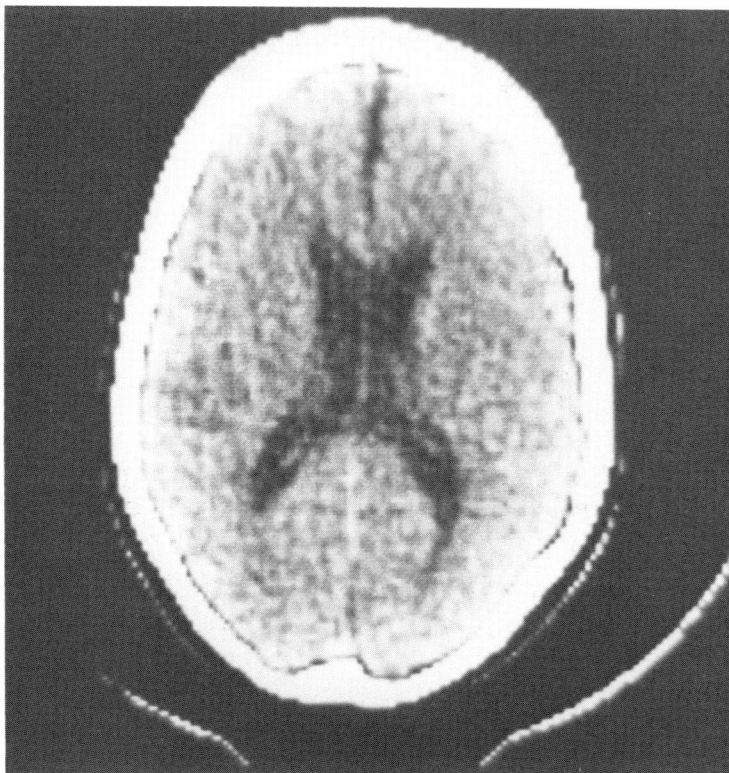

Figure 19   Normal CT scan: level of third and lateral ventricles.

detecting focal lesions. The most useful pointers to a positive scan result were headaches, focal signs, papilloedema and speech disorders; it is suggested that the presence of any of these represents a sound indication for a brain scan where dementia is of recent origin — that is, where the history is less than a year.

A CT scan does not, however, represent the last word in diagnosis; the precise nature of a lesion may need to be demonstrated by means of further specialized radiographic techniques, such as digital subtraction angiography (Meaney and Weinstein, 1986).

Measurement of cerebral atrophy

The degree of atrophy is assessed by measuring ventricular size and sulcal widening. Although both of these increase with age, it is still possible in most cases to distinguish between normal ageing and dementia. Where *normal ageing* is concerned, there is a gradual progressive increase in ventricular size from the first to the sixth decade followed by a dramatic increase in the eighth

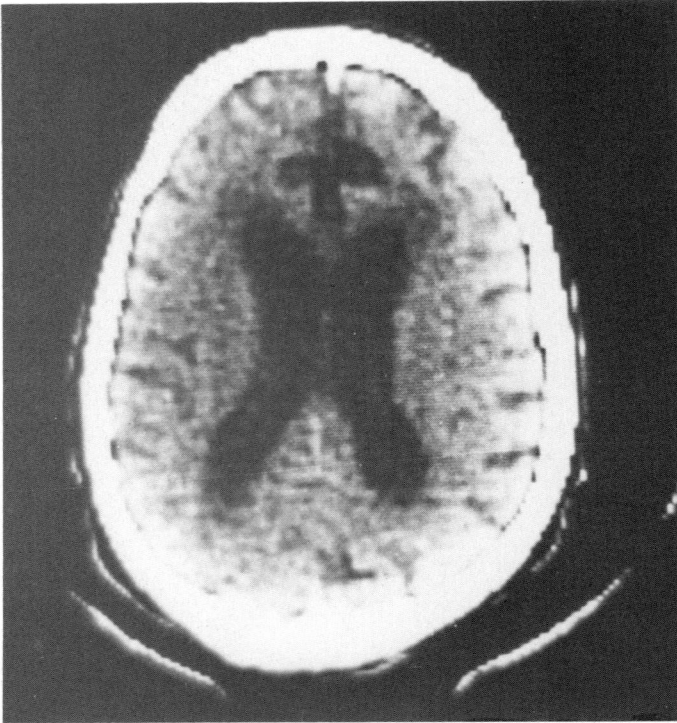

Figure 20   Gross ventricular enlargement in Alzheimer's disease.

and ninth decades, also with increased variability in the latter two groups (Barron *et al.*, 1976). Furthermore, in individuals over 60 there is an inverse relationship between performance on cognitive testing and ventricular size even where there is no clinical evidence of dementia (Jacoby *et al.*, 1980a); possibly this study population included subjects with 'preclinical' dementia. Where diagnosed *dementia* is concerned, however, Soininen *et al.* (1982) were able to separate patients with even moderate disease from age-matched controls. Demented patients differed from normals both in ventricular size and in sulcal width. But studies such as that by Jacoby *et al.* (1980b) have found rather more overlap between demented patients and controls; although there was a positive correlation between ventricular size and degree of dementia, there was a discrimination error of at least 17 per cent with slightly more false normals than false abnormals.

   It is doubtful, therefore, whether the sophisticated and expensive methods that have been employed to measure ventricular size, to take one index of atrophy, have much diagnostic value, since the index being measured is itself fairly insensitive; the literature in the area suggests that naked-eye rating of atrophy by an experienced clinician represents an equally good indication of the presence and degree of dementia. Sometimes 'Evans' ratio' is calculated

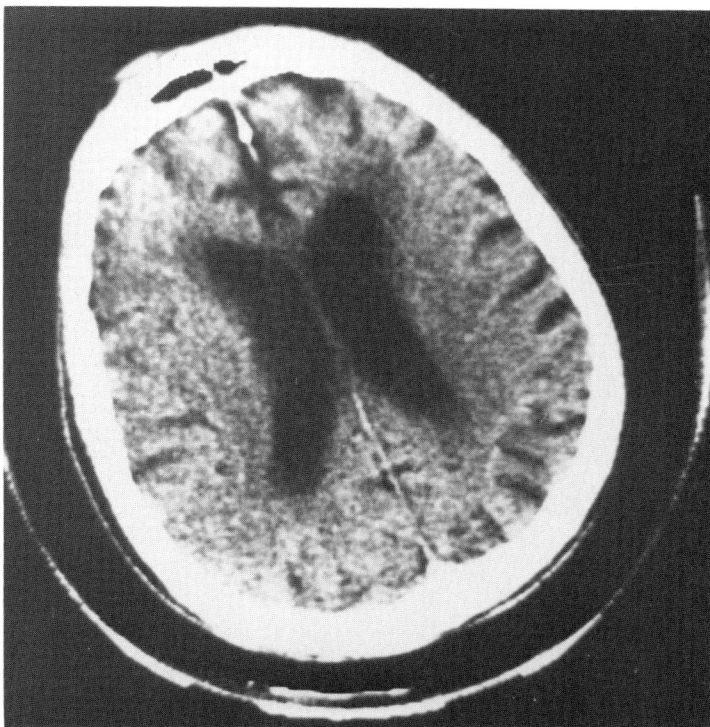

Figure 21   Progressive cerebral atrophy. The same subject as Figure 20, one year later; there is further cortical atrophy and ventricular enlargement.

(i.e. the distance between the tips of the frontal horns of the lateral ventricle divided by the maximum internal diameter of the skull), but this, too, is only a fairly blunt measure; Jacoby *et al.* (1980b) found that it did not correlate directly with the degree of impairment. A further complicating factor, as found by the same authors, is that elderly depressed patients tend to have 'atrophic' scans; they resembled the demented patients more than they did normals (Jacoby *et al.*, 1983).

Therefore the degree of cortical atrophy as seen on CT scanning is, in the diagnosis of dementia, only one factor to be weighed with others. It may be that serial scanning will be more helpful diagnostically than measurements at one point in time. Brinkman and Largen (1984: see below) found that scanning after a two-year interval discriminated reliably between normal ageing and cerebral atrophy.

Measurement of regional density

Naguib and Levy (1982a) measured regional density in a number of brain areas and found, from a two-year follow-up, that the patients who had died in the

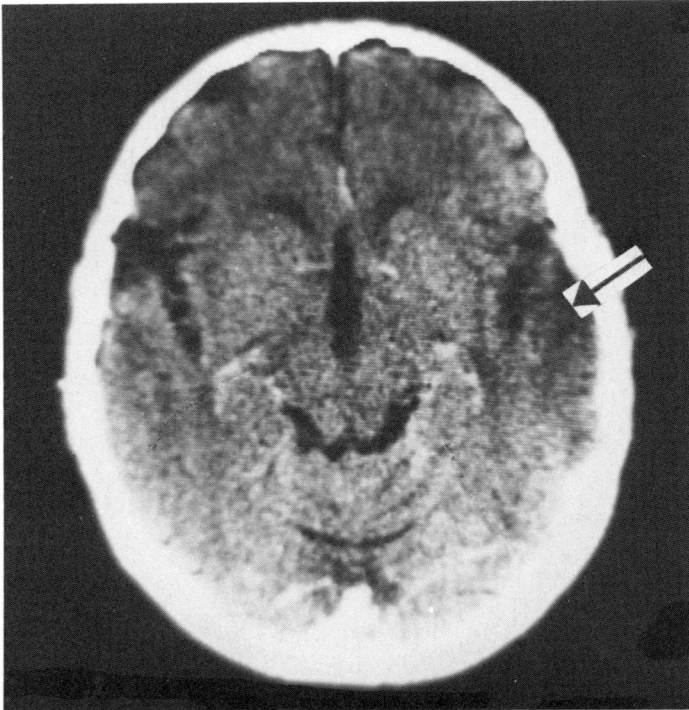

Figure 22   Left temporoparietal infarction (Case No. 1, p. 81).

interval had shown significantly lower density in the right parietal region than those who had survived. This accords well with McDonald's 1969 investigation which found that patients who performed badly on tasks involving parietal lobe function had a relatively poor prognosis and an increased risk of dying within a six-month follow-up period. It should be noted that, in the Naguib and Levy (1982a) study, measures of ventricular size and cortical atrophy were not found to have predictive value.

Naguib and Levy (1982b) examined the survivors from the first study and found that, although the number was small (10) there was a tendency for low density especially in the right parietal region to be an unfavourable prognostic indicator. Colgan (1985) followed up 48 AD patients who had been scanned on diagnosis and six months later. Measures of ventricular size did not show any correlation with Mental Test Score (p. 114), but there were correlations between regional density and some psychological measures (e.g. between right parietal density and score on the Digit Copying Test (p. 123), and low density in both parietal lobes appeared to predict a relatively short survival period; a longer-term follow-up is, however, necessary and is planned. As matters stand, measures of radiological density on CT scanning have not yet proved their predictive value over and above that of simple clinical tests, such as those in the Kew Cognitive Map (p. 117).

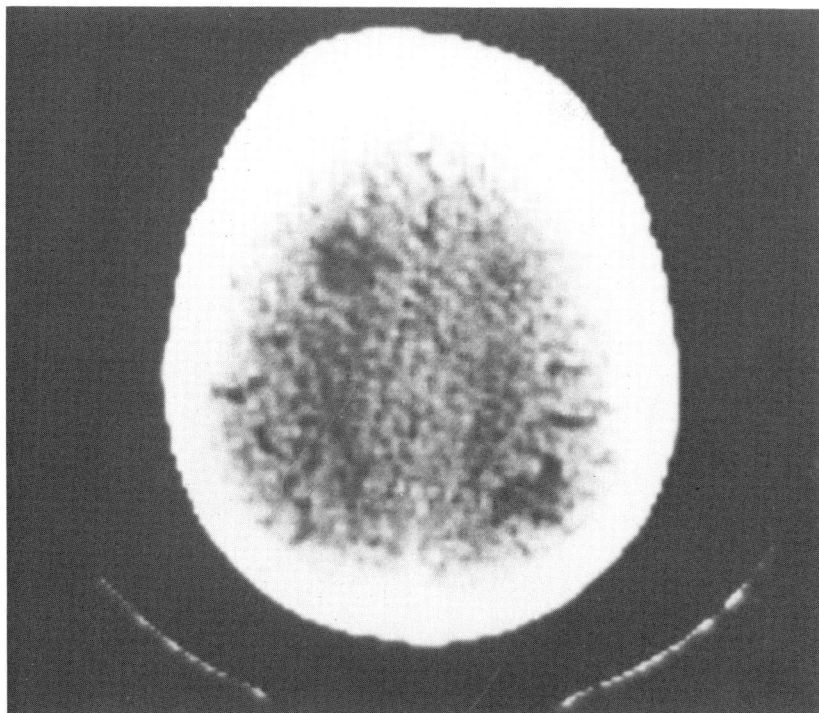

Figure 23 Multi-infarct dementia.

Serial measurement

It has been suggested that the factor which most clearly distinguishes AD from normal ageing is the *rate* of morphological change (figures 20 and 21). In a small pilot study Brinkman and Largen (1984) sequentially scanned five patients with probable AD, compared the rate of change over 15–35 months with that derived from previously published normative data (Barron *et al.*, 1976), and found a comparatively high rate of ventricular size increase in the AD group. It is of interest that the scans of two of the subjects would, on the basis of normative data, initially have been classified as being within the 'normal' range. Increase was, however, abnormally rapid in both patients, who appear to have shown unmistakable signs of dementia at the end of the study period. All of the scans were within the 'demented' range by this time; the study therefore does little more than confirm the fact that CT scanning is insensitive to early AD. The authors suggest that measurement of change over a longer period might provide a reliable means of diagnosing AD, and they propose two years — but this period does allow a great deal of time for clinical and other forms of observation; it is highly probable that the diagnosis will be apparent to all concerned by this time (as it was both at the beginning and at the end of the pilot study). It should be noted, finally, that the patients were aged under 65 at

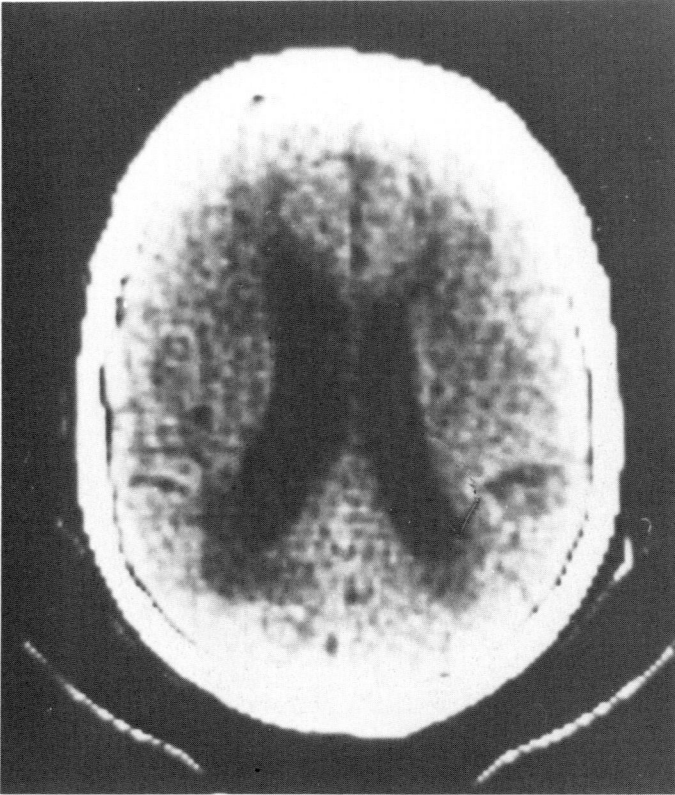

Figure 24   Multi-infarct dementia.

diagnosis, so the study does not fully deal with the problem of distinguishing between normal and abnormal ageing.

To sum up, the main applications of CT head scanning in the diagnosis of dementia are in:

  (a) Identifying a focal lesion; for example:
       (i) tumour (p. 134)
       (ii) infarct (Figure 22)
       (iii) subdural haematoma (p. 85)
  (b) Confirming a diagnosis of certain forms of dementia, especially;
       (i) multi-infarct dementia (p. 78; Figures 23 and 24)
       (ii) Huntingdon's chorea (p. 90)
       (iii) Pick's disease (p. 89)
       (iv) normal pressure hydrocephalus (p. 86; Figures 26)
  (c) Helping to confirm a diagnosis of established AD (Table 24; Figures 18, 20 and 21)

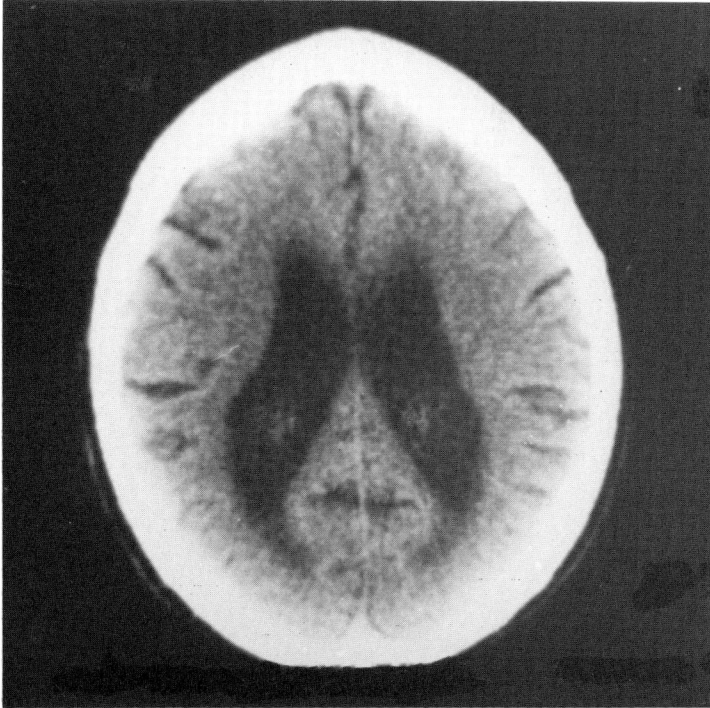

Figure 25   Gross ventricular enlargement and cortical atrophy (Case No. 6, p. 000).

Table 24.   The CT scan in Alzheimer's disease

Measure	Appearance
Cortical atrophy	Early: Blunting of extremities of horns of lateral ventricle (Figures 20, 21) Coarsening of sulcal pattern, esp. at vertex (Figures 18, 20) Late: Enlargement of all ventricles (Figures 20, 21, 24) Widening of all sulci (Figures 20, 21, 25) (False positive and false negative rates are about 20%)
Regional density	Generally reduced; right parietal density most consistent and predictive of survival. Measures do not necessarily correlate with cognitive ability
Serial change	Rate of increase in ventricular size appears strongly to discriminate AD patients from normals (Figures 20, 21)

NUCLEAR MAGNETIC RESONANCE (NMR) IMAGING

The EEG is a record of electrical activity, and the CT scan is a measure of tissue size and density; the NMR scan is a measure of biological activity. Nuclei with

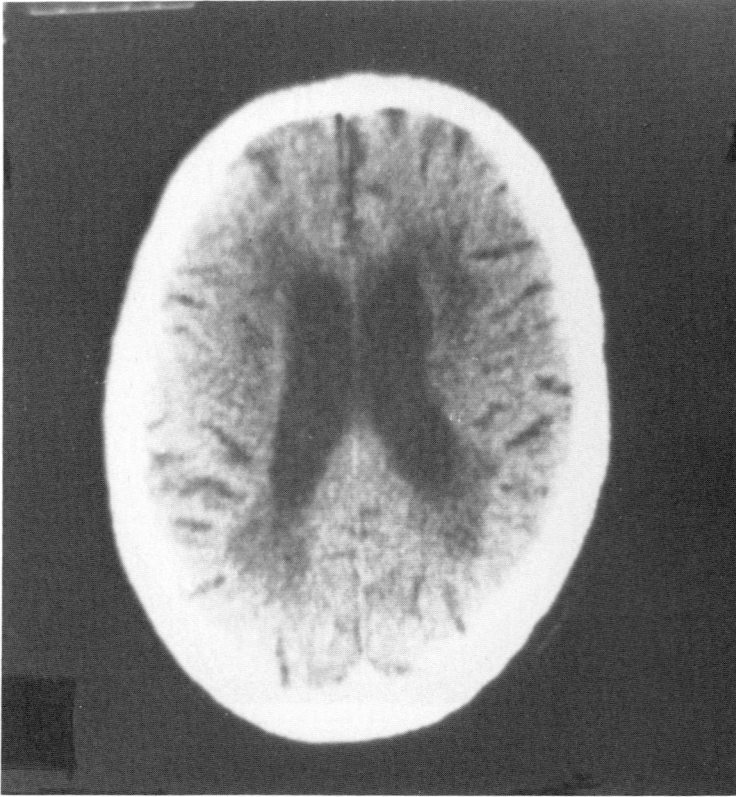

Figure 26   Ventricular enlargement and periventricular oedema in normal pressure hydrocephalus.

an odd number of nucleons (protons and neutrons) have an intrinsic magnetism that makes each such nucleus a magnetic dipole — a small bar magnet (Shulman, 1983). The ^{1}H proton, which is the nucleus of nearly all naturally occurring hydrogen atoms, and the ^{31}P nucleus, the nucleus of all phosphorus atoms, come into this category.

In NMR scanning two electromagnetic fields are applied: first, a strong magnetic field that brings about alignment of all dipoles and, second, a range of electromagnetic frequencies at each of which a specific population of nuclei will resonate, or 'flip' out of alignment. Therefore it is possible, for example, to visualize ATP activity (of particular value in detecting cerebral hypoxia in the newborn (Cady *et al.*, 1983)), and to reveal the distribution of water and lipids by mapping out that of hydrogen nuclei; these have special application in the diagnosis of stroke and tumour. The information available from CT scanning can also be obtained — ventricular size, ventricle–brain ratio and sulcal width (Eastwood *et al.*, 1985).

The information is reconstituted as 'slices' in the same way as the CT scan, but NMR has advantages over the former both in the greater amount of information that can be obtained, in the absence of bone shadow, and in the sharper differentiation between tissues of different densities. The patient, moreover, is not exposed to ionizing radiation and the technique is therefore theoretically eminently suitable for serial examination of the same subject. At present, however, NMR imaging is a slow procedure requiring bulky and expensive equipment.

The application of NMR scanning to the detection of localized lesions is fairly self-evident. What of the diagnosis of dementia — in particular, AD? The question is mainly whether the technique will enable detection of disease before the stage when structural damage is evident.

Besson *et al.* (1985) have identified the 'spin-lattice relaxation time' (T_1) as a parameter which might be sensitive to early AD. This is the rate of realignment with the static field after disturbance and it reflects, among other things, the amount and distribution of free water (T_1 in free water is relatively very high). The authors found T_1 to increase with the severity of dementia, with T_1 results in all areas significantly greater than in controls. The measure did not discriminate between patients with AD and MID, but it was possible to make the distinction by measures of protein density in the white matter; proton density was significantly greater in AD patients than in MID patients, who did not differ from controls.

The mechanisms underlying these differences are not yet clear. It should also be noted that the patient population in the above study were all in long-stay hospital beds and thus doubtless severely demented. The value of NMR scanning in the diagnosis of early dementia, or even dementia of moderate degree, remains to be proven.

POSITRON EMISSION TOMOGRAPHY (PET)

This requires inhalation or injection of radionucleides and the use of a cyclotron. The principle is that an isotope emits positrons when a positron and an electron collide; this radioactivity is measured and used to construct an image arranged in slices, as with other techniques. The radionucleide is often deoxyglucose; it passes into the brain in the same way as glucose but, after phosphorylation, metabolism is stopped and the deoxyglucose is trapped. The isotope can then be imaged, providing a relative measure of glucose metabolism.

PET scanning yields a more precise localization of stroke damage than do other techniques. Ramsay (1984) has summarized the other diagnostic benefits of PET scanning. By demonstrating reduction of glucose metabolism rate, ammonium isotopes may be used to measure blood flow; this may change with time following a stroke, indicating prognosis. In Huntingdon's chorea a decrease of biological activity in the caudate nucleus has been shown more impressively than is the anatomical shrinkage of the structure of CT scan, and in epilepsy a hypermetabolic area is revealed during the interictal phase in or surrounding the focus.

144

Where AD is concerned, there is a possibility that changes in neurotransmitter activity can be demonstrated and that serial measurement of other metabolic activities may elucidate the process of early neuronal destruction. This application at present would only have research value; such enormously expensive procedures are a long way from being useful clinically or widely available.

It is possible to sum up the value of psychological and other specialized diagnostic tests in dementia fairly briefly. In general, they confirm and quantify; they are of value principally in the diagnosis of the less common forms of dementia. Where diagnostic validity in AD is concerned, *there has to be a general conclusion that formal, technical or expensive tests can still add little or nothing to the judgement of a methodical clinician equipped with no more than a pencil and paper.* But it must be added that this is something of a theoretical position; practice may vary, but many clincians, myself included, would consider it ethically doubtful to rely purely on clinical judgement even in what appears to be a classic case of AD. The patient still deserves the time-honoured benefit of the doubt and, even if elderly, should be screened for systemic disease that might be at least contributing to his condition. If the patient is younger or the dementia is untypical (mainly in the ways outlined on p. 135), then a much more thorough investigation, usually including a CT scan, is indicated.

But the clinician is himself an expensive resource! He needs to employ his time with the patient to the best advantage, using questions and simple tests of proven value to probe specific areas (e.g. as outlined in Table 22), as distinct from following a long and unvarying history and mental state examination scheme in the hope that, by the end of it all, something worthwhile will emerge. To repeat — dementia is a latent condition, detectable only by challenge (Thompson, 1985); passive information-gathering is likely to prove uninformative.

SUMMARY

The clinical diagnosis of dementia is a three-stage process. First, remediable causes of confusion have to be sought; even where the patient is suffering from an underlying dementia, the treatment of 'acute-on-chronic' confusion may improve his general condition substantially. Elements in the patient's history that indicate a toxic confusional state are a brief or fluctuating course and the presence of associated features suggestive of extracerebral disease. Many confusional states arise from self-neglect; alcohol abuse is often an occult element, and sometimes confusion in an elderly patient may be an effect of medically prescribed drugs. Otherwise, acute confusional states in the elderly are usually pulmonary or cardiovascular in origin and can be diagnosed on routine physical examination. Other conditions that should be excluded routinely are urinary tract infection, diabetes and hypothyroidism.

Second, functional disorder needs to be distinguished from organic disorder. Uncertainty in this area is minimized if a psychiatric diagnosis is seen to be represented not by a single symptom (such as memory loss) but by a syndrome made up of a fairly consistent group of functional impairments which together identify it. Depressive illness, anxiety states or schizophrenia all have well-defined features, and there is only a small amount of overlap with each other and with the organic disorders.

Third, dementia is not simply a diagnosis of exclusion; AD in particular needs to be diagnosed on *positive* findings, like other syndromes; a safe diagnosis requires that the clinician elicit signs indicating disease in all or most of the cortical areas usually affected. These are especially: signs of frontal lobe disease (e.g. personality change, dysphasia), of temporal lobe disease (e.g. failure to establish items in long-term memory) and of parietal lobe disease (e.g. failure of sensory discrimination and apraxia). Methodical examination can distinguish between functional and organic disorder and between focal and diffuse disorder; 'localizing signs' can be detected on mental state examination just as they can on neurological examination.

Formal mental tests fall into two broad categories: the 'brief' tests that are normally used by a clinician and those that are applied by a psychologist. Both types are likely to be of value only in so far as they address specific questions; to confirm a diagnosis of AD, psychological testing in essence replicates the clinical examination in more detail, mapping out cognitive function in a number of defined areas. A small group of measures in this category, taken together, is likely to discriminate satisfactorily between dementing patients and normal elderly; it is unlikely that any single measure can do so. This applies equally to automated psychological testing, which may offer a modest advance in terms of standardization and test–retest reliability, mainly by eliminating 'observer effect'.

The EEG may be of use in the detection of early dementia, in particular in distinguishing it from affective disorder. But it is not helpful in the diagnosis of small lesions and it is vulnerable to the effect of drugs. The measurement of evoked potentials may be more useful than the spontaneous EEG, especially in the measurement of change over time, but it has not yet been established whether changes in any of the evoked potentials represent purely organic disease.

CT scanning is extremely helpful in detecting focal pathology and in the diagnosis of the less common forms of dementia (i.e. where damage is in some degree selective). It is insensitive to change in early AD, at which stage there is a high incidence of both false positives and false negatives.

NMR and PET imaging provide records of biological activity as well as of tissue size and density, and both can be of value in the diagnosis of small lesions and, where AD is concerned, may have research value in identifying the sites and nature of the primary pathological events. Such techniques would therefore be most effectively used at present in the examination of elderly patients who are mentally normal on standard clinical criteria; routine use in the diagnosis of the demented would be redundant and wildly uneconomic. As matters stand, in the diagnosis of dementia a clinician has few diagnostic tools more sensitive than his own eyes and ears.

CHAPTER 6

Drug treatment of dementia

This chapter, like most of the others, deals principally with Alzheimer's disease. The less common forms of dementia have been described separately; many of these, to a greater or lesser degree, respond to individual forms of therapy. But the world knows that there is no cure for Alzheimer's disease. How, then, does one treat the untreatable?

In the event, there are three possible lines of drug therapy in AD, and in almost any case at least two are likely to bring about some clinical improvement. First, certain conditions that frequently occur secondarily to the dementia, and which substantially worsen the patient's condition, can be diagnosed and treated. Second, there are drugs which may improve the underlying cognitive disorder ór at least there are drugs for which such a claim is made; these are claims that will be evaluated. Third, even where cognition cannot be improved, some of the troublesome symptoms associated with the demented condition may be subject to drug control.

'EXCESS DISABILITIES'

This term was introduced by Brody et al (1971), and is used here as a collective term for the conditions which may complicate dementia but which may in themselves be treatable. A high proportion of demented people come to medical attention, perhaps in a casualty department, because of an acute medical illness or in the wake of some social catastrophe (Dove and Dave, 1986; Fraser and Healy, 1986). The prevalence of physical illness among the demented is high (Copeland et al., 1975; Bergmann et al., 1978; Peck et al., 1978), and the AD-induced cognitive impairment may not be the main problem. An elderly woman with some degree of dementia can manage remarkably well at home without knowing the day, month or year, the name of the prime minister, or almost anything else that forms part of a standard cognitive test. Provided, that is, that she does not freeze, starve, fall downstairs or is not the cause of fire, flood, battle or explosion — all of which have been unfortunate realities at some time or another in my experience. But very many demented patients also suffer grievously from the more mundane hazards that arise from being confused, alone and unsupported.

We have already dealt with the extracerebral diseases which commonly cause confusional states; it is assumed that a patient who presents with apparent dementia has been examined and screened for these. This section proceeds a little further, to focus on some conditions which are frequently seen in patients with established dementia and which are sometimes caused by the dementia, but which in themselves are treatable. They can conveniently be divided into physical disorders and psychiatric disorders.

Physical disorders

Malnutrition

The prevalence of nutritional disorders in the elderly in the UK is at least 7 per cent (Department of Health and Social Security, 1979). Malnutrition will most directly cause handicap in the demented elderly by predisposing to pressure sores or fractures. Where the elderly in general are concerned, the nutritional deficiencies that have been most frequently observed are: vitamin C deficiency (Andrews et al., 1969), sometimes causing scurvy, and with an incidence in industrial areas of 1 per cent (Basu and Schorah, 1982); folate deficiency, leading to macrocytic anaemia (Sneath et al., 1973); and thiamine deficiency, leading to Wernicke's encephalopathy (Exton-Smith, 1980; Perkin and Handler, 1983).

The elderly with poor mobility, who are confined to their homes, or who have chronic disease (especially oral or intestinal), are clearly at special risk of malnutrition; the demented are also a high-risk group (Hancock et al., 1985; Greer et al., 1986). Calcium deficiency predioposes to fracture, especially to fractured neck of femur in the elderly (Parfitt, 1983); patients with fractured neck of femur occupy 40–50 per cent of orthopaedic beds (Schorah and Morgan, 1985). Reduced plasma protein levels also appear to predispose to fracture, as does vitamin D deficiency, which is encountered most frequently in the housebound elderly (Exton-Smith, 1984). Measures preventive of bone loss have been described by Passeri and Palummeri (1984). General living activities should include a proper diet, movement, physical exercise and exposure to sunlight. The diet should contain on average 1 g of calcium per day, and therefore be rich in milk, cheese, eggs and fish. Both smoking and excessive alcohol consumption damage bony tissue and should be avoided in individuals at risk. Vitamin D supplementation may also be needed; it has recently been shown, in fact, that for a group of institutionalized elderly twice-annual vitamin D supplementation was necessary in order to maintain serum level above the threshold associated with osteomalacia (Davies et al., 1985).

The effects of vitamin C deficiency are well known. The earlier signs of clinical scurvy are bruising, behavioural changes and lethargy. Unfortunately, dietary intake of vitamin C by the elderly both in the community (Munro, 1982) and in hospital (Millard et al., 1984) is often unacceptably low. Even in patients without clinical scurvy, vitamin C may be necessary to promote the healing of pressure sores (Taylor et al., 1974a, b), and to enhance the immune response (Kennes et al., 1983). Millard et al. write that, although two centuries have passed since the value of citrus fruits in the prevention of scurvy was recognized by mariners in primitive boats, there is still inadequate appreciation of the need for vitamin C supplementation for the elderly, especially those in institutions. The group found that a daily glass of orange juice was usually sufficient to maintain vitamin C status. Truswell (1985) lists other rich sources of vitamin C: blackcurrants, green peppers, green vegetables and potatoes. Vitamin C is easily destroyed by cooking, so vegetables should be cooked lightly and quickly. The vegetables should be added to water that is already boiling, since boiling inactivates the enzymes that would in turn partially destroy vitamin C during the process of cooking.

Folic acid and thiamine deficiency are common in elderly people with a high alcohol intake, especially if nutrient intake is poor; these deficiencies, together with their results (as above), unfortunately appear to be on the increase (Schorah and Morgan, 1985). *Potassium deficiency* is a common cause of 'acute-on-chronic' confusion; it may occur rapidly following vomiting or diarrhoea and it is well recognized as a consequence of diuretic intake. This last is not the result purely of potassium loss in the urine, but of a change in renal handling of potassium (Morgan, 1981); therefore, potassium levels of patients receiving treatment with diuretics require checking even if the patient has been taking standard doses of oral potassium. Potassium deficiency is also commonly seen following a cerebrovascular accident (Judge, 1968). *Iron deficiency* is also common in the elderly (DHSS, 1979), and is a frequent cause of anaemia; it usually results from poor dietary intake or gastrointestinal disease. Routine iron supplementation in the elderly is not indicated, but the diet should include liver, meat and fish, the best sources of iron; absorption of iron is enhanced by vitamin C (Truswell, 1985).

Dehydration may also contribute to confusion in the elderly; it is most commonly seen following fever, vomiting or diarrhoea; it may be detected on clinical examination or by the finding of raised plasma proteins, sodium, haemoglobin and urea.

Examination of a patient with dementia, then, should always include some note of nutritional status. Anaemia, weight loss and dehydration are recognized fairly easily; other evidence may be: ankle swelling (from hypoproteinaemia), gum haemorrhages, bruising, purpura or rashes, the last most commonly on the legs, suggesting scurvy. Reddening of the 'pressure areas', especially the sacral area, are a danger sign of incipient pressure sores.

Schorah and Morgan (1985) emphasize that most of the common nutritional deficiencies in the elderly are not related to financial considerations and can be alleviated by simple and usually inexpensive dietary modifications, which they list (Table 25).

Table 25.   Diet in the elderly
(Simple dietary modifications that could improve the intake of nutrients in the elderly)

Improving intake of specific nutrients
Fruit juice, fortified instant potato (vitamin C)
Fortified cereals (B vitamins)
Margarine, milk, cheese (vitamin D, calcium)
Discourage overcooking
Discourage prolonged food storage   (vitamin C, folic acid)
Improving protein/calorie intake
Milk, cheese
Complete liquid foods
Lunch clubs, meals on wheels

(Reproduced from Schorah and Morgan (1985) by permission of the authors and Update–Siebert Publications Limited).

Hypothermia

It is considered that about 10 per cent of old people are at risk of developing hypothermia (Fox *et al.*, 1973); dementia is a common precipitating condition, as are malnutrition, poor mobility and myxoedema. The demented are especially at risk because of inability to respond rapidly to cold stress, and hypothermia in this group does not necessarily occur only in the winter (Lye, 1985). But it is naturally most common in the colder months, and in patients who live in old housing with poor insulation; often about 30 per cent of the income of old people needs to be spent on heating during winter. Certain drugs also predispose to hypothermia, as does alcohol. Unfortunately, the drugs associated with hypothermia are often given to the elderly demented for insomnia, and include phenothiazines (commonly chlorpromazine or thioridazine) and benzodiazepines. Other predisposing drugs are barbiturates, imipramine, narcotic analgesics and reserpine.

Hypothermia is always a possible cause of a sharp worsening of confusion in a demented patient, especially one who lives alone or in unsatisfactory circumstances. He may have become apathetic or have lost the ability to dress and undress, and may sit in a chair all night instead of going to bed. At the time of examination there may not necessarily be cold extremities; the best area to test is the abdominal wall (Lye, 1985), and the possibility of hypothermia needs to be confirmed by means of a rectal temperature reading. It should be noted in particular (p.104) that most cases of hypothermia in the elderly are associated with other acute conditions, such as chest infection (Collins, 1983).

Trauma

A considerable number of the elderly mentally ill are admitted to hospital following some form of trauma; we (Fraser and Healy, 1986) found the proportion to be about 10 per cent. Fracture was the most common form, but demented patients are also frequently admitted to hospital following burns.

Demented patients who have suffered trauma need joint management in hospital by the psychiatrist and geriatrician (or surgeon). Continuing liaison is the only management style likely to prove rewarding where such difficult management and rehabilitation problems are concerned (p. 188).

Visual and hearing disorders

These are usually easier to recognize than to treat, but such defects can strongly predispose to psychiatric disturbance in the elderly and can worsen the effects of existing disorders, such as dementia (Ruben and Kruger, 1983). These defects have particular relevance to the pathogenesis of paranoid symptoms and hallucinations (p. 104) but also to states of apparent confusion. On one occasion when a patient's ears were syringed and on another when a hearing aid was provided I have seen the 'dementia' disappear as suddenly and memorably as if a switch has been pressed. But such instances are rare, and defective sensory input is more likely to contribute to confusion than to cause it; although the incidence of deafness in the demented is high, it is no greater than that in age-matched normals (Herbst, 1982). Nevertheless, assessment of hearing and vision should always form part of the examination of a demented patient.

Psychiatric disorders

Depression

There is a high prevalence of depression in patients with multi-infarct dementia (p. 78), and a somewhat lesser prevalence in those with Alzheimer-type dementia (Roth, 1983).

Depression is still, however, common in the latter group. In the early stages of the illness, in particular, the cognitive deficits are overlaid with sadness, apathy and pessimism; this is, of course, most evident where the patient retains a degree of awareness of his handicap, and it is most prevalent in patients of somewhat higher intellectual capacity and those who are still trying to follow some form of occupation, even if only part-time.

Diagnosis may be easy or it may be extremely difficult. Roth (1983) has emphasized the primacy of 'organic' factors, which must be sought and described first (as outlined on pp. 106–113) before even a tentative diagnosis of dementia is made. Subsequently, pointers to superadded depression are *consistent* mood change (as distinct from emotional lability), the biological signs of depression (such as early waking, loss of appetite, constipation, incontinence or psychomotor retardation) and, in general, functional impairment which is greater than one would expect from the dementia alone. For example, a patient with impairment of memory for recent events and some degree of expressive dysphasia but with no significant dyspraxia as revealed on drawing tests, and who is not washing, dressing or feeding himself, or who is doubly incontinent, is most probably depressed. The depression is not always as evident as this, but where there is some suggestion of depressive overlay —

often indicated by apathy and overdependence — it is strongly recommended that the patient be given a trial of an antidepressant; it must be emphasized that a diagnosis of dementia in some degree does not contraindicate treatment of affective symptoms. Dramatic benefit may result, and what was originally a major catastrophe or handicap can sometimes be reduced to little more than an inconvenience.

Case No. 9
Mrs I is aged 62 and was referred because of severe memory impairment. She had given up her part-time job because she could no longer find her way to work and (worst of all for her) she had been forced to give up her membership of a distinguished choir because she forgot to attend rehearsals, forgot her music and words, and was repeatedly losing her books. She had given up all her interests and no longer went out; she sat at home all day staring out of the window, and her husband had to do the housework.

Mental state examination indicated undoubted AD, but in view of her apparent depressive symptoms she was treated with mianserin 30 mg daily.

Her behaviour altered rapidly over the course of only two to three weeks. She resumed her interest in the choir, persuaded her husband and friends to take her to and from rehearsals, and spent hours at home learning her music and copying it out in easy-to-read form for use in rehearsals and performances; she also supplemented her memory with a diary and maps.

After about two months the mianserin was reduced and the patient relapsed into something like her original condition, so she is now having long-term maintenance therapy with what she and her husband call the 'singing tablets'.

Case No. 10
Mr J, aged 70, was a distinguished historian who had recently given up writing altogether because of rapidly progressing AD. His memory is substantially impaired, and a prominent feature is a severe degree of nominal dysphasia which affects both his writing and his speech. His incessant groping for words and the long circumlocutions that he needs to substitute for even simple words are painful to witness. (Incidentally, an extremely vivid example of just this phenomenon is portrayed in the dementing ex-professor in Kingsley Amis's *Ending Up*). Like Mrs I, Mr J became increasingly withdrawn and apathetic. He was treated with dothiepin and there was an overall gain in activity and alertness; with the help of his dictionary, his wife, and Roget's *Thesaurus* he began writing articles again.

Neither of these patients is in any degree better in terms of measurable cognitive function, but both have been able to gather the initiative (with, it should be noted, the help of a willing spouse) to compensate in some degree for their handicaps. It may be said that such improvements are transient; the dementia is bound to 'catch up' in the end. Logically one would expect so, but long-term evidence either way is lacking; where these and other patients are concerned, something has indisputably been gained in the medium term, and the interplay of neurotransmitter activity in AD is still so poorly understood that no treatment which substantially improves a patient can be discounted, no matter how transient one expects that the improvement will be.

The question of which antidepressants are suitable for elderly patients has been examined in detail elsewhere (Montgomery, 1982; Fraser, 1984). As a general principle the more strongly anticholinergic antidepressants such as imipramine and anitriptyline are not recommended for elderly patients, in particular the elderly demented. They are in themselves liable to cause confusion, probably because of central anticholinergic activity, although clinical experience indicates that the greater risks are of peripheral anticholinergic side-effects, such as cardiac arrhythmias or postural hypotension, sometimes leading to falls and fractures. Mianserin and dothiepin are safer antidepressants, especially for outpatients, but even then only with reliable supervision. An elderly depressed person who lives alone is probably best treated as either an inpatient or a day-patient.

Electroconvulsive therapy (ECT) may sometimes be indicated, even in a patient with some degree of dementia, if the depressive symptoms are severe or life-threatening; there might, for example, be anorexia with an immediate risk of dehydration or pressure sores. Naturally such a patient's age and overall prospects have to be taken into account, but ECT can at times be life-saving in such circumstances. There is no firm evidence that ECT worsens dementia, and, on occasions, cognitive impairment which is due to depression may be relieved (Fraser and Glass, 1980). But ECT does *not* improve the demented other than in cases of undoubted and severe depression.

It should be noted, finally, that a depressed and deteriorated patient who is unfit for ECT can be given antidepressants by injection or infusion; this measure is probably underused, and it can also be life-saving.

Paranoid states

Delusions of persecution are extremely common in early dementia; typical patterns have already been described (p. 107); most commonly, the patient has lost or forgotten things and (logically enough from his point of view) is convinced that malign forces have been at work. The distinction from paraphrenia is made only by careful cognitive testing (p. 106); the physical causes of paranoid states (p. 102) have also to be borne in mind.

In contrast to functional paranoid states, those induced by dementia are rarely improved by medication. The best remedies are practical ones. Where the patient lives alone, the strongly contributory effect of sensory deprivation is often evident; hearing and visual defects should be identified and treated as far as possible, and some form of impact on the patient's isolation is called for — perhaps in the form of regular visiting or day-care; with the additional companionship, these paranoid fears often become less prominent. Where a patient lives with her family, the family members will often benefit from an explanation of just why their relative makes her paranoid accusations; one golden rule is that they should not attempt to 'put her right' by arguing, since this only makes matters worse. 'Have it your own way, then, Mum', is often the formula which turns away wrath; the matter is likely to be abandoned, at least for the time being. Where paranoid ideas are productive of great excitement, regular doses of a tranquillizer such as thioridazine can have a dampening effect, although the delusions themselves will probably remain. Relatives can reasonably be told that such paranoid states are commonly transient; a much more amiable phase commonly follows.

Anxiety

Similar considerations apply to the treatment of anxiety symptoms. These are often prominent in the early stages of a dementing illness, when a patient may retain sufficient insight to worry about his failing mental powers and, in particular, to feel frightened about the possibility of further decline and about what the future holds for him. As with paranoid states, practical measures (e.g. additional help or a change in living circumstances) are much more likely to be helpful than the use of tranquillizers, which, even in small doses, can cause acute-on-chronic confusion and ataxia (Tinker, 1979; Campbell *et al.*, 1981; Prudham and Grimley-Evans, 1981; Swift, 1982). But it must be stressed that anxiety symptoms in the elderly are much more often indicative of a mixed state in which depression predominates than they are of 'pure' anxiety (a relatively rare condition), and such mixed states often respond very satisfactorily to antidepressant treatment (Nyström, 1967), even in the presence of some degree of dementia (Fraser and Glass, 1980). Depressive features can be elicited on methodical mental state examination; in cases of doubt, a measure such as the Hamilton Rating Scale (Hamilton, 1960) can be useful.

DRUG TREATMENT OF THE COGNITIVE DEFECT

Whether this is yet possible is a matter for considerable doubt. There are many ways in which the mental condition of a demented person may improve, and some of these can certainly be the outcome of treatment with the appropriate drug; the question is whether any drug can have a directly beneficial effect on cognition (e.g. memory and language functions) in AD, or whether all drugs which bring about benefit act without exception by way of a positive effect on mood and alertness. Such effects (as indicated above) are not to be discounted, but hints in promotional literature that dementia might be 'reversed' (Sandoz, 1978) or that the demented might be 'caught early' (Cox *et al.*, 1978) are highly tendentious and require acceptable proof.

This section will examine some of the claims that certain drugs are effective to a greater or lesser degree in alleviating cognitive impairment in AD; these drugs fall into three general categories. First, there are those active within the cholinergic system, such as lecithin or physostigmine; this group has already been described in the section dealing with the 'choline hypothesis'. Second are the vasodilators — such as cyclandelate, which has a direct action on vascular smooth muscle; the object is to increase cerebral blood flow and thus improve function. Third are the 'cerebral activators', which have a less specific or mixed action; ergot derivatives are the best-known drugs in this category.

Vasodilators

Drugs which can be classified as 'pure' vasodilators exert their effect on smooth muscle; since both AD and multi-infarct dementia are associated with reduced cerebral blood flow (Hachinski, 1978; Ingvar *et al.*, 1978), it might be expected that a drug which dilated cerebral arterioles would prove to be of clinical benefit. But it is now recognized that the reduced cerebral blood flow in AD occurs secondarily to the neuronal degeneration and the reduced metabolic activity; it is not the cause of the disease (Branconnier and Cole, 1977). Equally, relaxation of smooth muscle is unlikely to bring about any great benefit in MID, in which there is also extensive cell destruction (p. 79), although some slight improvement may be possible (see below). There have, nevertheless, been numerous trials of vasodilators in dementia; they have been reviewed in detail by Yesavage *et al.* (1979). Where the most commonly used drug in the group, cyclandelate, is concerned, the few studies which met acceptable research criteria found no benefit from the drug as compared with a placebo. Much the same was found to apply to other drugs in the group — papaverine, isoxsuprine and cinnarizine: the more exacting the research criteria, the less impressive was the drug's ability to bring about improvement. The authors criticize the design of most of the trials, in particular the lack of a placebo group in at least 50 per cent; to this can be added that there are extraordinarily weak diagnostic criteria, with a general failure to discriminate between dementia of Alzheimer's and of multi-infarct type. In fact, where a soundly-based diagnosis of MID is made, it is possible that some modest improvement may result from the use of, say, cyclandelate. Fine *et al.* (1970) found significant improvements in orientation, communication and socialization in a double-blind crossover trial, and Young *et al.* (1974) found slight improvements in memory, praxis and in some subtests of the WAIS (p. 121), and concluded that the drug had brought about a modest but real gain in ability to cope with everyday life. The question of clinical benefit therefore remains somewhat open where MID is concerned; however, there is no evidence to support the use of vasodilators in AD, especially as they may have unpleasant side-effects: flushing, nausea and rashes are common, and they may actually induce a 'steal' syndrome by their action on peripheral vessels, bringing about a reduction rather than an increase in cerebral perfusion (Leading Article, 1979b).

'Cerebral activators'

These are also known as 'mixed-action vasodilators', indicating uncertainty as to their precise mode of action; the standard-bearer of the group is dihydro-ergotoxine mesylate (DHE), a preparation of equal parts of three hydrogen-ated alkaloids of ergot; it is marketed in the UK as Hydergine. The substance was developed initially as a peripheral vasodilator, but it is now thought to have an effect on brain cell metabolism and is probably the most extensively studied and the most widely prescribed of all drugs for dementia. Its place in the management of AD has been examined in detail by McDonald (1982) and Goodnick (1985).

DHE probably does not augment cerebral blood flow (Meier-Ruge et al., 1978); some of its major effects are within the catecholamine and serotonin systems; it is, for example, a potent blocker of alpha-1 and alpha-2 (presynap-tic) receptors. EEG effects are consistent with a serotonin agonist action; administration in the elderly leads to an increase in fast components and a reduction in total sleep time and REM sleep time. There are therefore certain similarities to the actions of the tricyclic antidepressants, which owe at least some of their therapeutic action to blockade of presynaptic alpha-2 receptors, leading to negative feedback and thus to increased release of amine into the synaptic cleft (Green and Costain, 1981).

At cellular level, animal studies have indicated that DHE has a blocking action on noradrenaline at the cell membrane, preventing release of enzymes which will break down adenosine triphosphate (ATP). It is reported that, as a result, there is reduction of excessive anaerobic synthesis of ATP, preventing cellular acidosis (Loew, 1980), and also that DHE reduces breakdown of cyclic AMP (the intracellular 'second messenger'; p. 57) and increases cerebral oxygen utilization (Meier-Ruge et al., 1978). Its action, like that of all the ergot alkaloids, is thus complex, and any therapeutic benefit cannot so far be related to activity within a single area.

The therapeutic benefits of the drug have been measured both directly by means of clinical assessment (using rating scales) and indirectly using EEG measures, mainly of changes in evoked potentials.

The results of many of the clinical studies have been summarized by Yesavage et al. (1979) and McDonald (1982). Both authors have selected mainly those studies which employed double-blind placebo-controlled techni-que. The formal measure of change was most often the Sandoz Clinical Assessment — Geriatric scale (SCAG), which is an 18-item scale measuring a wide range of behaviour. Only four items deal specifically with cognitive function; other items are, for example, 'anxiety', 'irritability' and 'depression' (Shader et al., 1974). Measures such as subtests of the WAIS have also been used (Shader et al., 1979).

The general pattern in trials of acceptable design is either of significant overall improvement or of significant improvement on at least some measures. In 18 out of 22 such trials, the improvement was considered to be of practical importance. The principal benefits were increased alertness and relief of depression. The question therefore is — bearing in mind the similarity of some of the actions of DHE to those of the tricyclic compounds — whether DHE acts principally (or purely) as an antidepressant. This possibility has been examined in two ways. Gaitz *et al.* (1978) isolated effects on 'cognitive function' from the other tests on the SCAG, and demonstrated a significant improvement, which is held to rule out a 'halo' effect due to antidepressant activity. But 'lack of self-care' (which is, of course, common in depression) is grouped with the cognitive features, and, in addition, the measures of memory on the SCAG are broad and impressionistic and would, contrary to the authors' assertions, be highly vulnerable to affective change. On an objective symptom check-list, the finding of independent cognitive improvement was not supported. Chudnovsky (1979) found that, over a period of six months, DHE brought about an improvement in 'mood depression' and 'interpersonal relationships' significantly greater than that of a placebo, but cognitive function was not significantly altered. A 'halo' effect might also apply to results on the WAIS, which were reported to be improved after 15 months' DHE therapy (Kugler *et al.*, 1978), since the drug appeared principally to improve performance on speed-dependent measures (McDonald, 1982).

Shader *et al.* (1979) compared DHE with imipramine and placebo in geriatric patients with impairment of both mood and cognition. There was significant improvement (on the SCAG) with both over the placebo after nine weeks of treatment, but not at seven weeks. Improvement occurred on items that measured mood but not in cognition; there were no significant differences between imipramine and DHE.

McDonald's general conclusion is that most studies of DHE indicate that it acts principally as a mood elevator and that there is no consistent evidence of improved cognition other than as a byproduct of affective change; the same difficulty applies to studies which measure alteration in evoked potentials (e.g. Exton-Smith *et al.*, 1983; Tecce *et al.*, 1983), since no form of evoked potential being measured at present appears to be invulnerable to affective disorder (p. 132).

Further assessment of 'cerebral activators' will require much more exacting standards than in the past. First, entry criteria will need to be improved; vague terms such as 'dementia', 'chronic senile cerebral insufficiency' and 'geriatric patients' (the latter not even a diagnosis) are fairly usual; even studies which deal specifically with AD do not in general set out diagnostic requirements. An exception is the study by Exton-Smith *et al.* (1983) in which patients with MID were screened out by means of the Hachinski Ischaemia Score (p. 82); in this study improvement in event-related potential was observed in only two of five AD subjects, and neither of these showed any clinical improvement. This group believes, however, that recommended doses of DHE may be too low, and work is continuing with higher dosages.

Second, where the assessment of change in dementia is concerned, measurement will have to be of the functions known specifically to be affected in the form of dementia under study, especially AD (p. 106). A general improvement in a demented patient is always to be welcomed, but one must know which type of patient will respond to a particular drug.

The same applies, in general, to trials of other drugs in the 'cerebral activator' category, such as naftidrofuryl (Praxilene), pyritinol and pentifylline (*Drug and Therapeutics Bulletin*, 1984), which will not be dealt with separately here.

So what place have these drugs, in particular DHE, in the management of AD? On the positive side, DHE is inexpensive and has a low incidence of side-effects. Those that have been reported are sublingual irritation, gastrointestinal upset and bradycardia (Goodnick, 1985). In patients with early dementia some overall improvement, principally in mood and alertness, may be expected. It may, however, be three or even six months before clear benefit is apparent (Gaitz *et al.*, 1977). Generally, one would agree with Hollister (1983) that a clinician who wants to do his best for a patient with early dementia, and who is something of an optimist, ought to give a trial of a drug from this category, though without making any promises to the patient or his relatives. Giving such drugs is, of course, futile in cases of moderate or severe dementia, and where symptoms such as apathy, sadness and lack of energy or initiative are prominent, it is better to give a trial of an antidepressant.

SYMPTOM CONTROL

A report by a working party of the Royal College of Physicians (1981) into organic mental impairment in old age concluded that, where therapeutic possibilities in Alzheimer-type dementia were concerned, 'research into symptom control is as important in the short to medium term as fundamental investigation of the causes of SDAT is in the long term'. There is, of course, some overlap between the symptoms of disorders which complicate dementia, such as depression, anxiety and deficiency syndromes, and those which can be regarded as symptoms of the depression itself, such as wandering and incontinence. However, the distinction can generally be made. It is assumed that the clinician will have excluded prominent secondary medical or physical syndromes and also, in the case of established dementia, dismissed the use of 'cerebral activators'. But there are still a number of ways in which the patient might be improved. Many of them will be discussed in the following two chapters; this section asks whether any pharmacological measures can help in 'symptom control'. We will mainly consider the two features, common in the demented, which cause the greatest amount of difficulty and distress to relatives and other carers: incontinence and behaviour disturbance.

Incontinence

Incontinence, whether double or single, is the one symptom that above all contributes to low status and morale both among the demented and those looking after them. It is a symptom which will often on its own ensure that a patient with AD spends the remainder of his days in a 'dementia ward' rather than in a more domestic establishment or in his own home. Staff on wards for the demented spend about one-quarter of their time mopping-up (Exton-Smith *et al.*, 1975), and incontinence laundry and other services for the demented cost the National Health Service about £250,000 annually. The prevalence of urinary incontinence in those aged over 65 is about 12 per cent, and of faecal incontinence about 3 per cent; the majority of the incontinent elderly are in some degree demented (Campbell *et al.*, 1985; Tobin and Brocklehurst, 1986). The prevalence of incontinence in the demented is around 40 per cent in patients aged 75–79 and 50–55 per cent in those aged 80 and over (Gilleard 1981; McLaren *et al.*, 1981; Campbell *et al.*, 1985).

Incontinence in the late stages of any debilitating illness may sometimes be unavoidable (although even then it can be managed with the minimum of discomfort and distress for all concerned), but it is not otherwise an inevitable part of dementia, especially of AD. Thorough investigation is always indicated; the clinician must therefore be familiar with the conditions which cause or favour incontinence, and must evolve an orderly system for excluding or treating them. Two common causes of urinary incontinence have already been described (pp. 101 and 102): urinary tract infection (often a cause of double incontinence) and diabetes. Drugs are also a major cause of incontinence; those most likely to be responsible are diuretics, hypnotics and sedatives. Any acute illness can be a temporary cause. Constipation or impaction is a frequent cause of double incontinence in the elderly; diagnosis is usually made on abdominal or rectal examination and on a plain bowel X-ray. Prostatic enlargement in the male is also a possibility.

Depression may also be a cause of double incontinence, often in association with constipation. The other (the often self-evident) factors which tend to precipitate incontinence are a change to an unfamiliar environment, immobility and inadequate staffing or poor design in institutions.

Most elderly demented people with urinary incontinence have an underlying degree of bladder instability; Overstall *et al.* (1980) put the figure for detrusor instability at 57 per cent and for outflow obstruction at 13 per cent. In 7 per cent the cause was an atonic bladder; in 21 per cent, miscellaneous causes operated (infection or drugs, for example). We will not deal in detail here with the mechanisms of bladder function and the changes that lead to incontinence; there are lucid explanations by Garland and James (1978), Malone-Lee (1984) and Overstall (1984). In brief, the typical defect is loss of inhibitory control of the sacral reflex, resulting in excessive detrusor activity; this may be confirmed by means of a cystometrogram. But bladder instability and the causes of incontinence listed earlier are not mutually exclusive; it is rarely possible to attribute incontinence to a single cause in the demented elderly; in a study of 65 old people with incontinence, Campbell *et al.* (1985) found that a combination of factors — for example, poor mobility, diuretics, infection and confusion — most often led to incontinence.

The causes of incontinence in the demented elderly are listed in Table 26, with the warning that more than one usually applies. They are given not in order of frequency but in the suggested order in which the various possibilities

Table 26.   Common causes of incontinence in the demented

Drugs (esp. tranquillizers/hypnotics, diuretics)
Diabetes
Urinary tract infection
Constipation or faecal impaction
Outflow obstruction (e.g. prostatic enlargement, carcinoma of bladder or prostate)
Systemic infections
Pelvic tumour
Depression
Immobility
Unfamiliar surroundings
Detrusor instability

are best excluded; investigations, as well as routine screening (p. 104), should include a bowel X-ray. A cystometrogram may be helpful where a cause cannot be identified or a patient does not respond to treatment as expected (Overstall, 1984).

Where management is concerned, impaction will probably require repeated enemas; continence is commonly regained following disimpaction (Garland and James, 1978; Tobin and Brocklehurst, 1986). A bladder retraining programme in less demented patients, especially females, can also be remarkably effective (Jarvis and Miller, 1980).

Certain drugs may be useful in the treatment of detrusor instability; most are essentially anticholinergic and act largely by inhibiting smooth muscle contractions. Their use is reviewed in detail by Malone-Lee (1984). *Imipramine* and *amytriptyline* have been used effectively in the treatment of urinary incontinence; the value of imipramine is better supported in the literature. The actions of imipramine are complex, and, in addition to blocking bladder contractions, it appears to have local anaesthetic properties and an effect on sleep profile, all of which taken together make it especially effective in the treatment of nocturnal enuresis, usually in a dose of 10–25 mg; the single night-time dose may also be effective against daytime incontinence, although sometimes an additional morning dose may be needed. The side-effects of tricyclic drugs in the elderly are well recognized (e.g. postural hypotension and cardiotoxicity), but they are largely dose-related and these small amounts tend to be well tolerated. Imipramine is therefore recommended as the drug of first choice for bladder instability.

Emepronium bromide (Cetiprin) is also commonly used and is also an anticholinergic, but absorption of the drug is unreliable and there is a higher incidence of unwanted side-effects at therapetic dosage than with imipramine (e.g. paralysis of accommodation, dry mouth, postural hypotension and falls), but it may at times be effective where imipramine has failed.

Oxybutynin is a new and fairly potent antispasmodic agent with a direct action on smooth muscle and a fairly insignificant degree of anticholergic activity. It has been extensively evaluated in the USA and, to a somewhat lesser degree, in the UK (Cardozo and Stanton, 1979), where it is available on a named-patient basis only. It appears promising, but it will normally be prescribed only after the patient has been evaluated by a urologist.

Where all other measures fail, some form of incontinence aid may be required; there is now an extremely wide range and the clinician must seek specialist advice on what is best for a particular patient. Some large psychiatric hospitals now have an 'incontinence adviser', usually of the status of a sister or charge nurse; this member of staff will have received training in a urological unit; the system is highly recommended. Patients living at home can be provided with incontinence aids by the district nursing service (p. 181), or the patient's GP can refer to the specialist urological department; relatives can also receive advice from the Disabled Living Foundation (p. 208).

Behavioural disturbance

Symptoms falling into this general category — wandering, aggressiveness, restlessness or insomnia — are the most troublesome of all for those who care for the demented; even incontinence may be surprisingly well tolerated by comparison. Sanford (1975) found that sleep disturbance, restlessness and wandering were the symptoms most likely to determine an elderly demented person's admission to hospital. Argyle et al. (1985) also found that problems of behaviour were the least well tolerated by carers, although no single problem stood out as being the most liable to precipitate hospital admission. In general, relatives were worn down by a multiplicity of problems; wandering, restlessness and aggressiveness were usually reported as prominent difficulties.

Behavioural disturbance in the demented is usually fairly pervasive; problems such as sleep disturbance and daytime wandering and restlessness generally do not represent isolated symptoms which occur separately and can be treated separately. However, one can generally subdivide such disorders into two groups. First, where there is a 'driven' quality to the symptoms, which appear to arise from an abnormal mood state, usually anxiety or agitated depression. Second, where the symptoms appear simply to be the result of disorientation; the elderly person wanders out of the house and cannot find her way home, potters around at night making cups of tea or gets into the wrong bedroom or wrong bed (especially in an institution). Effective management depends in some degree in differentiating between these two categories of disturbance; the following plan for investigation and management is proposed.

First, is an abnormal mood state responsible? Initially one should have excluded *depression*, as outlined on p. 105. But diagnosis will naturally be most difficult in a patient with almost no verbal communication, although even severe dementia does not exclude the possibility of treatable depression. Pointers will be consistent mood change (as distinct from emotional lability) and the biological changes of depression — sleep disturbance, retardation, loss of appetite and weight, constipation. The same applies to anxiety, which will also present with the somatic features that are well recognized in patients of all ages (e.g. tremor, tachycardia, sweating, diarrhoea) but which is likely to be more directly related to a specific situation; there may be problems with managing at home, or the move to an unfamiliar environment might have proved frightening. The treatment of depressive symptoms has been described on p. 151, and the same principles apply even to the severely demented. Where *anxiety states* are concerned, tranquillizers should be avoided if possible since they are in themselves likely to contribute to confusion. But where sensitive and kindly attention to the patient and his environment are not enough, it is often possible to use such drugs effectively without worsening confusion. Benzodiazepines are generally considered to be unsatisfactory for daytime sedation (Briggs and Castleden, 1984; Overstall, 1982) although, contrary to medical opinion, many patients find them to be helpful and free of unwanted side-effects (Pinsker and Suljaga-Petchel, 1984). But thioridazine is now more frequently used, at least in hospitals; there is a lower incidence of side-effects than with benzodiazepines, and the side-effects commonly associated with the phenothiazines are rare, even in the elderly (Linnoila and Viukari, 1976).

The benzodiazepines may be used for night-time sedation, in which case it is best to use one of those with shorter half-lives, such as temazepam. Chlormethiazole is also satisfactory; it does not appear to accumulate (Exton-Smith and Witts, 1980) and is safe and effective in patients of this age-group (Nayal *et al.*, 1978). It has also, when used during the day, brought about improvement in demented patients in terms both of several behavioural indices and of EEG patterns (Dall, 1982). The drug is contraindicated in liver disease as it is extensively metabolized in the liver; one frequent side-effect is also unpleasant nasal irritation, though this is less common in older people, probably due to partial atrophy of the nasal mucosa.

In summary — although well-designed clinical trials in the area are few, the consensus from most is that thioridazine is the drug of first choice in the demented elderly for tranquillization both by day and by night, with chlormethiazole as the second choice, perhaps in the unusual event of phenothiazine-type side-effects.

Then, is the mood disorder essentially one of *emotional lability*? This is essentially one of the 'release phenomena' resulting from frontal lobe disease: the emotions are changeable and incongruous, the patient is unpredictable, there is extreme restlessness and unprovoked aggression, and there are likely to be other signs of frontal lobe disease, such as deterioration of self-care or, possibly, 'primitive' reflexes (p. 109). Such patients can be most difficult to manage, and in my experience the greatest problems arise in the case of the younger AD patient who is still physically fit and who can be persistently overactive and destructive.

Medication of some kind is usually necessary; it is suggested that, before major tranquillizers are used, anticonvulsant drugs are given a trial. Drugs in this category have proved most effective in controlling disturbed behaviour in both adults and children with brain damage; sulthiame has been the most extensively used and tested, and has proved effective even where phenothiazines have failed (for a review, see Moffat *et al.*, 1970). There has been no major trial of the drug in the brain-damaged elderly, but in some patients, especially the younger group of AD sufferers, I have found it at times extremely effective in rendering the patient more tranquil (and even euphoric) without at the same time inducing an unacceptable degree of sedation. Sulthiame will shortly become unavailable in the UK; carbamazepine is recommended as an alternative. Otherwise, recourse is to the phenothiazines (usually thioridazine or chlorpromazine) or chlormethiazole. Haloperidol can be most effective in calming a very disturbed patient, but it is generally unsuitable for continued use because it accumulates rapidly and can bring about heavy sedation or gross extrapyramidal side-effects within a disconcertingly short space of time.

Finally, is the behaviour disorder of the second or more 'benign' type — that is, fairly contented wandering or pottering as a result of disorientation? There is really no medication that will help here; tranquillizers are likely to do no more than make the confusion worse, or lead to falls or total immobility. There is in fact no offence in an elderly person's harmlessly exploring her environment; the fault is more often in the designs of homes or other institutions that do not allow the demented the wander with impunity. An example might be a local authority home which does not have an enclosed garden and is open to a main road. In a mental hospital, we have been able to 'open' two wards for the severely demented by means of access to a large grassy area with a wooden fence; in the area there are rustic benches, a raised goldfish pond and an area for gardening. Wanderers can stroll at will (weather permitting), as distinct from remaining sedated, incontinent and a prey to pressure sores in the ward armchairs. Where a patient is at home, attendance at a day centre may keep him occupied, and he will often, as a result, sleep better at night. But if some night sedation is after all unavoidable, thioridazine is probably again the best choice.

Other symptoms

Many symptoms that occur in association with AD, such as parkinsonism and fits, are direct results of the brain damage and may often be effectively treated with drugs; others, such as pressure sores, contractures or venous stasis and thrombosis, are secondary and are often the result of mismanagement. Discussion of treatment in this area properly belongs in a textbook of geriatrics — but it should be said that many of the severely demented require joint management by a psychiatrist and a geriatrician; at the very least, any doctor dealing with the demented should have training in geriatric medicine or some form of regular geriatric contact, since treatment and preventive measures in the ill elderly are constantly being improved. The days when the demented were cared for, often by part-timers, in the back wards of poorly equipped mental hospitals, should be passing. Many of the most serious chronic problems that occur in the demented can be avoided by good team management and they are generally much more easily prevented than treated. Doctors are often taken to task for keeping the elderly mentally ill alive 'artificially'. One is usually presented with the hypothetical case of the elderly lady who is demented, deaf, half-blind and doubly incontinent, with painful pressure sores and a chest infection. Do we give an antibiotic and (perhaps) prolong a wretched existence or do we allow her to die (perhaps) quickly and peacefully? There can be no satisfactory answer; it is the wrong question. It would be much better to ask, *'Need the patient have got into such a condition in the first place?'* In many instances — probably most — the answer is, 'No.'

SUMMARY

There are three potentially rewarding lines of drug management in Alzheimer's disease; most also apply in some degree to other forms of dementia.

First, symptoms within the category of 'excess disabilities' can be treated. These are conditions which are superimposed on the dementia and which create major illness or handicap. They may be physical disorders (often resulting from isolation and neglect) or psychiatric disorders (especially depression). The positive approach in management consists of identifying such conditions at the outset, since it is often they rather than the underlying dementia which are responsible for a patient's becoming hospitalized. Subsequent treatment can lead to a great improvement in the patient's overall condition (even though his cognitive status is unaltered) and can prevent long-term institutionalization or heavy dependency.

Second, there are drugs which may improve the patient's cognitive state. The most commonly used are the ergot mesylates, but the effects are modest, and the probability is that such drugs act primarily as mood elevators, with secondary effects on attention and alertness. These improvements are not to be discounted, although where clear depressive symptoms are evident it is likely that an antidepressant will be more effective.

Where additional illness has been treated, and cognition cannot be improved, the third principle is that of 'symptom control' — that is, management of the features of the demented state which commonly make life intolerable for both a patient and those who care for him. *Incontinence* is not an inevitable symptom of dementia and its cause must be investigated; urinary tract infection and faecal impaction are, for example, commonly missed and strongly predispose to incontinence, as do also depression, immobility, unfamiliar surroundings and certain drugs, especially diuretics and sedatives. There is usually in addition a degree of detrusor instability. Drugs of the anticholinergic group may help, but because incontinence in the demented usually results from a combination of factors, medication is only an adjunct to intelligent overall management of the patient, with particular attention to mobility.

Behavioural disturbances fall into two broad categories. First, there are those which arise from an abnormal mood state — depression, anxiety or emotional lability resulting from frontal lobe damage. Effective symptomatic treatment with drugs may be possible in this group. Second, there is the type of 'behavioural disturbance' which results principally from disorientation and in which an abnormal mood state is not prominent. This is best managed by providing the right environment and support; drugs are rarely helpful.

Finally, a large number of the chronic problems of the demented, those that fill hospitals, are secondary; dementia is not as a rule preventable, but many of its serious complications are.

CHAPTER 7

Other forms of therapy

This chapter will deal with measures that fall more or less within the category of 'psychological treatments'. One question is, of course, whether psychotherapy will revive dead or dying brain cells. No — but we have already seen that there is a complex pattern of symptomatology and deterioration in dementia; the cognitive impairment is only one problem among many. There are claims, it is true, that certain techniques will indeed improve cognitive functioning — memory and orientation, for example — and we shall examine these. But emotions such as despair, paranoia, apathy and helplessness strongly colour the typical picture of 'senile dementia', and this applies both to the patient and to those looking after him; here there may be the strongest case for techniques that are essentially psychotherapeutic. These cannot, however, be more than adjuncts to the treatments that have been described earlier; there is no clinical evidence that would support their use as alternatives.

A number of authors have reviewed the literature on psychotherapy with the demented. Barns *et al.* (1973) quote from Allison's *The Senile Brain* (1961):

> 'Whatever may be said in favour of it, old age is a losing game. We must, therefore, focus attention on the ways of ensuring that points in the game are not given away unnecessarily.'

Examples from the two types of therapy common in the area are reviewed. First, some distinctly military 'reality orientation' techniques in which the patients are assembled in front of a blackboard and 'drilled' in the correct day, date, time, names of staff members and other facts about their daily lives. The authors' conclusion is that the technique 'should be used at all times by anyone who has contact with elderly patients'. The second and complementary technique is rather more soft-centred, but still involves 'certain prescribed attitudes'; for example, 'kind firmness' and 'active friendliness'. In this latter regimen the doors of the patients' rooms, or their beds, may be docketed in accordance with the prescribed attitude; for example, green for 'active friendliness' or blue for 'passive friendliness'. It is suggested at the end of the review that 'senility could be reversed' by means of such techniques, and that such forms of stimulation 'could be curative', but no supporting evidence whatever is presented. This does not matter so much in the case of measures that are kindly and humanitarian, but evidence is rather more necessary where regimens not invariably agreeable to the patient are being imposed.

Muslin and Epstein (1980) adopt a more psychoanalytical viewpoint; the papers they review are generally exploratory and impractical; they quote with disapproval the eminently rational view of Ginzberg (1950) that, 'if with younger individuals the main task is to help them adapt to environmental difficulties, it is the other way around with elderly patients — we must try and adapt the environment to them'.

A detailed and searching review by Gotestam (1980) examines the literature on psychoanalytic psychotherapy with the elderly published since 1930 and on behaviour therapy since 1968. Of the former group he concludes that, '. . . after 40 years of treating the aged individual with psychotherapy, there are only two experimental studies that can support claims of its efficacy. And of the two studies, one was poorly run and the other was not carried out on psychiatric patients'. (The two studies in question are Wolff (1963) and Godbole and Verinis (1974).) There were rather more positive results with behavioural techniques, especially those directed to 'target' symptoms. Token economy systems were shown to enhance continence (Grosicki, 1968) and walking (MacDonald and Butler, 1974).

Miller (1977) examined in considerable depth the concept that dementia may be susceptible to psychological manipulation. The work reviewed deals mainly with environmental change and begins with studies such as those of Sommer and Ross (1958) and Cosin et al. (1958), who found a general enhancement of behaviour in the demented where chairs in a ward were grouped in circles and around tables as distinct from being placed in a long line. Studies of the 60s and 70s evaluated the benefit of discussion groups, behavioural reinforcement techniques, and communal activities and games such as bingo; all of these brought about increased 'purposeful activity' — for example, talking to other staff and patients and using ward provisions appropriately. When the various measures were withdrawn, behaviour reverted to its baseline level. At this time 'reality orientation' techniques were introduced (and will be dealt with separately). In short, the principle here was of sensory stimulation; deteriorated abilities such as memory and orientation would be reawakened and exercised. Miller found a general consensus that there is, again, some benefit while these therapies are being applied, although there is no enduring alteration.

So are such techniques, often laborious and time consuming, worthwhile? This is the question we will now critically examine, although there has to be a general principle that no measure which contributes to the well-being of a demented person is to be despised — as in the case of the more 'medical' treatments. The results from some may be minimal, but as with other serious diseases for which there is no 'cure', *progress in the medium term is likely to come from the cumulative effect of a number of measures, each of which in itself offers only modest benefit*. The proviso is only that the results from any treatment must be in reasonable proportion to the time and effort expended on it; ideally, too, it should be capable of being integrated with other care measures. The following sections first discuss individual and group psychotherapy and then 'stimulation' techniques such as reality orientation.

PSYCHOTHERAPY

Psychotherapy is impossible to define (Wolff, 1973), but its *object* is, one might suggest, the alteration of an individual's view of himself and his environment by means of his encounter with another person. Where the elderly demented are concerned, psychotherapy is best seen not as a form of treatment which is either given or withheld like a pill; a psychotherapeutic style can run like a thread through all contacts between a patient and his doctor or other staff. A demented patient has lost, or risks losing, his self-esteem to a catastrophic degree. If in hospital, he has lost his home, his place in the world and his identity, and he may now be dependent on others for the most basic or intimate procedures. It follows that every contact with the patient must be managed in such a way as to preserve his self-worth, even if he is being given a bath, an injection or an enema, and he must be addressed with the respect and given the dignity that his age demands. The doctor should address the patient as 'Mr X' or 'Mrs Y', never by a first name or by diminutives, and shake hands when they meet. (A very wise and elderly psychiatrist once told me that the only way to communicate with a psychotic was to talk to him 'like an ordinary person', and the same should apply as far as possible to the demented.) Perhaps there will be a rather different relationship with the nursing staff, who spend much longer with the patient, but one would then expect that such informalities as the use of first names would be mutual.

This definition of psychotherapy doubtless would not appeal to the specialist, who would say that it amounts to nothing more than kindly and sensitive handling — but even these do require some knowledge of a demented person's mental processes and, based on this, a degree of thought and imagination. To take an extreme but sadly common example, almost nothing is more detrimental to a person's self-esteem and sense of identity than to dress him up, like a November guy, in ill-fitting and cast-off clothes — which still is the routine on admission to many mental hospitals. Patients' own accounts, their emotions and their behaviour, and their relatives' reactions, testify to the sense of despair and depersonalization that comes from wearing someone else's cigarette burns. A certain awareness of the part played by self-esteem in mental health would lead to the avoidance of such blunders.

It is also necessary to have some understanding of the way in which the world is perceived by a demented person. As indicated earlier, there is a fairly common pattern of progression from a bewildered and anguished phase, in which the patient is aware of his gradual loss of contact with the outside world, to one in which he is more tranquil but where normal person-to-person contact is virtually lost. What is in the mind of demented Mrs Jones? She cannot tell us, but anyone who spends sufficient time talking to her will discover that she lives in an inner world made up almost exclusively of her memories; she is aware of us somewhere out on the rim of this world — young, strangely clad people making unintelligible sounds, rushing hither and thither like figures in an old film, shouting and gesticulating at her; she wonders what all the fuss is about. Her personal time-capsule is almost intact; King Edward is still on the throne, Baldwin is the Prime Minister, Mother is making dinner in a long-since bombed terrace house, the other children are . . . somewhere, she is not quite sure at the moment. But some things are very strange. 'There's this woman comes up to me and says something about being my daughter. I may have seen her before, I may not — but what nonsense, how can *I* have a daughter? Now she's crying . . . Silly girl.'

'Transference', as pointed out by Goldfarb and Turner (1953), can have its own meaning where dealings with a demented person are concerned; one may have to take an essentially 'filial' role (or whatever role is assigned) and make whatever contact is possible from there. There are healthy and virtually intact areas even in the most demented, and it is possible to make contact with them even though the patient's main sources of identity and self-worth are likely to be located in the remote past. This is why techniques such as 'reminiscence groups' have proved so acceptable to the elderly; contact with the patient is aided by a variety of artefacts relating to his earlier years — local photographs, postcards, books, songs. The demented, too, often have long and fascinating tales to tell about life during both World Wars.

Within the family (and the great majority of demented people either live with their families or are visited by them) it is often well understood that the patient is 'living in the past' — indeed, the futility of arging and lecturing is often better understood than by professionals. The older person can often maintain a major role as the keeper of family lore, the one who passes on special and private knowledge to the younger generations. Townsend (1957) and others have written about the unique bond that can exist between the very old and the very young. A. and S. Sampson (1985) observe how often grandparents and great-grandparents can find a common bond with the young outside the rational, competitive world of the intervening generations. 'The tricks of memory in old age,' they write, 'conspire to bridge the long divide to childhood, as old people find they can remember events seventy years ago much more easily than the happenings of the previous week.' The concept of a second childhood, say the authors, exists much more positively and interestingly than in the sense of senility or dependence.

BEHAVIOURAL TECHNIQUES

Reality orientation

Reality orientation depends on an assumption that the failing mental capabilities of a demented person can be stimulated and exercised; the idea is appealing, and the technique has gained great popularity both in the USA and in the UK, where one can hardly find a self-respecting psychogeriatric ward without its 'reality board'. Reality orientation programmes were instituted by Folsom in 1965 and are described in detail in his papers of 1967 and 1968 and by the American Psychiatric Association in 1969. It is suggested that, because the older patient has withdrawn from his contacts and his environments, parts of his brain have ceased to function, and that this process may be reversed (a) by constant stimulation and repetitive orientation to his environment and (b) by placing him in a group of people, contact with whom will diminish his isolation. Thus, unused neurological pathways may again become effective.

Reality orientation (RO) therefore takes two general forms. First, 'classroom RO', in which there is intense cognitive training for about half an hour daily; the patients are presented with such items as the day, date and place, usually on a board, and they are actively rehearsed by the therapist. The other form, which has been called 'twenty-four hour RO', introduces orientation training into all staff–patient contacts. Instead of simply calling a patient for lunch, the nurse might say, 'It's twelve o'clock, Mrs Smith, time to get ready for lunch', or 'It's three o'clock in the morning, Mrs Jones. Are you having trouble sleeping?'

The earlier literature on RO did not make a distinction between demented and other elderly patients; the first controlled trial of the efficacy of RO as applied to the demented was by Brook et al. (1975). A room was equipped with interesting and stimulating material — boards with magnetic letters with the day, date and so on, a clock-face, coloured illustrations of everyday objects, books and newspapers. Eighteen patients with a diagnosis of dementia were assigned to either an experimental or a control group. The experimental group were actively encouraged to use the material in the room, going through the items on the board and rehearsing the use of everyday objects. The other group were also brought into the room, and were allowed to use the material if they wished, but they received no active encouragement from the therapists. There was a marked improvement in the group where staff gave encouragement, but not in the control group. They became more talkative and alert, and almost all cases of incontinence improved. The less deteriorated patients benefited most. Improvement was measured by means of nurses' ratings; rating was 'blind', but the rating instrument is not described and there is no indication that cognition was improved; it is not especially surprising that patients were stimulated and enlivened by this unusual degree of staff attention.

Woods (1979) tested a hypothesis that improvement as a result of RO is principally brought about through reinforcement — that is, as a result of staff reward and encouragement following desired responses. All patients in the study were mildly cognitively impaired. There were three groups: in one there was formal RO, in another a discussion group in which inappropriate contributions were accepted, and the third group were untreated controls. There was careful assessment on a variety of measures of cognition and behaviour. The RO group improved significantly on the Wechsler Memory Scale and behaviour rating scales, and there was a trend towards improvement on a memory and information test; the other groups did not improve. The author suggests that some of the symptoms of demented people may fall into the 'learned helplessness' category. After the repeated trauma of failing at tasks that were once very simple, they may adopt a helpless non-responding position; RO may ease the patient out of this position by helping him to make successful answers once more. It is concluded that staff encouragement is all-important and that the wrong form of attention is possibly worse than no attention at all.

Hanley *et al.* (1981) tested class RO and ward orientation training in groups of demented patients in hospital and in an old people's home. Class RO brought about some improvement in orientation but the results were modest in proportion to the time and effort spent in training the therapist and in providing the therapy; there were no improvements on measures of behaviour. However, ward RO — practical training in finding one's way about the ward, often reinforced by notices and signposts — was extremely effective in improving orientation, notably in time.

Holden and Woods (1982) have provided a detailed and realistic assessment of RO. There is a general conclusion that information presented simply and attractively has distinctly positive effects on orientation (as it does anywhere else), and also that there are in general gains in staff and patient morale, though these are less easy to demonstrate. RO is not a novelty; the authors say that they have come across many staff who have been using RO-type techniques with the elderly for years. The aim for the demented patient has to be limited, although it is not to be forgotten that the demented do have some learning capacity; this, however, requires the aid of external cues, such as clear and colourful signs indicating, say, the toilet, the dining-room or the patient's bed.

Miller (1977), who also stresses the practical value of such cues, goes on to deal sensitively with the patient who is 'happily demented' — who is to all appearances contentedly established in a hospital ward or an old people's home for life. RO will not enable her to leave, so why bother her with techniques which will bring her out of her 'twilight world' and into the realities of old age with all its losses and infirmities? Why intervene? The answer is essentially that any contact with an elderly demented person represents some form of 'intervention'. It may be constructive or damaging. There must be no question of imposing techniques on a patient who is reluctant or in whom they might cause distress; the object is to nurture and encourage, not to force. The patient is provided with opportunities and given a choice; the demented are rarely given choices.

Normalization

This more or less means what it says; normality represents for the elderly person a continuation of previous patterns of living. Therefore, where possible, previous interests, styles of living and preferences (e.g. for clothes, possessions, tasks) are to be fostered; Miller (1977) examines the concept in some detail. It originates from the area of mental subnormality; the demented, like other mentally handicapped groups, may be physically fit and active and do not necessarily need to be surrounded by the trappings of a hospital ward. Nor do they need to be in large sex-segregated institutions far from population centres where staff make every decision about their daily lives. They can equally well be cared for in domestic-scale establishments near their familiar environments and their relatives. Present-day economics will, however, severely delay the provision of these smaller units, but it is perfectly possible to apply 'normalization' principles even in mental hospital wards by thoughtful use of furnishings, partitions, pictures, seating, magazines and newspapers; indeed, one can capitalize on the very 'disadvantages' of a large institution by colonizing the adjacent outdoor space, as described on p. 163.

Other forms of therapy — art, music, reminiscence therapy (Woods and Britton, 1985) — for the demented have been described. Others are introduced from time to time. Marr (1983) writes of 'bibliotherapy', in which patients are encouraged to share their pleasure in books, poetry and pictures. But just what is 'therapy'? The skilled musician who regularly plays and sings with some of my demented patients told me that if I am to refer to her sessions as 'music therapy', then the next item on the programme could equally well be called 'lunch therapy'! Well, if lunch improves as a result, why not? More seriously, there is no magic in any particular form of patient contact. Any skill can be utilized in finding and addressing the positive and healthy areas within a patient; the means will vary between patients as it will between therapists. There is certainly a risk of elevating very simple and commonsense measures into mini-sciences, sometimes incongruously, but (provided they can be integrated with other care measures and are acceptable to the patients) this is infinitely preferable to pessimism and neglect. It is worth repeating the proposition that the treatment of dementia is likely to advance as a result of the sum of modest benefits rather than as the result of a single major 'breakthrough'.

Finally, while it may seem hardly possible to make direct contact with the most severely demented patients, who may thus seem 'untreatable', one can still 'treat' the patient's *context*, the place where he is. This brings one back to the normalization principle, the provision of an acceptable domestic environment in what is likely to be the patient's permanent home. Models of terminal care have been much publicized in the last few decades, but they have rarely been applied specifically to the demented (though 'continuing care' is a rather better term for this group). It is a pity, since *terminal or continuing care provision for the demented must be in no way inferior to that available to other groups of patients*. This should be a guiding principle for the 80s and beyond. There are, of course, some differences in the management of the severely demented and that of, say, cancer sufferers, the main one being that there cannot be the same degree of emotional and verbal contact with patients in the former group. But those who care for the demented are still in the main serving *families*, and staff morale and satisfaction can be greatly enhanced by making the unit a warm and welcoming place for the patient's children, grandchildren and others of his extended family. In one dementia ward a scrap-book project (with pictures and cuttings relating to the earlier part of a patient's life) has been used with splendid results; this involves all of the family and makes visiting-time more enjoyable; it also provides the staff with a more complete, 'three-dimensional' view of the patient.

The 'quality of life' for the severely demented in hospital is scarcely accessible to objective measures, but for those who must have such a measure, here is one. Ward A is long, stark, poorly lit and drably painted; the walls are bare and the atmosphere is permeated with the faint odours of urine and disinfectant. The patients are ranged in lines against the walls in aluminium chairs, half-covered with white blankets; they are being 'commoded' one by one. Loud 'pop' radio plays all day. In Ward B there are pictures and murals; there are colourful curtains and an open french window leads into a small enclosed garden with rustic furniture and a raised goldfish pond covered with water-lilies. Inside, the armchairs have been arranged in circles around tables or by the television set; there are books and magazines on the tables. There is music, but it is unobtrusive: a tape of 'golden oldies'.

Neither ward is imaginary. The question is: in which ward do the patients wail endlessly, loudly and piercingly, and in which are the patients almost all receiving tranquillizers? The answers can be easily guessed.

SUMMARY AND CONCLUSIONS

Drug treatment and conventional medical and nursing care are incomplete therapies for the demented. Psychological techniques can bring additional benefits; these are usually modest, but so also, unhappily, are those of most drugs, and it is generally the case that a patient will be improved by a combination of a number of measures, each of which would bring about little change by itself.

Formal psychotherapy is not helpful in the management of dementia, but a psychotherapeutic style can enhance all staff–patient contacts, with particular emphasis on the repair and maintenance of a patient's self-esteem; it can begin with the quite rare expedient of the doctor's shaking hands with the patient and greeting him formally by name, and continue with courtesy and the preservation of a patient's dignity during nursing procedures. Every patient has inner healthy areas from which he can give something, and the search for these can be a most rewarding task both for the patient and the person caring for him; often they are located in the distant past.

Reality orientation is the most favoured of the techniques which have been applied in order to stimulate the failing mental capabilities of a demented person; unhappily, orientation cannot be 'taught', and blackboard techniques are generally ineffective. But 'twenty-four hour RO' can bring about some improvement in ward orientation, although the technique is little more than a formalization of commonsense measures to help the patient find his way around the ward with large and colourful cues. However, a formal system can bring about increased staff engagement and will in general enliven and improve the ward atmosphere.

Nearly every sensitively applied medium for making contact with a patient will bring its own rewards. It is sometimes asserted that demented patients are most happy left as they are, but this is an argument of which one must be wary; many groups of people have at various times been described as 'happy as they are' (the reader can think of his own examples), and if such a view had always prevailed then medicine and society would have made precious little advance in the past few decades. On the other hand, the patient, in his last few years, is not to be bullied or regimented; he is to be given opportunities, stimulation and encouragement to engage in his immediate world, that is all.

Treatment is not only to be applied to the patient but also to his context; for better or worse, he will in some degree mirror his surroundings. Patients in long-stay wards should be managed in settings which are in no way inferior to those provided for patients in other terminal care establishments. There are means by which the spirit that animates the hospice movement can permeate even the 'back wards' of a mental hospital.

CHAPTER 8

Services for the demented

The previous chapter dealt largely with the demented in hospital or in other institutions. But more than four-fifths of the demented live at home (p. 30). Because of their dementia, all are in some degree handicapped, and therefore certain supports are necessary in order for them to live lives that are as normal and as satisfying as possible. This structuring is not only part of the treatment of a demented patient; sometimes, since we have so few effective drugs, it *is* the treatment.

There is now a large literature describing and evaluating the care of the demented in the community. Before long the dementia wards of the large mental hospitals may close for ever, and therefore even the most severely affected will have to be cared for either in their own homes or in various types of local unit. Exactly which type is a question which we shall examine later but, as this chapter is essentially one for the practical clinician, it will not deal in detail with the growth and philosophy of community care for the demented but will consist largely of a factual description of the services that are available at present, how they are best made use of and how they are developing. On many occasions a patient has to enter an institution because of a single symptom, such as incontinence, when, did the family or GP but know it, the service that could have enabled the patient to live at home was readily available. Our 1987 study (Van der Cammen *et al*.) revealed serious deficiencies in the utilization of services, partly because the patient's needs had not been accurately diagnosed but more usually because of a simple lack of information. Unhappily, when a demented patient is admitted to hospital it is often the case that the 'excess disabilities' of his condition (p. 147), which would at one time have been remediable, have advanced to a degree where he is no longer able to regain the *status quo* and is permanently entrenched in a state of high dependency.

Case No. 11
Mrs K has been demented for five years; she lived alone. Her relatives did their best for her, bringing in all her meals and cleaning her flat, but she spent all day and most nights in the same armchair; now she has painful contractures of both knees and hips and, in spite of intensive physiotherapy, she cannot regain

mobility. She will need to go to a home which accepts chairbound residents, but there are very few of these, and she had been in a psychiatric ward for over a year.

Case No. 12
Mrs L set her flat on fire; she had been poorly supervised, and an accumulation of paper litter had probably been responsible. Now she is homeless and also, because of smoke inhalation, she sustained severe tracheal burns and has a tracheostomy. She will continue to need full nursing care.

While it is not unusual for accidents to lead to hospital admission (p. 150), more usually relatives and neighbours are gradually worn down by the demented person's symptoms (p. 161) and it is frequently the case that, even if the patient is improved following admission to hospital, the store of good will that had previously existed has long since been depleted. Macmillan (1960) found that, when the demands on a family exceeded a certain level, irreversible rejection occurred, and further help was of no avail.

Many of these difficulties can be avoided. Townsend (1957) showed that lack of social supports was more likely to determine admission to an institution than was illness; the elderly who remained in hospital were also at the time most likely to do so for purely social reasons (Amulree *et al.*, 1951; Graham, 1954), yet all but a tiny proportion of relatives and neighbours were willing to care for the elderly person, given appropriate help. This was confirmed by Bergmann *et al.* in 1978; regrettably the intervening period had seen no improvement in the provision of services. A heavy burden of care tended to fall on the relatives of the demented person (44 per cent were considered to make 'excessive demands') and help 'was not readily forthcoming'. The prospects for the demented living alone were even more bleak; the risk of institutionalization or mortality within a year was 81 per cent. A preventive approach to dementia, the authors write, does not have to await further fundamental aetiological research; there are already means by which the demented could be 'treated', and deterioration prevented, by mobilization of adequate supportive resources in the community.

The case of high-quality community care of the demented is thus most persuasively made, as it has been made by others, but next the much-used and rather enigmatic phrase 'community care' needs to be defined. Care in the community, or by the community? L.B. Hunt, Senior Medical Officer at the DHSS, defines community care as 'the provision of alternatives to long-term institutional care for the chronically sick or those suffering from long-term handicaps of disability' (1985). The definition (and indeed the whole paper) is disappointingly negative; migration of patients and staff from institutions — or avoidance of admission in the first place — must be seen as options that will enable the patient to receive an improved quality of care and of life, not an equivalent one (and sometimes a worse one). De-institutionalization has no virtue in itself; it does not even save money (Opit and Shaw, 1976).

E.D. Acheson, Chief Medical Officer at the DHSS (1985) examined 'that over-used word Community' and writes that the term has taken on an ethos of virtue which makes for clouded thinking; he suggests that it is best to refer to a 'domiciliary care policy' if the object is to maintain as many of the elderly frail as possible in their homes. But there will inevitably be some for whom an adapted institutional environment may be preferable.

The present chapter is not limited to a description of community care provisions; it deals factually with services available to the demented both at home and in institutions. But the emphasis is on the demented person at home; this is usually the first point of contact, and it is at this stage that preventive measures can be most effectively applied.

DOMICILIARY CARE: THE PROVISIONS

The general practitioner

The primary care physician is, or should be, the key figure in the diagnosis and management of the demented person at home. Unhappily, dementia, though a serious illness, is frequently dismissed as an inevitable consequence of ageing and a problem of little concern to doctors; although there are now many GPs who carefully assess and manage their demented patients, the present trend towards the 'multidisciplinary team' carries the risk that the demented may be again 'de-medicalized' and that the diagnosis and management of an elderly person with brain disease may again be seen as a matter that can be dealt with equally by a doctor or by a member of one of the paramedical professions. Skilled though such colleagues may be, this will not do; one cannot imagine patients suffering from any other form of illness being managed in this way, or that any would improve as a result. But — going back one stage — patients with dementia are, more often than not, unknown even to their GPs (Williamson *et al.*, 1964; Foster *et al.*, 1976). Murphy (1985) cites more recent studies which indicate that this situation has scarcely improved, and also that, when the relative brings the problem to the GPs attention, the response is often unhelpful. A report of 1984 by the Surrey Council for Mental Health found that 38 per cent of people who consulted their GP with a memory problem were told that nothing could be done, and that the symptoms were due to age (Murphy, 1985). It was rare for the GP to alert domiciliary services, and patients passed on to the psychogeriatrician were almost never investigated first.

Yet it has been shown that, with adequate initial assessment, the condition of many patients can be improved (Foster *et al.*, 1976; Van der Cammen *et al.*, 1987). But it is necessary, to begin with, that the GP is aware of dementia where it exists. It is calculated in the 1981 Report of the Royal College of Physicians that, on average, each GP will have about 25 patients suffering from dementia, of whom half will be severely demented. The report recommends that all practices should possess an age/sex register, and that the population especially at risk for dementia (i.e. those over 65) should be subject to some form of regular screening. Staff such as health visitors have been shown to be effective, when trained, in identifying possible mental illness in an elderly patient.

Next it is necessary that the GP himself employ some form of screening of elderly patients who might consult him for reasons other than loss of memory; the Abbreviated Mental Test Score (p. 115) would be suitable for this. Some additional training or contact with specialists in the area is likely to make him more aware of the treatable causes of memory loss; many of these can be identified and treated without referral elsewhere.

Third, the GP will be the main provider of services, either from the resources of the primary care team or in partnership with a specialist or with the social services. He is the only person who holds all the patient's (and his family's) records; he is locally placed and therefore, ideally, will be familiar with local provisions and how to obtain appropriate specialist help. It is he, too, who is ideally placed to press for improvements where these services are defective. All of this applies equally to the intractibly demented; it is still the GP who is best placed to co-ordinate the 'treatment' that consists in providing the necessary supportive structures for a demented old person.

The psychogeriatrician

A psychogeriatrician is a consultant psychiatrist with a special responsibility for the elderly mentally ill; the Department of Health and Social Security (1975), the Royal College of Physicians (1981) and the Health Advisory Service (1982) have all recommended that at least one consultant psychiatrist in each health district should have such responsibility, although by 1981 only about one-third had made appointments. A detailed survey by Wattis *et al.* (1981) identified 106 consultants with a 'special interest' in the elderly; 39 were working full-time with the elderly, 52 more than half-time and a further 15 were running clearly defined psychogeriatric services. It was striking that the consultants were relatively young (mean age 45) and that more than half had started work with the elderly in the past five years; the evolution of psychogeriatrics as a subspeciality, the authors write, is therefore a very new major development in British psychiatry. Similarly, in the 1985 parliamentary debate on Alzheimer's disease (p. 3), the Under-Secretary of State reported that there now appeared to be no difficulty in interesting able psychiatrists in taking up the psychiatry of old age and in accepting special responsibility for the elderly; this, which has largely been due to enthusiastic leadership, is certainly a factor to be set against the many gloomy forecasts about dementia. But there is still a serious lack of training opportunities (Blessed, 1986); the number of psychogeriatric senior registrar posts in the UK needs, at the very least, to be doubled (Arie, 1985).

The majority of psychogeriatricians, incidentally, treat all new mental illness in patients aged 65 and over — though styles vary — but the management of patients with AD will inevitably be the major concern. In addition to his clinical responsibility, he needs to educate medical and other colleagues, and in particular to help with the co-ordination of the many services for the elderly mentally ill. Arrangements by which responsibility for the elderly is shared by a number of consultants whose main work is with younger patients tend not to work satisfactorily, since none is likely to have a sufficient degree of familiarity and contact with the local services of the elderly; a psychogeriatrician functions by 'making the system work' as much as he does by conventional clinical means.

It must be said again that practice varies greatly, but a psychogeriatrician will generally work with a team of staff who also have a special responsibility for the elderly — for example, a psychologist, a social worker, a community psychiatric nurse and an occupational therapist. Referral will almost always be from the patient's GP and, as recommended earlier, diagnosis in the first instance is a matter for the consultant — who will probably need to examine and screen the patient in an outpatient department. Continuing responsibility thereafter has to be carefully allocated. Stirling (1985) has warned against the 'multidisciplinary trap'; that is, if it is uncertain who has the necessary skills to deal with a patient then responsibility is shared in the hope that, given such a spread of professional ability, the patient will somehow get the help he needs. Following diagnosis, when a treatment and support 'package' has been arranged, the patient is best assigned to a team member who will then be the 'key worker' and who will continue to visit the patient under the supervision of the specialist or the GP. Responsibility for the patient should be handed back to the primary care team as soon as possible, although in practice the key worker is often shared by both groups — for example, a geriatric visitor working from a community health clinic. This does not matter; indeed, sometimes the arrangement can be ideal, making for better continuity — provided that the key worker is clearly identified and has easy access to both GP and specialist.

Psychogeriatrics, though maintaining contact with its parent discipline psychiatry, has developed to a large extent in parallel with the geriatric service, and a psychogeriatrician will usually work in close association with his physician colleagues; there is substantial overlap between the demented and the physically ill (Copeland et al., 1975), and some facilities for joint management are highly desirable; even if they are not, there must be ease of access by one service to another and there must also be education of the physician and the psychiatrist in each other's disciplines (Arie, 1977). The organization of joint provisions is dealt with in more detail on p. 188.

A psychogeriatrician is appointed by the district health authority and usually contacted by the patient's GP.

The community psychiatric nurse (CPN)

The community psychiatric nursing service has evolved from small projects of the 1960s; there are now 3000–4000 CPNs working in the UK. It is not known exactly how many work with the elderly, but the majority of well-established psychogeriatric services have CPNs attached (Health Advisory Service, 1982). The Royal College of Physicians Report of 1981 refers to the most valuable role which the CPN plays in maintaining the elderly demented in the community, supporting relatives, advising on medication, and helping to settle and monitor in their own homes patients already known to the psychiatric service. The CPN will also, on occasion, initiate referral to a specialized service.

A CPN requires as a minimum a Registered Mental Nurse qualification and experience at staff nurse level. Formal CPN courses are now being established in addition, but are not yet mandatory (Brooker and Beard, 1984; Skidmore, 1985; these two articles deal in detail with the organization and development of community psychiatric nursing).

CPNs may be based in a hospital, but they are now more often based in local health centres or clinics; a CPN team will consist of the CPNs based at perhaps two or three local centres and will often include at least one member with special responsibility for the elderly. This member should meet regularly (weekly or fortnightly) with the psychogeriatrician to discuss their joint patients; this contact is one of the most worthwhile that the latter will make in terms of maintaining the demented elderly at home.

The 1982 Health Advisory Service document recommends that there be two to six CPNs for the elderly in a health district with an elderly population of 30,000.

CPNs are employed by the district health authority. Referral systems vary. Some CPNs take referrals only from psychiatrists, but many operate an 'open' referral system. In the latter system the majority of referrals in practice come from GPs, but anyone can contact the service — including the relatives or the patient himself. Most large clinics or health centres either will have a CPN attached or will be able to give information about the service. However, although referral may come from any source, CPNs do not operate in isolation any more than do other staff working with the elderly, and there will be close collaboration with the GP and (if appropriate) the psychogeriatrician, especially if the patient is receiving medication.

The geriatric visitor (GV)

This service grew from small beginnings in the former London Borough of St Pancras in the 1950s. An unusually high proportion of elderly people in the area lived alone (as they still do) and the Medical Officer of Health, in association with Age Concern, engaged a small number of SRNs to carry out a pilot project with particular emphasis on regular visiting and supervision of this group. The service was found to meet a huge need, and in the London Borough of Camden there are now over 40 GVs, each with a case-load of about 200 individuals or couples, and the service has spread nationwide. As the GV service is part of the health visitor service, however, the elderly in some districts are looked after by a 'generic' health visitor.

A large part of the GV's work is with the demented; his purpose is to supervise, advise and prevent. For example, a GV might visit a patient who has recently been discharged from hospital, or a person with dementia who is at risk of self-neglect, in order to ensure that complications such as malnutrition or hypothermia are avoided. The GV will call upon a specialist service where this is indicated and can also advise on local provisions, such as day centres. He does not, strictly speaking, 'treat' patients; this is the province of the district nurse. The line of distinction with the CPN service is not very clearly drawn; either service can adequately supervise a demented person, and it is often a question of availability. Or it may be clear that either physical or psychiatric problems predominate. But the involvement of two or more nursing services simultaneously (not uncommon) is by all means to be avoided! (Fortunately, the present rather confusing system is likely to change soon with the establishment of managed and integrated neighbourhood nursing services (DHSS, 1986).)

GVs are employed by the district health authority and based in local health centres or clinics; many teams operate an open referral system, but most referrals come from GPs or hospital consultants (or hospital nurses, when a patient is about to be discharged). Therefore a GV may be contacted either through a doctor or directly, when he will call and assess an elderly person's needs.

The district nurse

The district nurse will deal with a demented person when some form of continuing treatment is required; this could, for example, include the management of incontinence and the provision of necessary aids, although a GV may also arrange this. Therefore, the district nurse is likely only to have an *ad hoc* involvement with a demented patient, but the reference is made since doctors dealing with the elderly are commonly uncertain about how the different categories of home nursing relate to each other and exactly what can be expected from each.

Traditionally the district nurse works closely with the GP and is usually based in a health centre and less usually in a local clinic; contact is normally through the GP.

Other professional staff closely allied to the medical and nursing professions can be called upon to help maintain the demented person at home. For example, an occupational therapist can assist a patient with the tasks of daily living, and can often perform a most valuable function in taking a hospitalized demented person to his home for assessment and retraining, sometimes on several occasions, in preparation for discharge. Some health districts have a community occupational therapist who will provide continuing supervision and help over longer periods.

A physiotherapist is especially concerned with mobility problems; again, many districts have a community service.

The contribution of the clinical psychologist is less well defined; many districts are without a specialist psychologist for the elderly. Indications are that a psychologist can help particularly in supporting the carers of the demented (Gilleard, 1984; Woods and Britton, 1985); the psychologist may meet the family regularly and help them towards an understanding of the emotional needs of the demented person and of how they can be met from the family's own resources. He can also help with behavioural management in a number of ways — for example, if aggression or incontinence are problems.

Social Services

The social worker

A social worker may be a member of the specialist psychogeriatric team; otherwise the psychiatrist or GP will work with a social worker based in an area or neighbourhood office. The majority of social workers are now employed by local authorities; none is now employed by health authorities. The most effective system is generally that of the specialized social worker (Health Advisory Service, 1982). The social worker assesses the needs of patients living at home, and provides and co-ordinates the necessary services. The following services are typically available to the elderly.

Home helps

Individuals needs are assessed by the home help organizer. Of all agencies, the home help spends the greatest amount of time with the patient. She may well be the first to notice and report any change in the patient's condition; because of the extended contact time, as distinct from the briefer visits of the GV or district nurse, it is probable that the home help maintains more of the elderly mentally infirm at home than does any other community service (Gilleard, 1984).

Meals on Wheels

These are provided to housebound or mentally confused people who are unable to cook for themselves and who do not have a daily hot meal cooked for them by friends or relatives. In most areas they can be made available on seven days a week.

Good neighbours

These are volunteers who visit the patient regularly and who help with simple tasks such as shopping, or who help the patient to get in and out of bed, or to wash and dress. They are paid a small honorarium for their services.

The incontinence laundry service

This service will call daily; it normally requires a doctor's recommendation.

Luncheon clubs

These are sometimes provided in co-operation with voluntary bodies. They are mainly a means of ensuring that the patient has a hot meal daily (meals on wheels are not provided for those able to attend a local luncheon club), but they also have a valuable social function. Most provide additional activities such as games or film shows.

Day centres

Many patients with mild dementia will benefit from attendance at day centres and luncheon clubs, especially if daytime supervision is required for a patient whose relative is at work during the day. There are a few day centres which cater specifically for the more severely confused, and in these there are extra staff and increased supervision; there may also be a resident or visiting nurse who can administer daytime medication and attend to other nursing needs. Such centres can be extremely valuable, being the key element in maintaining at home severely demented people who would otherwise be in long-stay wards. A psychogeriatrician is well advised to 'adopt' such a centre where it exists, and to visit regularly.

RESIDENTIAL CARE

Sheltered housing

In most areas there are 'sheltered' or 'supported' housing schemes for the elderly. These developments are defined, in one borough, as 'purpose-built housing designed for elderly people, so that they live independently as part of the community . . . with a resident warden who can provide assistance and advice when it is needed'. They are self-contained flatlets with warden supervision which varies in degree; there is usually daily visiting by the warden, an intercom and alarm system, and sometimes a bleep system. These flatlets are generally for people with some form of illness or disability, including dementia, but who are able to care for themselves with the help of support services (such as those described above).

They are not as a rule suitable for people with moderate or severe dementia or for those who need a lot of practical support, although in some areas there are 'special' sheltered housing schemes for those who need rather more assistance; in these schemes care assistants are available in the mornings and evenings to give residents extra help with, say, cooking, washing or dressing. There are usually two full-time wardens in such special schemes and, with this additional support and also, where necessary, regular nursing visits and the provision of incontinence aids, people with a moderate degree of dementia can often be maintained indefinitely in the community.

In a few areas there is a 'peripatetic warden' scheme, where a warden regularly visits and supervises elderly tenants in what is otherwise standard council accommodation.

Several voluntary groups also run supported housing schemes; information is generally available from a local social services office.

Local authority sheltered housing schemes are usually administered by the housing department; referral is normally initiated by a doctor or social worker, but the elderly person or his relatives can apply directly to a district housing office.

It has been suggested that sheltered housing and other residential care schemes may be overused; some people with only a limited or single disability that could be dealt with by domiciliary services may be unnecessarily committed to an 'institutional' model of care, with the sacrifice of privacy and independence that this entails (Eley and Middleton, 1983). A study by Butler (1982) found that many provisions were irrelevant to patients' needs; for example, about half of the residents in his study had tied the alarm bell out of reach. He draws attention to the inflexibility of domiciliary services which lead to the move of people to these 'new institutions' — for example, meals on wheels that can be provided on only five days a week, and day centres that will take a patient only once or twice weekly. But this pattern has of late tended to improve for the better (as indicated above), and Eley and Middleton's conclusion that residential care schemes 'at best over-provide for a minority at the expense of greater numbers in need' overstates the case. There are intangible benefits of sheltered housing; elderly people with memory loss usually welcome the additional sense of security and companionship — while privacy is also maintained — especially in inner city areas.

Private sheltered housing units also exist; indeed, the last few years have seen an unprecedented surge in the commercial development of housing schemes for the elderly, and several thousand flats are being built annually, with a target of 15,000. The optimum size of development is generally considered to be about 15 flats; prices range from medium to fairly expensive. Flats in the higher price category offer a garden, a garage, a range of electronic aids and a 'secretary' rather than a warden. Age Concern (p. 205) has published a pamphlet called *A Buyer's Guide to Sheltered Housing*, and at least one UK house agency specializes in sheltered housing.

Local Authority homes for the elderly

These were defined in Part 3 of the National Assistance Act of 1948 and are often referred to as 'Part 3 accommodation'. The term is not a happy one and is often misheard or misunderstood; elderly people, or their relatives, have been known to ask indignantly why they are not good enough for 'class 2' or even 'class 1' accommodation! Unfortunately an 'old people's home' sounds even less acceptable; the term 'residential home', in spite of being tautologous, usually goes down better, but the imagined stigma of 'going into a home' is something that anyone dealing with the elderly has to confront regularly; indeed, with its air of finality, it is usually more feared than going into hospital.

Part 3 homes are 'primarily a means of providing a greater degree of support for those elderly people no longer able to cope with the practicalities of living in their own homes even with the help of the domiciliary services' (DHSS and Welsh Office, 1977). The following paragraphs will not deal in detail with residential care for the elderly but will examine current provisions in so far as they serve the demented.

A Part 3 home is not an extension of the hospital service, and it is not planned or staffed to accommodate the severely mentally or physically ill. Some local authorities specifically exclude the demented from their homes, but in practice all homes for the elderly have demented residents, diagnosed or undiagnosed; careful examination of the populations of some homes (p. 31) have shown that the proportion of such patients can be alarmingly high. In general, Part 3 homes will not exclude applicants suffering from a degree of confusion; people considered unsuitable are generally those with problematic behavioural symptoms of dementia or severe incontinence; one local authority, for example, excludes 'elderly persons who, following assessment and treatment, remain hostile and aggressive to a degree beyond that which could be tolerated by other residents' or who 'remain uncontrollably doubly incontinent'. A tendency to wander may also exclude an elderly person although, as pointed out earlier (p. 163), the fault is often in the design and location of the home.

Many of the other problems are remediable and, although specialist medical assessment of prospective residents has been recommended (DHSS and Welsh Office 1977), this almost never takes place. The Division of Old Age Psychiatry of the Royal College of Psychiatrists has taken up this issue and also recommends strongly that all residents be fully assessed, either before or shortly after admission, by a doctor with special experience in geriatric medicine or the psychiatry of old age. Their 1985 document sets out detailed guidelines for assessment and urges that specialists in the elderly institute discussions with their social services colleagues at local level as to how these medical examinations can be instituted and how good collaboration can be maintained.

The doctor, it should be added, must ensure that a person entering a Part 3 home will not actually receive a lesser degree of care than he would at home. It is an unfortunate irony that, for example, the nursing (and incontinence) services available to people at home are not necessarily provided in residential care, so the patient not uncommonly deteriorates and in due course enters hospital. Given that there are increasing numbers of ill and confused people in local authority homes, the solution is of course to build adequate supporting services into the system. But the question arises — and has been much debated — whether specialized homes should provide for the confused or whether such a policy of 'segregation' is undesirable. Meacher (1972) strongly advocates that the elderly mentally infirm be accommodated in the same homes as mentally intact people; this policy is, however, impractical. The demented and frail require expert medical and nursing care and, unhappily, expertise in the area (and the necessary finance) does not exist in such abundance that it can be distributed among the 12 or more homes (in the public sector alone) which may exist in a typical health district. The non-segregationist viewpoint appears on the surface good and humanitarian, but in practice failure to provide specialist residential care results in the demented being 'segregated' in mental hospitals. Yet many of the demented now in such institutions could be accommodated either in specialist and properly staffed local authority homes or in NHS nursing homes for the elderly mentally ill. There are probably at present no examples of the former type of provision, and planning for NHS nursing homes for the elderly commenced in the UK only in 1984; however, as the mental hospitals close, they will almost certainly represent one of the types of care for the future.

Admission to a Part 3 home is arranged on the application of a social worker and with the agreement of the matron of the home. But it should be borne in mind that a local authority home is not the only or even the least expensive option, and there is a strict means test which takes all disposable property into consideration; therefore the doctor or the patient's relatives are well advised to 'shop around'. Social workers will on occasion fail to co-operate, for ideological reason, in the move to a home in the 'private sector', with the deplorable result that the patient remains in a mental hospital, but all social services area offices are obliged to keep a list of such homes in their area, and advice can also be obtained from Counsel and Care for the Elderly (p. 207).

Grants from the DHSS may be available in order to enable people of insufficient means to live in private residential or nursing homes (see also below).

Nursing homes

These are for people who are mentally or physically infirm; some are specifically for the demented, while others will accept those who are less severely demented but who have physical problems (e.g. incontinence or poor mobility) which would disqualify them for a Part 3 or other residential home. The great variety of types of nursing home — almost all owned by private organizations or charities — makes detailed description impossible; it can simply be said that a doctor dealing with the elderly should make himself familiar with what is offered by such homes in his own area. Proper utilization of these services can make for a huge reduction in unnecessary bed occupation and in the length of waiting-lists for admission (Fraser and Healy, 1986).

Nursing home care is, however, expensive. The current DHSS grants are higher than those for people in residential homes, but they probably never meet the full amount. So some 'topping-up' is required, and at present it appears that local authorities are not permitted to provide these additional amounts, although funding arrangements are constantly being altered and vary from one area to another. NHS nursing homes for the elderly physically and mentally infirm are badly needed.

Information about nursing homes in a given area is available, again, from a local social services office or from Care and Counsel for the Elderly.

Adult fostering

Adult fostering schemes are available in an increasing number of areas, and they can sometimes prove ideal for elderly confused people; single women, married couples or families can provide domestic-style support for elderly people who might otherwise be in old people's homes or dementia wards. Such schemes are managed and supervised by the social services.

HOSPITAL SERVICES

The District General Hospital (DGH)

It is by way of the casualty department, the outpatient department or the wards of the DGH that many (perhaps most) of the demented make their first contact with the psychogeriatrician, and it is also in these settings that their dementia is often first diagnosed. It is also in the wards of the DGH that we discover one of the most problematic elements of dementia — 'bed-blocking' by the elderly confused with a build-up of waiting-lists (the bane of psychogeriatric practice) and loss of beds to the acute services.

Liaison psychiatry (broadly, the management of psychiatric illness in patients occupying general hospital beds) has been an influential element in psychiatry for over a decade now, but the need to apply liaison principles specifically to the elderly has only recently been emphasized (Junod, 1981; Bassuk *et al.*, 1983; Lipowski, 1983). One such liaison scheme has been evaluated by Fraser and Healy (1986); the patients were 100 consecutive new referrals to a psychogeriatric service from the acute wards of an inner city teaching hospital. A doctor from the psychogeriatric team was assigned specifically to elderly patients in the acute beds, the principal aim being where possible to assist the ward staff with the treatment and discharge of the patient without any intervening transfer; the doctor also had a special brief to become familiar with services for the demented in the local community. Patients were transferred to psychiatric beds only if their period of physical treatment had come to an end and there was no alternative placement or if they had become, for some reason, unmanageable in the acute ward.

Fifty-seven of the patients suffered from some degree of dementia (43 were clinically AD, 10 were MID and 4 were alcoholic dementia).

The liaison project, besides bringing other benefits, was successful in virtually eliminating bed-blocking in the DGH; by the end of the study period there were no patients awaiting transfer from the acute wards, and the mean waiting time for transfer had been reduced from eight to two weeks. There were no patients in the community awaiting transfer either at the beginning or at the end of the study. These figures can be set against those from an adjacent health district where there was no psychiatric service to the DGH; here there was a waiting-list of 45 patients. Fourteen of these were occupying acute beds; the average time that the inpatients had spent on the waiting-list was two and a half years.

The days of such unacceptably long waiting-lists will be over only when adequate district-based psychogeriatric services are established and when the demented in acute wards are assessed and treated in co-operation with the general physicians or geriatricians. The DGH provides, and will continue to provide, a substantial service for local patients with dementia, especially as many demented patients are physically ill with a high potential mortality (our study showed 22 per cent within six months) and, as the dementing population ages, its numbers will inevitably include a greater proportion of the physically ill and frail. Therefore the mental hospital, the traditional setting for the care of the demented, will become even less appropriate than at present, since these hospitals are in general inconveniently sited and do not have the staff or facilities to manage a patient population which is very dependent physically. Liaison and shared care schemes in district general hospitals are two of the necessary new models.

The psychogeriatric assessment unit

In 1970 the DHSS gave specific encouragement for the development of assessment units within geriatric departments for which geriatricians and psychiatrists would have joint responsibility. It was proposed that approximately 15 beds would be provided for a total population of 250,000. Only a comparatively few such units have been established, but there have been several other and smaller collaborative projects between geriatricians and psychiatrists (Royal College of Physicians, 1981). At present about 20 services have joint assessment units, but several more are in the planning stage (Wattis *et al.*, 1981). Subsequent reports and documents have also recommended the provision of joint units (DHSS, 1975; DHSS and Welsh Office, 1978; Royal College of Physicians, 1981; Health Advisory Service, 1982) although with a shifting emphasis, now more on joint *management* as distinct simply from 'assessment'. Copeland *et al.* (1975) studied 160 patients entering geriatric and psychiatric units and concluded that the usefulness of joint assessment units in avoiding misplacement was dubious. There might indeed be positive disadvantages to an elderly patient who was admitted to one ward and transferred later to another. There would be a break in nursing care; also, availability of assessment beds might encourage inadequate preadmission assessment.

  The Rising Tide (Health Advisory Service, 1982) examines a number of models of co-operation between geriatric and psychiatric departments, and finds potential virtues in all of them. But some form of co-operation there must be, and it is likely that the ill elderly who are treated in a setting where specialist resources have not been pooled will lose out in one respect or another. And it is also likely that joint assessment units will turn out to provide much less than expected if they are to be the only setting for co-operation between geriatrician and psychiatrist; the provision of such units will probably turn out to be no more than a stage in the development of a fully integrated service for the elderly. With the increasing life-span of both the demented and the non-demented, the distinction between 'psychogeriatric' and 'geriatric' will become increasingly blurred; already the 1975 DHSS recommendation that a patient can be assigned to one service or another after four weeks' assessment looks unrealistic. Following discharge, a patient will of course have to become the responsibility of one consultant, but Arie (1983) aptly points to the episodic nature of psychogeriatric care; periods of treatment are episodes in a continuum of care, and a patient is often a 'geriatric' case on one admission and a 'psychiatric' case on the next.

In our own unit we have extended joint management to a small number of patients who need continuing hospital care. These are generally the demented who suffer from immobility or other chronic physical handicaps or illness; there is a distinct need for a few beds of this type, and the need will become more prominent, so it is likely that this model of care will also come to represent part of an adequate service for the demented.

The psychogeriatric day hospital

An earlier section dealt with day centres. A day hospital is different in two fundamental respects: first, it is administered by a health authority and, second, most patients are attending for courses of treatment that will last for a finite period — as distinct from the more open-ended arrangement that is usual at a day centre. However, some day hospitals accept elderly patients on a long-term basis and, in practice, about half of the patients at a psychogeriatric day hospital are likely to be demented in some degree (Hassall *et al.*, 1972) although the proportion varies enormously (Reichenfeld, 1983; Gilleard, 1984) and the discharge rates for this group are very low (Arie, 1979).

It is recommended (Health Advisory Service, 1982) that every psychogeriatric service should provide day hospital places in a proportion of two or three per 1000 population aged 65 and over. But provision is very uneven. In 1981 one-quarter of psychogeriatric services had no day hospital and the average number of day places per 1000 elderly was less than one (Wattis *et al.*, 1981). Psychogeriatric day hospitals are still being evaluated, however, and it is not certain whether such a provision can be regarded as an essential part of medical care for the demented. It depends very much on what services already exist, and to what extent they can be utilized; for example, collaboration by a psychogeriatrician in the running of a local authority day centre for the elderly confused (p. 183) may be preferable to the setting up of a separate establishment. This arrangement has proved highly effective in one area (Camden); also, the confused who require physical management can be treated in a geriatric day hospital, in co-operation with the geriatric service. But such arrangements are not always possible, so specialist psychogeriatric day care may have to be provided. Whatever the precise arrangements, it is generally taken as indisputable that day care in an attentive and stimulating environment will (a) enable monitoring and treatment of the patient's psychiatric and physical needs, (b) provide an alternative to social isolation or hospital admission, and (c) support carers who are able to manage a patient at home provided that he is looked after for some part of the day; carers may also be offered some form of group support.

But there are limits to day care; the daily task, for example, of helping a confused patient to dress, prepare for transport and (perhaps reluctantly) enter an ambulance, may turn out to be more taxing than were the original problems. It has been suggested, in fact, that day care for the demented does not provide an alternative to hospital care for more than a small proportion of patients; for most it represents an enrichment of the supporting services that already exist. Where some patients are concerned, day care does either delay the need for hospital care or shorten its duration (Greene and Timbury, 1979; Jones and Munbodh, 1982) but these benefits, where measurable, have appeared disappointingly modest. On the other hand, the value of a day hospital cannot altogether be measured. Gilleard *et al.* (1984b) have examined the question: 'How much difference does a day hospital make?' and conclude that such questions are unanswerable, since no agreed criterion of success exists. The group assessed the impact of day hospital care on the demented patient's family and found that day care was generally seen as helpful and positive — although for the majority of patients the outcome was a stay of six months or less followed by hospital admission. The benefits were likely to be maximal where the carer anticipated advantages from attendance and foresaw few problems of adjustment and acceptance by the demented person. The corollary is, unhappily, that an offer of day care is unlikely to be helpful where the attitude of carers is negative at the outset; it represents largely a means through which existing goodwill may be expressed, not a means of bringing about any radical changes. Thus Gilleard *et al.* rightly emphasize that workable decisions can be made only where there is co-operative decision-making between professional and family carers.

Continuing inpatient care

Most aspects of long-term hospital care for the severely demented have been examined in earlier sections. The most common style is still the 'dementia ward' of the mental hospital and, although there may be many disadvantages in terms of location and staffing, it is generally possible to transform such wards into attractive and humane places for confused old people (p. 163) and at least some are likely to remain in existence for many years to come. But they should be supplanted as soon as possible by the second and third styles of continuing care.

The second style is that of joint management by psychiatrist and geriatrician (p. 188), and is primarily for the demented who are, in addition, severely physically ill or infirm.

The third style, not yet established within the NHS, is that of the nursing home for the severely demented (but who are not, generally, severely physically ill on admission). Such homes will probably open within the next few years, as the mental hospitals close. A group in one health district (Bloomsbury), planning for the closure of two mental hospitals, is seeking to provide nursing homes on principles that include the following:

(a) The homes will be for residents with a diagnosis of senile dementia who have lived locally and who are unsuitable, because of the degree of their dementia, for accommodation in a social services facility and who cannot adequately be supported in their own environment by domiciliary services.

(b) Each will be of domestic scale, with possibly 20 residents.

(c) They will provide permanent homes for people who will not be moved if their condition deteriorates, unless a serious medical condition dictates a stay in hospital.

(d) The environment should offer personal privacy to the residents, with sufficient space to receive family and friends in private if desired.

(e) Each resident will have their own clothes that are appropriate to their age, and in line with their tastes and expectations of friends and peers.

(f) The residents will have access to skilled professional help, including help with everyday skills such as eating and dressing.

(g) Where possible, family and friends will be encouraged to take part in activities with the resident.

(h) Wherever possible, residents will be involved in choices about themselves and their environment; otherwise, someone who knows them well should act on their behalf.

(i) The environment will be as safe as possible, without being restrictive; each home will, for example, have an exclosed garden.

Such homes will best be sited in close proximity to a DGH, so that expert medical and paramedical care is readily available. The main risk that could follow from these slightly idealistic guidelines would be of demented patients finding themselves housed in a number of scattered units, each not having quite the necessary amount of expertise available to it. With careful selection of a site and in order to ensure the best use of local services for the elderly, the average health district would probably be best served by two such nursing homes, each with approximately 20 places.

Finally, the demented must not gravitate to long-term hospital (or nursing home) care by default, but only following a positive decision that a particular ward or other setting is the one in which an individual can best be cared for. How can one ensure this? One unit (in St Pancras Hospital) has established a 'continuing care panel' made up of a consultant, a senior social worker and a senior nurse. The patient is presented to the panel by the senior registrar who has been responsible for his care in the acute ward, and who makes out a 'case' for continuing care based on needs which could not be met in any other way. The patient is then either accepted for continuing care or 'referred back' on the grounds, for example, that the patient could be managed adequately by means of domiciliary services. This system has led to greatly improved utilization of continuing care beds and has thus cut back sharply on waiting time for transfer of patients who genuinely need such beds.

MINIMUM REQUIREMENTS FOR A SERVICE TO THE DEMENTED

These are derived from the Report of the Royal College of Physicians on Organic Mental Impairment in the Elderly (1981) and the Health Advisory Service report, *The Rising Tide* (1982). They are for a health district with a total population of 200,000 and a population aged 65 and over of 30,000. As the service will almost inevitably include patients with functional illness, the figures for this group are given as well.

(a) Functional illness:
  (i) 15 acute beds
  (ii) 5 new long-stay beds
  (iii) 20 day places
(b) Dementia:
  (i) psychogeriatric unit: 30 beds
  (ii) psychogeriatric long-stay: 75–90 beds
  (iii) day places: 90
(c) Consultant time:
  15 sessions
(d) Non-consultant medical staff:
  (i) trainees: 25 per cent share of total in psychiatry
  (ii) senior registrars: 25 per cent share of total in psychiatry
  (iii) clinical assistants according to availability and deployment
(e) Secretarial staff:
  1.5–3 secretaries, with additional secretarial time for a day hospital
(f) Community psychiatric nurses for the elderly:
  2–6 CPNs
(g) Social workers for the elderly:
  1.5–3 hospital based

These figures represent bare minima and are extremely modest. In addition, the service should have available the expertise of occupational therapists, physiotherapists and a psychologist; these would probably be shared with either the geriatric or the general psychiatry service.

SUMMARY

An essential element in the management of dementia is the supporting structure we can provide in order to allow the demented to maintain a satisfactory quality of life either at home or in some acceptable form of residential care; sometimes this is the only form of treatment we can offer. The effectiveness of such supports depends heavily on their timely provision; unfortunately, there is a low level of diagnosis and awareness of dementia; the condition is commonly undetected until it has reached an advanced stage, at which time the patient is likely either to be permanently rejected by his carers because of behavioural problems or to have developed serious physical complications. In both cases, hospitalization is usually necessary, and it is often permanent.

Contacts between an elderly person and his GP or other member of the primary care team should include some form of screening for memory impairment; there are a number of suitable brief tests. Although most demented people will benefit from assessment by a specialist team, the primary care team is best placed to provide and co-ordinate the community care 'package' in the longer term. Some staff, however, may be effectively shared by both teams.

The domiciliary care of the demented fails because of poor utilization of existing services as often as it does because the services themselves are poor.

Relatively simple provisions (of which the patient or carer is frequently unaware) may make not only for the avoidance of hospitalization but also for an unexpected degree of improvement in the patient's quality of life; many of the services available to old people at home have been described.

There is a wide spectrum of residential care establishments for the elderly, in theory reflecting the range of handicap among the demented, from sheltered housing schemes to nursing homes. But the biggest single group of elderly in residential care is in local authority homes, and in these there are many demented people whose needs are not fully recognized and the access of such homes to nursing and specialist services is poor. Although 'segregation' of the demented in homes that offer a relatively high degree of support is an unpopular option, it is in practice the best way to utilize scarce resources and to avoid permanent hospitalization.

The district general hospital fills a central role in the diagnosis and management of the demented; it is commonly the first point of contact between a demented person and a specialist psychiatrist. Liaison with the acute services here will prevent the accumulation of 'bed-blockers' and the appearance of waiting lists.

Adequate treatment of demented patients also requires ready access to a geriatric service. In many health districts there are joint assessment units, but, with the increasing age and frailty of the demented population, these are inadequate as the sole point of co-operation between the psychiatrist and geriatrician; joint management is increasingly necessary, and some patients will need joint continuing care. A well-designed selection process can ensure that patients are placed in continuing care wards not by default but only if these are the settings where their needs will be most adequately met.

The mental hospital is unlikely to be the future setting for the continuing care of most demented patients — who should be considered separately from other groups of patients for whom mental hospitals may still be appropriate. The severely demented will often best be managed in appropriately staffed nursing homes sited in close proximity to the acute services.

CHAPTER 9
Legal aspects of dementia

Patients with a diagnosis of dementia are, by definition, in some degree suffering from impaired ability to make major decisions, for example about their medical treatment, their living circumstances or the management of their finances. Others have to make these decisions on their behalf, but who? In the event, any doctor who deals with demented people has to participate willy-nilly in such decisions, and there are only a few clear guidelines; psychogeriatrics, as a young subspecialty, has not altogether got to grips with, say, the status of 'informal' demented patients in locked wards, the question of consent to treatment or the matter of who is ultimately to be responsible for the finances of a demented patient. There are a number of legal instruments, but they do not cover all or even most sets of circumstances, and this includes the 1983 Mental Health Act; the existence of the demented elderly is only now being acknowledged in discussion documents. Some statutory help and guidance is available in the area of patients' finances, although the use of such provisions as the Court of Protection and the much more restricted power of attorney tends to be poorly understood. The present chapter will indicate the ways in which the best use is made of these and will also set out some principles that may help with management in the deeply clouded areas which, in one way or another, concern the rights of a demented person. Does Mrs Jones have the 'right' to remain at home in a state of squalor and self-neglect, refusing hospitalization, residential care and domiciliary services — or does she have the 'right' to the best possible treatment in a psychogeriatric ward, whether she wants it or not? Again, who decides?

Legal or quasi-legal decisions about patients fall into two general categories — first, those that specifically concern treatment (including hospitalization), and then those that have to do with a demented person's affairs and property. They are best considered separately.

ADMISSION AND TREATMENT

Most demented people agree to receive treatment and, if necessary, to be

194

admitted to hospital. Whether or not a demented patient is capable of giving 'informed' consent is a question which is rarely raised — fortunately, since, if it were, very little psychogeriatrics would be practised! Where routine procedures are concerned, stated or implied consent by a demented patient is normally taken as valid. In the event of any challenge the defence would usually be that of clinical necessity. A discussion paper published by the Mental Health Act Commission (1985a) deals with the matter of consent by informal incapable patients and the conclusion is that no radical change in practice is necessary. Where such a patient's attitude to treatment is 'neutral', treatment may be given, although good practice requires two safeguards. First, the doctor should discuss the proposed treatment with relatives or close friends of the patient and should evaluate their views and also attempt to find out what the patient's former attitudes to the proposed treatment would have been. Second, he should 'give due weight to the observations and opinions of other persons, of any discipline, who are involved in the medical treatment. But the ultimate responsibility will nevertheless remain his'.

These recommendations refer to what one might call 'routine' treatments; treatments such as ECT are subject to separate provisions (p. 197). They are not legally binding, and simply formalise what is done in most cases anyway. In practice, the difficulty is rarely with the patient who consents to treatment or who is neutral about it, but is, of course, much more commonly with the patient who refuses treatment.

Case No. 13
Mrs M is 84; she has been widowed for 20 years and is moderately demented. She rarely leaves the house, spending most of the day and night in an armchair; she does not go to bed and rarely washes or changes her clothes. She is abusive to the home help and district nurse; she eats her meals on wheels intermittently, she does not pay her gas bills and she is, from time to time, disconnected. At other times she leaves the gas on. She is incontinent, and various odours permeate the block of flats. But she refuses to go into hospital or (even more vehemently) any kind of 'home'. Something, say her neighbours, must be done (a familiar greeting to any psychogeriatrician).

Case No. 14
Or there is Mrs N, who patrols her block of flats nightly, tapping on doors and ringing bells, asking the same questions over and over, asking the way, sometimes wandering into the street in her nightclothes. It is a disgrace, the doctor is told by neighbours and relatives, that 'they' won't do anything. Why can't they 'put her somewhere'(But Mrs N is moderately fit and well nourished; her flat is warm and fairly comfortable, and she professes herself quite happy to potter around as she is doing; she does not want to leave her home.)

Situations like these can involve the interests of a considerable number of people; it is a useful rule in such circumstances for the doctor, faced with conflicting demands, to remind himself of just who his patient is. As in other parallel circumstances (where the patient is very young, for example), *the doctor is not the agent of any third party*; he is not engaged to carry out the wishes of the next of kin (or the neighbours, or anyone else) but to act in the best interests of the patient. Naturally he will do his best to be helpful to relatives and neighbours, but a demented person cannot be removed compulsorily from his home simply because he lives in circumstances that are less than ideal or because other people are being inconvenienced. A decision to admit compulsorily will, as with other patients, be taken on the grounds of risk — either that the patient himself is likely to deteriorate (usually as the result of physical illness or self-neglect) or that the health and safety of other people are being endangered, because the patient represents a fire hazard, to take one example. The decision will naturally depend on information and opinions from a number of other people; where a patient appears to be at risk because of refusal to accept necessary treatment (and 'treatment' here can be taken to include the full range of domiciliary services), then it is often best to call a case conference; normally the specialist, the GP, the social worker and the patient's next of kin would attend; the patient, if capable of expressing his views, should also have the opportunity of doing so. Neighbours or others who have views about the patient might also be invited, but the rules of confidentiality need to be observed; it is too often the case that a person's medical details come to be treated as public property just because he is elderly and demented.

The purpose of a case conference is to allow the fairly speedy exchange of information and, if the patient is not to be admitted to hospital, to make a clear allocation of tasks for the patient's care and supervision at home. What is important is that a named person (perhaps a geriatric visitor) should be responsible for visiting the patient at regular intervals and for informing the GP or consultant of any change in his condition.

If a patient is to be admitted compulsorily, three Acts apply — the Mental Health Act 1983, the National Assistance Act 1948 and the National Assistance (Amendment) Act 1951.

The Mental Health Act 1983

The provisions of the Act will not be described in detail; the reader is referred to the Act itself, to the DHSS memorandum of 1983 and to Bluglass (1983). It can be said only that in most cases where demented patients are admitted compulsorily to hospital, section 2 of the Act will be employed. The application for admission is made by the next of kin or an approved social worker and supported by the written recommendations of two doctors (usually the GP and the specialist) on the grounds that the patient is suffering from mental disorder of a nature or degree which warrants his detention in hospital for assessment (or assessment followed by medical treatment) for at least a limited period, and that he ought to be so detained in the interests of his own health or safety or with a view to the protection of other persons.

The patient may be detained in hospital for 28 days. The Act supersedes the 'admission for observation' of the 1959 Act; 'assessment' implies more active intervention in order to form a diagnosis and to plan treatment (DHSS, 1983; McFarlane, 1983). Treatment following admission is still, however, subject to consent (Bluglass, 1983), except as a matter of urgent necessity (Mental Health Act 1983, section 62). Otherwise treatment without consent requires that the patient be detained under section 3 of the Act, and there are additional requirements for certain specified treatments such as ECT (section 58). But in practice the objection of a confused elderly person is usually to hospitalization rather than to treatment, and the need for detention under section 3 very rarely arises. In cases of doubt, the doctor should seek advice either from the Mental Health Act Commission (p. 209) or from his defence society.

The National Assistance Act 1948

This is the same Act under which 'Part 3 accommodation' was established (p. 184). Section 47 of the Act gave the medical officer of health the power to apply to a magistrate for the compulsory removal to hospital or other suitable place of persons who:

(a) are suffering from grave chronic disease or, being aged, infirm or physically handicapped, are living in insanitary conditions and

(b) are unable to devote to themselves, and are not receiving from other persons, proper care and attention.

The medical officer was required to certify that removal was necessary 'in the interests of any such person . . . or for preventing injury to the health of, or serious nuisance to, other persons'. The patient could be detained for up to three months.

The 1948 Act, however, required that the MOH give seven days' notice to a court of summary jurisdiction before removal could be authorized. In 1951, amending legislation was introduced by Dr Alfred Broughton MP, who had been dismayed by the plight of an elderly woman in his constituency (Gray, 1980). She had fallen, refused to go to hospital, and had lain on the floor for the statutory seven days. During this time she developed a pressure sore, contracted tetanus in the sore and died shortly after admission. A Private Member's Bill was passed without difficulty and became the National Assistance (Amendment) Act 1951. The 1948 grounds for removal still stand but the amendment allows for compulsory removal to be effected immediately if necessary in the interests of the patient, provided that the opinion of the MOH (now the community physician) is supported by that of another registered practitioner; the period of detention in such a case is only three weeks.

The main practical difference between the Mental Health Act and the National Assistance Act is, therefore, that the latter allows compulsory removal on the grounds of physical illness, health hazard or serious nuisance. Placement is usually in a general or geriatric hospital, but sometimes in an old people's home. However, the latter is dependent on the local authority's agreeing to accept the patient, and some local authorities will not accept section 47 patients as a matter of policy. Indeed, it is very questionable whether a person who is suffering serious illness or self-neglect should be admitted anywhere but to a hospital.

Section 47 is of limited usefulness, poorly understood and now infrequently used (Gray, 1980; Norman, 1980). An example of its use was in Case No. 5 (p. 97), where a confused diabetic patient was admitted to a general hospital, but the Mental Health Act could equally well have been employed; the latter Act does not specify that a patient be admitted to a psychiatric ward, and confused elderly people are often best treated initially in a general or geriatric ward or, ideally, in a joint psychogeriatric unit. As we are dealing here specifically with the demented, it generally follows that the patient's inability to care for himself is the result of mental illness, so the Mental Health Act would serve in most cases to secure admission. If there is any doubt the patient should be referred to the local community physician, but section 47 now tends to be employed only with great reluctance and in the direst of circumstances.

The demented patient in hospital

Case No. 15
Mr O has been admitted 'voluntarily' for assessment; he is probably suffering from dementia of moderate degree and he is disorientated, noisy and restless. His relatives have departed and he insists on leaving the ward and going home, even though he does not know his address. He is banging on the (locked) doors and rattling the handles. As a voluntary patient, does he have the right to leave?

Case No. 16
Mrs P is severely demented and has been in a continuing care ward for several years. She has never expressed a wish to come into hospital, although she appears contented. But she is moderately fit physically and, if the doors were unlocked, she would certainly wander out and would not find her way back. She, also, is a 'voluntary' patient.

The case of Mrs P is common (indeed, almost the rule on long-stay wards), while that of Mr O is rare. But many demented patients attempt or ask to leave the ward; can they legally be prevented? As matters stand, it is all a question of degree. When a patient is making repeated and single-minded attempts to leave the ward, where it is unsafe for him to do so, and where he cannot be persuaded to stay, then The Mental Health Act will certainly apply. The family, of course, must be consulted and ideally a member of the family (as distinct from a social worker) should make the application; this can represent an important act of participation in the patient's management and can lead to a very worthwhile sense of joint responsibility.

The case of Mrs P is much less simple. There was an old convention that certain patients with a failure of autonomy due to illness or handicap but who did not 'refuse to go into hospital or be taken there by relatives or friends' (Speller, 1971) could be placed in a 'not unwilling' category and regarded more or less as informal. But Gostin (1975) has written that 'the patient is not making an informed consent to admission if he does not fully understand his informal status'. And 'not unwilling' has no standing in law; patients are either formal or informal and there is no intermediate status. Thus the position of informal demented patients in locked wards remains deeply uncertain. The Mental Health Act Commission (1985b) has briefly considered such 'de facto' detention; it is considered that it can at present be justified under common law (i.e. on the grounds of necessity), but it is possible that in due course some form of guardianship will be proposed. However, the question is not in the end to be resolved by devising yet more legislation and yet more styles of compulsion, but by designing environments where locked doors are generally unnecessary (as outlined on p. 163) and which are acceptable to the patient and to his family. The clinician should ask himself whether it is the unacceptability of the hospital environment that is determining compulsion in any case; it often is.

But the locked dementia ward will unhappily be with us for some time to come. The best advice I have been given is that, since the doctor is caring for a patient on behalf of his next of kin, his responsibility is therefore to care for the patient in all respects as would a wise relative. Therefore, for example, a door would not be left open if the patient were placed at risk as a result, or the patient could be restrained from behaving in a way that would cause injury to himself or anyone else; such restrictions could again be justified under common law. The present situation is far from ideal, but the 'wise relative' principle is one that can be commended until we have greatly improved the general circumstances in which we treat demented patients.

PATIENTS' PROPERTY AND AFFAIRS

The great majority of demented people are helped informally with their affairs by their relatives; both the patient's capacity to give consent and the relatives' good faith are generally assumed unless there is evidence to the contrary. Where there is no next of kin, the affairs of a demented person can be managed by an officer appointed by the Director of Social Services or, if the patient is in hospital, by the hospital's patients' affairs department. In more complex circumstances — usually where there is severe incapacity or large sums of money are involved — there are three legal instruments that may be used to safeguard property, although the value of one of them is very restricted.

Powers of Attorney

A power of attorney is a form of agency, and its general principles lie in common law; the Powers of Attorney Act 1971 has defined the form and effect of powers of attorney. Fundamental to them is the agency principle that an act by a person's agent is in general to be treated as one by the person himself (Law Commission, 1983). A power of attorney is thus a formal arrangement whereby one person gives another authority to act on his behalf and in his name. Generally speaking, anyone who is capable of entering into a valid contract can be the attorney. The document, a form of which is appended to the 1971 Act, is drawn up by a solicitor and signed by the donor, dated and witnessed. The attorney is commonly a near relative, but may also be a friend, a solicitor or a bank; in fact, there are very few exclusions. The power of attorney may, however, be limited in specific ways, and there are certain functions that cannot be delegated, such as the execution of a will and consent to treatment (McFarlane, 1983).

The principal (i.e. the donor of the power of attorney) must be capable of understanding the nature and effect of the contract at the time that he makes it; furthermore, loss of mental capacity by the donor has the effect of automatically revoking the power of attorney, which then becomes void. So it will be seen that the power is inoperative in the very circumstances against which it is commonly created. Therefore, while it is conceivable that a mildly demented person could be capable of granting a power of attorney, it is of course the case that dementia is progressive; so a relative of a demented person should be advised to take advantage of new legislation and seek an 'enduring' power of attorney.

Enduring powers of attorney

In a working paper of 1976 and a subsequent report, *The Incapacitated Principal* (1983), the Law Commission recommended that, since the existing law was unsatisfactory, a person of sound mind should be permitted to grant a power of attorney which would survive his subsequent mental incapacity. This would be termed an 'enduring power of attorney'. A Bill was presented, but became law only in 1986; the main difficulty was the building in of adequate safeguards. Under the Enduring Powers of Attorney Act 1985 a donor can now appoint someone who will continue to manage his affairs (within limits that he may specify) should he subsequently become mentally incapable. He must, of course, be capable at the time of granting the power. The agreement does not require a solicitor and the 'prescribed form' is set out in the Act; however, legal assistance is highly advisable, since some of the regulations are complex.

An existing power of attorney cannot, incidentally, be converted into an enduring power because the two take completely different forms.

If the person granted the enduring power of attorney believes that the donor is becoming mentally incapable, he must apply to the Court of Protection (see below) to have the power of attorney registered; he is also required at the same time to notify the donor and the donor's close relatives of his application so that, if they wish to, they can lodge objections. Any dispute will be settled by the Court of Protection. After registration, the attorney will have wide powers to manage the donor's financial affairs, and the donor cannot then revoke them without the court's confirmation. It is envisaged that the enduring power of attorney will to some extent replace receivership under the Court of Protection, which takes longer to arrange and is relatively expensive.

The Court of Protection

The Court of Protection is an office of the Lord Chancellor's Department and is responsible for managing the property and affairs of those who are incapable of managing them for themselves; this is usually done by appointing a receiver. The majority of those whose affairs are being managed by the court are elderly people suffering from dementia; at present the affairs of about 20,000 people are in the court's hands, and about 5000 new cases come under its jurisdiction every year (Royal College of Psychiatrists, 1985b).

The procedure is that a person who wishes to take charge of the affairs of someone who is demented (usually a relative) seeks a receivership from the court on his behalf. He may approach the court either directly through its Personal Application Branch (see Appendix) or through a solicitor. Where possible, the court will appoint either a relative or a close friend as receiver and will give preference to a person holding a power of attorney. Otherwise the court may appoint as receiver the Principal of the Management Division, or another suitably qualified person, such as a solicitor, accountant, or Director of Social Services.

The court's jurisdiction extends only to those who are incapable of managing their affairs because of mental disorder; medical evidence is therefore necessary before the court can act, except in an emergency — in which case the court may make an interim order. Medical evidence is given by means of completing form CP3. The certifying doctor may be either the person's general practitioner or any other registered medical practitioner who has examined the patient. Helpful notes on completion now accompany the form; more detailed guidance is provided by MacFarlane (1985).

The receiver must submit detailed accounts to the court annually; the patient may also be visited by a Lord Chancellor's Visitor. There are various categories of 'visitor' and fairly detailed provisions. A 'medical visitor' may visit patients about whom there is insufficient or conflicting evidence in the initial application or where testamentary capacity is in doubt. The court also has the power to make a will on a patient's behalf, if necessary. However, although a patient's affairs may be in the hands of the Court of Protection, he may still be of testamentary capacity (see below). If a doctor is satisfied that the patient has testamentary capacity, he will certify this to the court, who will authorize the preparation of a will by the solicitors concerned. The doctor who found the patient capable will be asked to act as one of the witnesses to the will. But if he is in doubt, he is advised to refuse to give an opinion in favour of capacity (MacFarlane, 1985), in which case a Lord Chancellor's medical visitor will examine the patient and report. If testamentary capacity cannot be established, the court may make a 'statutory' will for the patient, following a hearing at which interested parties may attend or be represented.

On some occasions a patient may apply to come out of the court's care; this is an application for an order 'determining' the proceedings of the court. A doctor is then required to certify that the patient is again capable of managing his affairs; in cases of doubt, a further opinion must again be sought from a medical officer. As most patients under the court's jurisdiction are suffering from organic brain damage, orders to determine proceedings are in practice very seldom sought.

A working party of the Royal College of Psychiatrists reviewed the working of the Court of Protection and published a report in 1985. Among its recommendations are:

(a) There should be two medical certificates in support of an application for the appointment of a receiver, including one from a medical practitioner appointed under section 12 of the Mental Health Act 1983 (i.e. a doctor recognized 'as having special experience in the diagnosis or treatment of mental disorder').

(b) The certificates should be scrutinized by the Lord Chancellor's medical visitors.

(c) The first visit to a patient after the appointment of a receiver should be carried out by the medical visitor, except for patients in NHS hospitals or local authority accommodation.

(d) The court should review the necessity for the continuation of a receivership after an initial period of two years on the basis of a certificate provided by the patient's medical practitioner and subject to scrutiny by the Lord Chancellor's medical visitors.

The requirements for medical certification and also for review would therefore be much more stringent, and more in line with those of the Mental Health Act; there is at present much too great a disparity between the rules that safeguard a patient against a limited period of loss of liberty and those that safeguard him against permanent loss of control of all his finances and possessions.

Testamentary capacity

In law, for a person to be capable of making a valid will he must be in possession of 'a sound disposing mind' at the time he executes the will (Sanders, 1984). Evidence regarding testamentary capacity is usually given by a medical witness, but it may come from any source. In the event of any dispute, a court will often, for example, call evidence from independent witnesses who have observed the patient's behaviour around the time that the will was made. For a person to be of sound disposing mind the following conditions have to be satisfied (Rentoul and Smith, 1973; Sanders, 1984):

(a) The testator should know what a will is.

(b) He should have a reasonable idea of the amount of money and property at his disposal.

(c) He should know to what persons he would reasonably be expected to leave his possessions, and the claims of each. The law recognizes 'moral' claims as well as the claims of close kinship. The claim, for example, of a friend or distant relative with whom the patient has lived in his last years could possibly outweigh that of a son or daughter who has visited him infrequently.

(d) His mind should be free of any delusions or obsessions which would pervert his judgement in disposing of his property. The presence of, say, paranoid ideas would not in itself invalidate a will, but the patient should be free of any disorder 'which would influence his mind in disposing of his property in such a way as would not have been done if his mind had been sound' (*Banks* v *Goodfellow*, 1870).

(e) He should not, in the making of his will, have been subject to undue influence. This is defined as persuasion brought to bear on a testator who is, usually because of physical or mental illness, too weak to resist, with the result that the will is no longer 'the offspring of his own volition' (Sanders, 1984).

When the doctor has been satisfied on the above points, the will is read to the testator, signed or marked by the testator, and then signed by two witnesses in the presence of each other and of the testator; the doctor may or may not be one of the witnesses. But it should be remembered that if a doctor witnesses the will of a person who is not his patient (a friend or neighbour, for example) he equally has a duty to satisfy himself as to testamentary capacity; in the event of any subsequent legal proceedings, he would certainly be called as a witness.

A diagnosis of dementia does not necessarily mean that a person is not of testamentary capacity. But if a doctor finds that he is not, then the person who has taken the initiative in will-making should be advised to apply to the Court of Protection in order to arrange receivership; the doctor will in due course report on a form CP3, as outlined earlier.

SUMMARY

The law does not deal specifically with the question of consent to treatment by demented patients; as matters stand, consent to routine diagnostic and treatment measures is generally taken as valid subject to certain safeguards; among these, consultation and co-operation with the next of kin are important.

Compulsory admission to hospital can be effected under the Mental Health Act 1983 or the National Assistance Act 1948. In the former case, the criteria for admission are exactly the same as for younger patients; the question is one of risk to the patient or others, arising from his mental illness. A demented person cannot be admitted compulsorily to hospital simply because he is causing a moderate nuisance or because he is living in less than ideal conditions. Admission is usually under section 2 of the Act but treatment (except in an emergency) is still subject to consent; compulsory treatment requires that the patient be detained under section 3 of the Act, and for certain treatments there are additional requirements.

The National Assistance Act has limited usefulness and is cumbersome in operation. It allows removal on the grounds of health hazard (to the patient or others) or serious nuisance. It applies largely to patients who are suffering from physical illness or self-neglect, but this is in practice usually the result of dementia, in which case the Mental Health Act would be applicable.

The status of the 'voluntary' demented patient in a locked ward is still undefined. In the uncommon instances where a patient is making determined and single-minded efforts to leave he should (if there is no alternative to hospitalization) be detained under the Mental Health Act. Where the majority of demented patients are concerned, the duty of the doctor is generally to act as would a wise relative, especially in protecting the patient against hazards. This often means a locked ward, but environments where the demented are treated can often be improved to the point where such restraints are virtually unnecessary.

The property and affairs of demented people are sometimes managed by the next of kin by means of a power of attorney, but this requires that the patient be capable of making the arrangements initially, and it automatically becomes void if at any time in the future he becomes incapable; the relative of an elderly or demented patient should therefore seek an enduring power of attorney or a receivership under the Court of Protection. The former arrangement will be preferable in most cases, but legal advice is necessary.

A demented patient may be legally capable of making a will, even one whose affairs are being managed by the Court of Protection. The testator should know what a will is, he should know what property is at his disposal and the claims of potential beneficiaries, he should be free of symptoms that would distort his judgement in disposing of his property, and he should not be subject to undue influence. A doctor, in whatever capacity he witnesses a will, must first satisfy himself as to testamentary capacity. If a patient is incapable, the Court of Protection has the power to make a 'statutory' will on his behalf.

Finally, the present chapter is intended only as a general guide. Advice in cases of difficulty should be sought from a lawyer, from the Mental Health Act Commission (p. 209), the Court of Protection (p. 207) or, by a doctor, from his defence society.

APPENDIX

Helping agencies

This is a list of organizations which may be able to provide help additional to that available from the statutory services. Only national bodies are listed; it should be noted that there are also numerous local organizations which provide help with elderly people; details can usually be found in a social services office or a public library.

Certain organizations for the elderly informed me specifically that they did not make provision for the demented; they have therefore not been listed because this section — like the rest of the book — is about dementia rather than about the elderly generally.

All the organizations listed are non-profit-making, being almost all registered charities. Many invite membership but, generally speaking, advice and information are given free of charge.

Age Concern England, Bernard Sunley House, 60 Pitcairn Road, Mitcham, Surrey CR4 3LL. Tel: 01–640 5431
Formed in 1940 and now comprising over 1600 local independent and autonomous Age Concern groups. Provides services to elderly people with the help of over 120,000 volunteers. Campaigns with and on behalf of elderly people, stimulates innovation and research, and works in partnership with both statutory and voluntary bodies; there are sister organizations in Scotland, Wales and Northern Ireland.

Services include day care, visiting, lunch clubs, family support, bereavement counselling and advice on health and financial matters. Mental health in old age receives special emphasis, and Age Concern now supports or disseminates information about a huge number of local projects — for example, day centres for the elderly mentally ill, relatives' support groups, reality orientation groups and care attendant schemes.

Age Concern's many publications include *Mental Health in Old Age: A Directory of Projects*, *Age Concern at Work* and *The 36-Hour Day: Caring at Home for Confused Elderly People*.

Alzheimer's Disease Society, 3rd Floor, Bank Buildings, Fulham Broadway, London SW6 1EP. Tel: 01–381 3177
Concerned with Alzheimer's disease and related disorders. There are numerous local branches providing support and information and a full-time counsellor can be contacted at Head Office. There are another ten offices throughout the UK. The aim of the Society is to increase public awareness of the disease and to promote better care. It encourages and funds research, maintains a Caring Fund to provide financial support, has compiled book-lists for lay and professional carers, publishes a newsletter for members, organizes conferences and symposia, and provides counselling on legal, social and family matters. Publications include a helpful and authoritative booklet: *Caring for the Person with Dementia: a guide for families and other carers*.

Association of Carers, First Floor, 21–23 New Road, Chatham, Kent ME4 4QJ. Tel: 0634 813981
Established to help bring the needs of carers to the attention of those who make the policies in health and social services departments. A carer is defined as 'anyone who is leading a restricted life because of the need to look after a person who is mentally or physically handicapped or ill or impaired by old age'.

Provides financial advice, help with equipment, assistance with holidays, group support and advice on the best use of statutory services; it also campaigns for their improvement. Publications include *Help at Hand*, a signpost guide for carers, which covers benefits, services and the emotional aspect of caring.

Association to Combat Huntingdon's Chorea, 34a Station Road, Hinkley, Leicestershire LE10 1AP. Tel: 0455 615558
Founded with the aim of promoting research, relief and treatment, disseminating knowledge about the disease, and providing information and support (including financial support when appropriate) to families and their associated professionals. There are 23 branches throughout the UK and local contacts elsewhere. Services include day centres, support groups and a small number of residential places in specialized units. Also raises funds, stimulates research and provides a large number of authoritative publications on Huntingdon's chorea. A recently published information sheet, for example, deals with new developments in predictive testing.

Centre for Policy on Ageing, 25–31 Ironmonger Row, London EC1V 3QP. Tel: 01–253 1787
The centre aims to promote informed debate about issues affecting older people, to stimulate awareness of their needs, to formulate and promote policies and to encourage the spread of good practice.

Is essentially a research, public education and grant-giving body rather than one which patients and their relatives can approach directly for advice. However, it maintains a large library on the social aspects of ageing and a residential homes advice team.

Two recent projects have a direct bearing on dementia. First, a survey of good practice across the entire field of mental illness in the elderly (now published as *Mental Illness in Old Age: Meeting the Challenge* by Alison Norman) and a study of small specialist units for dementia sufferers, to be published shortly.

Citizen's Advice Bureaux (National Association of Citizens Advice Bureaux, 115–123 Pentonville Road, London N1 9LZ. Tel: 01–833 2181)
The first Citizens Advice Bureau provided an emergency wartime service in 1939; there are now 937 bureaux nationwide; the bureau sees itself as 'the well-informed general practitioner of the social services, combining the roles of prevention, diagnosis and referral to the specialist consultant'. Staff could not advise specifically on dementia, but would advise on benefits for both carers and sufferers and help negotiate with social services where problems occurred. Over all, would principally be of assistance to carers.

Community Health Councils (Association of Community Health Councils, Mark Lemon Suite, Barclays Bank Chambers, 254 Seven Sisters Road, London N4 2HZ, Tel: 01–833 4456.)
Established in 1974 to represent the consumer within the NHS; there is a CHC in each health district, made up of both professional and lay members. The CHC's object is essentially to maintain and improve the quality of service and of facilities and to provide information on existing services. A local CHC may be especially helpful in instances where a service is felt to be poor or inadequate or where a patient or his relatives wish to pursue a specific complaint.

Counsel and Care for the Elderly, 131 Middlesex Street, London E1 7JF. Tel: 01–621 1624
Founded primarily to give advice on residential care; can be most helpful to elderly people or their relatives seeking places in private residential or nursing homes, although only a small number of such establishments provide for patients with dementia. Advice on specific homes is restricted to the Greater London area, but those who wish to live in homes elsewhere can be advised about appropriate sources of information.

Also advises on housing (e.g. sheltered housing), financial benefits, nursing care at home, temporary care, holidays or 'anything under the sun which may be worrying elderly people'. Financial asistance may be provided. Counsel and Care also has a wide knowledge of other charities which provide help for elderly people. Publications include numerous information sheets, mainly about accommodation and finance.

Court of Protection, 25 Store Street, London WC1E 7BP. Tel: 01–636 6877
See also pp. 201–202. The Court of Protection is an office of the Lord Chancellor's Department which exists for the purpose of protecting and managing the financial affairs and property of people who, because of mental

disorder, are unable to manage for themselves. The Court will send a useful explanatory leaflet (PN11) on request; other publications are a Receiver's handbook (PN6) and a leaflet EP(a) explaining the Enduring Powers of Attorney Act 1985 (p. 000).

Crossroads Care Attendant Schemes (Association of Crossroads Care Attendant Schemes Ltd, 94 Coton Road, Rugby, Warwickshire CV21 4LN. Tel: 0788 73653)
Both the name and the concept come from the popular UK television serial. An episode in which a solution was found to the problem of a young physically disabled man at home was translated into real life when ATV donated £10,000 to found a pilot scheme in Rugby.

There are now about 100 such schemes nationwide; the objective of the Association is 'to relieve stress in families or persons responsible for the care of disabled persons and exceptionally, in suitable circumstances, to help such disabled persons who live alone. Also to avoid, where possible, admission to hospital or residential care due to a breakdown or other failure in the household, and to work closely with existing statutory services'.

Some schemes include the demented; where they do, Crossroads attendants can be particularly helpful in visiting a patient whose carers go out to work during the day, thus enabling them to continue in employment.

Disabled Living Foundation, 380–384 Harrow Road, London W9 2HU. Tel: 01–289 6111
Terms of reference include all disabilities, mental, physical and sensory, together with multiple handicaps and the infirmities of age. Is concerned with those aspects of ordinary life which present particular problems to disabled people of any age. There is an information service which draws on a huge central bank and an extensive reference library. There are specific advisory services dealing with matters such as incontinence, clothing, visual handicap, and aids and equipment. Leaflets on all of these services are available and there is also a library resource list dealing with the elderly, including those with dementia.

Foundation for Age Research, 49 Queen Victoria Street, London EC4N 4SA. Tel: 01–236 4365
Does not directly provide advice for carers but its object is to improve the quality of life of the elderly by funding medical and scientific research into the ageing process and disabilities of the elderly, encouraging and enabling young people of ability to work with the elderly and co-ordinating information and research. There are groups of Friends nationwide, and at present the Foundation is funding over 50 research projects, some concerned with dementia.

Health Education Council, 78 New Oxford Street, London WC1A 1AH. Tel: 01–631 0930
Provides a wide range of information and advice concerning the elderly. Publishes a leaflet: *Home Care of the Elderly* and also *Who Cares?: information and support for the carers of confused people*. The latter in particular, clearly written by experts, is highly recommended. This and *Caring for the Person with Dementia* from the Alzheimer's Disease Society are the best booklets on dementia at present available.

Help the Aged, St James's Walk, London EC1R 0BE. Tel: 01–253 0253
Dedicated to improving the quality of life of elderly people in need of help both in the UK and overseas. Raises and grants funds towards community-based projects, housing and overseas aid. In the UK it provides or supports services such as day centres, minibuses, day hospitals, special housing schemes and hospices, and overseas is concerned with refugees, health-care programmes, self-help groups and liaison with other voluntary agencies. Help the Aged works closely with Age Concern; the emphasis of the latter is on providing services through local groups in the UK and of the former on fund-raising for projects both in the UK and abroad. The main office, together with numerous other centres, provides information and advice on all problems affecting elderly people. Publications (a catalogue is available) include *The Time of Your Life — a handbook for retirement* and *Recall* and *Do You Mind the Time?*, reality orientation programmes.

Mental Health Act Commission, Room 22, Hepburn House, Marsham Street, London SW1P 4HW. Tel: 01–211 8061
See also p. 199. The Commission was established in 1983 to protect the rights and interests of all patients detained under the Mental Health Act 1983, to receive and investigate complaints by or about detained patients, to arrange for 'second opinions' where required and to formulate a Code of Practice for the care and treatment of all mentally ill and handicapped persons.

The Commission will therefore deal with most queries from interested parties relating to mental health provision, but especially those relating to detained patients, compulsory treatment or patients' rights. It will also advise professional staff on the proper interpretation and use of the Mental Health Act 1983. It publishes an explanatory leaflet about the Commission; the other two main publications thus far are the draft Code of Practice (1985) and the first Biennial Report (1985).

MIND (National Association for Mental Health), 22 Harley Street, London W1N 2ED. Tel: 01–637 0741
Is concerned with all aspects of mental health, in particular with improvement of services, and will provide information and advice on all mental health matters. There are 190 local associations affiliated to MIND, and some of these provide help and support to those who care for the elderly. The comprehensive

publications list (No. 1, 1986) includes *Coping with Caring* (about dementia), *Home Support for Mentally Infirm Elderly People, What Next for Elderly People?* (including the mentally infirm), and *Who Cares about Relatives*, helpful and practical leaflet about relatives' support groups.

National Council for Carers and their Elderly Dependants, 29 Chilworth Mews, London W2 3RG. Tel: 01–724 7776
Objects are to provide advice, information and support for carers of the elderly, to give information about carers' needs to statutory bodies, to act as a pressure group on behalf of carers and to campaign for better benefits and services for carers. Provides an information and advice service, publishes a newsletter and supplies information about short-term respite care. There are about 50 local branches throughout the UK. Publishes useful leaflets on the common problems encountered by carers and the various kinds of help they can have. A comprehensive information pack is available.

Parkinson's Disease Society, 36 Portland Place, London W1N 3DG. Tel: 01–323 1174/5
Objects are to help patients and their relatives with the problems arising from Parkinson's disease, to collect and disseminate information about the disease and to encourage and provide funds for research. There are over 150 branches throughout the UK, and a quarterly newsletter. The Society provides a personal information and support service, and draws on the help of both medical and welfare experts. Helpful publications include *Parkinson's Disease: a booklet for patients and their families*, and *Parkinson's Disease Day-to-Day*, a practical guide to living with the condition.

University of the Third Age (In London: Langton Close, Wren Street, London WC1X 0HD. Tel: 01–833 4747)
An educational organization for retired people, with 150 groups throughout the UK. Provides a wide range of courses, and a recent development has been to include the housebound or those with limited mobility. Membership is available for a modest annual fee and members are sent details of all courses and meetings in their area.

U3A (as it is called for short) may appear to have little connection with dementia; it is, however, well worth listing here in view of the positive effect that learning and stimulation can have on mental health in old age.

REFERENCES

Acheson, E.D. (1985). That over used word Community! *Health Trends*, **17**, 3.
Adams, R.D., Fisher, C.M., Hakim, S., Ojemann, R.G. and Sweet, W.H. (1965). Symptomatic occult hydrocephalus with 'normal' cerebrospinal-fluid pressure, *N. Engl. J. Med.*, **273**, 117–26.
Adolfsson, R., Gottfries, C.G., Oreland, L., Roos, B.E. and Winblad, B. (1978). Reduced levels of catecholamines in the brain and increased activity of monoamine oxidase in platelets in Alzheimer's disease, in *Alzheimer's disease: Senile Dementia*

and Related Disorders (Eds. R. Katzman, R.D. Terry and K.L. Blick), Raven Press, New York.

Adolfsson, R., Gottfries, C.G., Roos, B.E. and Winblad, B. (1979) Changes in the brain catecholamines in patients with dementia of Alzheimer type, *Br. J. Psychiat.*, **135**, 216–23.

Adolfsson, R., Brane, G., Bucht, G., Karlsson, I., Gottfries, G.-C., Persson, S. and Winblad, B. (1982). A double-blind study with levodopa in dementia of Alzheimer type, in *Alzheimer's Disease: A Report of Progress in Research* (Eds. S. Corkin, J.H. Growdon, K.L. Davis, E. Usdin, R.J. Wurtman), Raven Press, New York.

Agate, J.N. (1960). Mental health of the ageing, *Geront. Clin.*, **2**, 65–67.

Agid, Y., Ruberg, M., Dubois, B. and Javoy-Agid, F. (1984). Biochemical substrates of mental disorders in Parkinson's disease, in *Advances in Neurology*, vol. 40 (eds. R.G. Hassler and J.F. Christ), Raven Press, New York.

Åkesson, H.O. (1969). A population study of senile and arteriosclerotic psychoses, *Hum. Hered.*, **19.**, 546–66.

Alfrey, A.C., LeGendre, G.R. and Kaehny, W.D. (1976). The dialysis encephalopahy syndrome: possible aluminium intoxication, *N. Engl. J. Med.*, **294**, 184–8.

Allison, R.s. (1961). *The Senile Brain*, Edward Arnold, London.

Alzheimer, A. (1899). Beitrag zur pathologischen Anatomie der Seelenstörungen des Greisanalters, *Neurol. Zentralbl.*, **18**, 95–6.

Alzheimer, A. (1904). Histologische Studien zur Differenzialdiagnose der progressiven Paralyse, *Nissls. Arbeiten*, **1**, 18.

Alzheimer, A. (1907). Über eine eigenartige Erkrankung der Hirnrinde, *Allg. Z. Psychiat.*, **64**, 146–8.

Alzheimer, A. (1911). Über eigenartige Krankheitsfalle des spateren Alters, *Z. Neurol. Psychiat.*, **4**, 36–85.

American Psychiatric Association (1969). *Reality Orientation. A technique to rehabilitate elderly and brain damaged patients with a moderate degree of disorientation.* American Psychiatric Association Hospital and Community Psychiatric Service, Washington DC.

Amster, L.E. and Krauss, H.H. (1974). The relationship between life crises and mental deterioration in old age, *Int. J. Aging Hum. Dev.*, **5**, 51–5.

Amulree, Lord, Exton-Smith, A.N. and Crockett, G.S. (1951). Proper use of the hospital in treatment of the aged sick, *Lancet*, **i**, 123–6.

Anderson, J.M. and Hubbard, B.M. (1985). Definition of Alzheimer's disease, *Lancet*, **i**, 408.

Andrews, J., Letcher, M. and Brook, M. (1969). Vitamin C supplementation in the elderly: 17 month trial in an old persons' home, *Br. Med. J.*, **ii**, 416.

Anthony, J.C., LeResche, L., Niaz, V., Von Korloff, M.R. and Folstein, M.F. (1982). Limits of the 'Mini-Mental State' as a screening test for dementia and delirium among hospital patients, *Psychol. Med.*, **12**, 397–408.

Argyle, N., Jestice, S. and Brook, C.P.B. (1985). Psychogeriatric patients: their supporters' problems, *Age Ageing*, **14**, 355–60.

Arie, T. (1977). Guidelines for collaboration between geriatricians and psychiatrists in the care of the elderly: a discussion paper for the Standing Joint Committee of the British Geriatrics Society and the Royal College of Psychiatrists, London.

Arie, T. (1979). Day care in geriatric psychiatry, *Age Ageing*, **8**, Suppl., 87–91.

Arie, T. (1983). Organization of services for the elderly. Implications for education and patient care — experience in Nottingham, in *Geropsychiatric Diagnostics and Treatment* (Ed. m. Bergener), Springer, New York.

Arie, T. (1985). Some current issues in old age psychiatry services. Paper presented at DHSS/Royal College of Psychiatrists conference, March 1985.

Austin, J.H., Rinehart, R., Williamson, T., Burcar, P., Russ, K., Nikaido, T. and Lafrance, M. (1973). Studies in ageing of the brain. III. Silicon levels in postmortem tissue and body fluids, *Prog. Brain Res.*, **40**, 486–95.

Baddeley, A.D. (1983). *Your Memory: A User's Guide*, Penguin, Harmondsworth.

Baddeley, A.D. and Warrington, E.K. (1970). Amnesia and the distinction between long- and short-term memory, *J. Verb. Learn. Verb. Behav.*, **9**, 176–89.

Baddeley, A.D., Sunderland, A. and Harris, J. (1982). How well do laboratory-based psychological tests predict patients' performance outside the laboratory? in *Alzheimer's Disease: A Report of Progress in Research* (Eds. S. Corkin, J.H. Growdon, K.L. Davis, E. Usdin and R.J. Wurtman), Raven Press, New York.

Baker, H.F., Rudley, R.M. and Crow, T.J. (1985). Experimental transmission of an autosomal dominant spongiform encephalopathy: does the infectious agent originate in the human genome? *Br. Med. J.*, **291**, 299–302.

Ball, M.J. and Nuttall, K. (1980). Topography of neurofibrillary tangles and granulovacuoles in patients with Down's syndrome: quantitative comparison with normal ageing and Alzheimer's disease, *Neuropath. Appl. Neurobiol.*, **7**, 13–20.

Ball, M.J., and Hachinski, V., Fox, A., Kirschen, A.J., Fisman, M., Blume, W., Kral, V.A., Fox, H. and Merskey, H. (1985). A new definition of Alzheimer's disease: a hippocampal dementia, *Lancet*, **i**, 14–16.

Ballinger, B.R., Reid, A.H. and Heather, B.B. (1982). Cluster analysis of symptoms in elderly demented patients, *Br. J. Psychiat.*, **140**, 257–62.

Banks v *Goodfellow* (1870). LR5 QB 549.

Barclay, L.L., Zemcov, A., Blass, J.P. and McDowell, F.H. (1985). Factors associated with duration of survival in Alzheimer's disease, *Biol. Psychiat.*, **20**, 86–92.

Barns, E.K., Sack, A. and Shore, H. (1973). Guidelines to treatment approaches: modalities and methods for use with the aged, *Gerontologist*, **13**, 513–27.

Barron, S.A., Jacobs, L. and Kinkel, W.R. (1976). Changes in size of normal lateral ventricles during aging determined by computerized tomography, *Neurology*, **26**, 1011–13.

Bartus, R.T. (1979). Physostigmine and recent memory: effects in young and aged nonhuman primates, *Science*, **206**, 1087–9.

Bartus, R.T. and Lambert, W. (1978). Aging in the rhesus monkey: specific behavioral impairments and effects of pharmacological interventions. Presented at XIth International Congress of Gerontology, Tokyo, Japan.

Bassuk, E.L., Minden, S. and Apsler, R. (1983). Geriatric emergencies: psychiatric or medical? *Am. J. Psychiat.*, **140**, 539–42.

Basu, T.K. and Schorah, C.J. (1982). *Vitamin C in Health and Disease*, Croom Helm, London.

Beardsley, J. and Puletti, F. (1971). Personality (MMPI) and cognitive (WAIS) changes after levodopa treatment: occurrence in patients with Parkinson's disease, *Arch. Neurol.*, **25**, 140–50.

Bedford, P.D. (1958). Discussion: intracranial haemorrhage — diagnosis and treatment, *Proc. Roy. Soc. Med.*, **51**, 209–13.

Bell, B.A. and Ambrose, J. (1982). Smoking and the risk of stroke, *Acta Neurochirurgica*, **64**, 1–7.

Bendheim, P.E. and Bolton, D.C. (1985). Alzheimer's disease: is there evidence of an infectious cause? *Geriat. Med. Today*, **4**, 93–102.

Berg, L., Danziger, W.L., Storandt, M., Coben, L.A., Gado, M., Hughes, C.P., Knesevitch, J.W. and Botwinick, J. (1984). Predictive factors in mild senile dementia of the Alzheimer type, *Neurology*, **34**, 563–7.

Berger, B., Escourolle, R. and Moyne, M.A. (1976). Axones catécholaminiques du cortex cérébral humain — observation en histofluorescence de biopsies cérébrales dont 2 cas de maladie d'Alzheimer, *Revue Neurol.*, **132**, 183–94.

Bergman, H., Borg, S., Hindmarch, T., Ideztiom, C.M. and Mutzell, S. (1980). Computerized tomography of the brain and neuropsychological assessment of male alcoholic patients, in *Addiction and Brain Disease* (Ed. D. Richter), University Park Press, Baltimore.

Bergmann, K. (1969). The epidemiology of senile dementia, *Br. J. Hosp. Med.*, **2**, 727–32.

Bergmann, K. (1977). Prognosis in chronic brain failure, *Age Ageing*, **6**, Suppl., 61–9.

Bergmann, K., Foster, E.M., Justice, A.W. and Matthews, V. (1978). Management of the demented elderly patient in the community, *Br. J. Psychiat*, **132**, 441–9.

Bernheimer, H., Birkmayer, W., Hornykiewicz, O., Jellinger, K. and Seitelberger, F. (1973). Brain dopamine and the syndromes of Parkinson and Huntingdon. Clinical, morphological and neurochemical correlates, *J. Neurol. Sci.*, **20**, 415–55.

Bernouilli, C., Siegfried, J., Baumgardner, G., Regli, F., Rabinowicz, T., Gadjusek, D.C. and Gibbs, C.J. Jr (1977). Danger of accidental person-to-person transmission of Creutzfeldt–Jakob disease by surgery, *Lancet*, **i**, 478–9.

Berrios, G.E. and Brook, P. (1984). Visual hallucinations and sensory delusions in the elderly, *Br. J. Psychiat*, **144**, 662–4.

Besson, J.A.O., Corrigan, F.M., Foreman, E.I., Eastwood, L.M., Smith, F.W. and Ashcroft, G.W. (1985). Nuclear magnetic resonance (NMR). I. Imaging in dementia, *Br. J. Psychiat.*, **146**, 31–5.

Bielschowsky, M. (1903). Die Ziele bei Impregnation der Neurofibrillen, *Neurol. Zentralbl.*, **22**, 997–1006.

Bird, E.D. and Iversen, L.L. (1977). Huntingdon's chorea — post-mortem measurement of glutamic acid decarboxylase, choline acetyl-transferase and dopamine in basal ganglia, *Brain*, **97**, 457–72.

Birkett, D.P. (1972). The psychiatric differentiation of senility and arteriosclerosis, *Br. J. Psychiat.*, **120**, 321–5.

Blessed, G. (1986). Survey into the availability of higher specialist training in the psychiatry of old age, *Bull. Roy. Coll. Psychiat.*, **10**, 88–9.

Blessed, G. and Wilson, I. (1982). The contemporary natural history of mental disorder in old age, *Br. J. Psychiat.*, **141**, 59–67.

Blessed, G., Tomlinson, B.E. and Roth, M. (1968). The association between quantitative measures of dementia and senile change in the cerebral grey matter of elderly subjects, *Br. J. Psychiat.*, **114**, 797–811.

Bleuler, E.P. (1911). *Dementia Praecox or the Group of Schizophrenias*. (Trans. J. Zinkin), International Universities Press, New York, 1950.

Blocq, P. and Marinesco, G. (1892). Sur les lésions et la pathogénie de l'épilepsie dite essentielle, *Semin. Méd.*, **2**, 445–6.

Bluestein, H.G. (1978). Heterogenous neurocytotoxic antibodies in subacute lupus erythematosus, *Clin. Exp. Immunol*, **35**(2), 210–17.

Bluglass, R. (1983). *A Guide to the Mental Health Act 1983*, Churchill Livingstone, London.

Böck, E., Kristensen, V. and Rafaelson, O.J. (1974). Proteins in serum and cerebrospinal fluid in demented patients, *Acta Neurol. Scand.*, **50**, 91–102.

Bockman, J.M., Kingsbury, D.T., McKinley, M.P., Bendheim, P.E. and Prusiner, S.B. (1985). Creuzfeldt–Jakob disease prion protons in human brains, *N. Engl. J. Med.*, **312**, 73–8.

Boller, F., Mizutani, T., Roessmann, U. and Gambeti, P. (1980). Parkinson's disease, dementia, and Alzheimer disease: clinico-pathological correlations, *Ann. Neurol.*, **7**, 329–335.

Bondareff, W. (1983). Age and Alzheimer disease, *Lancet*, **i**, 1447.

Bonita, R., Scragg, R., Stewart, A., Jackson, R. and Beaglehole, R. (1986). Cigarette smoking and risk of premature stroke in men and women, *Br. Med. J.*, **293**, 6–8.

Bowen, D.M. (1980). Biochemical evidence for selective vulnerability in Alzheimer's disease, in *Biochemistry of Dementia* (Ed. P.J. Roberts), Wiley, Chichester.

Bowen, D.M. (1981). Alzheimer's disease, in *The Molecular Basis of Neuropathology*, (Eds. R.H.S. Thompson and A.N. Davison), Edward Arnold, London.

Bowen, D.M. and Davison, A.N. (1977). Selective vulnerability of neurones in Alzheimer's disease, *Br. J. Psychiat.*, **131**, 319.

Bowen, D.M., Sims, N.R. Benton, S., Haan, E.A., Smith, C.C.T., Neary, D., Thomas, D.J. and Davison, A.N. (1982). Biochemical change in cortical brain biopsies from demented patients in relation to morphological findings and pathogenesis, in *Alzheimer's Disease: A Report of Progress in Research*, (Eds. S. Corkin, J.H. Growdon, K.L. Davis, E. Usdin and R.J. Wurtman), Raven Press, New York.

Boyd, W.D., Graham-White, G., Blackwood, G., Glen, I. and McQueen, J. (1977). Clinical effects of choline in Alzheimer senile dementia, *Lancet*, **ii**, 711.

Bradshaw, J.R., Thompson, J.L.G. and Campbell, M.J. (1983). Computerised tomography in the diagnosis of dementia, *Br. Med. J.*, **286**, 277–80.

Braham, J. (1971). Jakob-Creutzfeldt disease: treatment by amantidine, *Br. Med. J.*, **iv**, 212–13.

Branconnier, R. and Cole, J.O. (1977). Senile dementia and drug therapy, in *The Aging Brain and Senile Dementia* (Eds. K. Nandy and I. Sherwin), Plenum Press, New York.

Brandenburg, W. and Hallervorden, J. (1954). Dementia pugilistica mit anatomischen Befund, *Arch. Path. Anat.*, **325**, 680–709.

Breitner, J.S.C. and Folstein, M.F. (1984). Familial Alzheimer disease: a prevalent disorder with specific clinical features, *Psychol. Med.*, **14**, 63–80.

Briggs, R.S. and Castleden, C.M. (1984). The therapeutics of senile dementia, *Geriat. Med. Today*, **3**, 61–77.

Brinkman, S.D. and Largen, J.W. (1984). Changes in brain ventricular size with repeated CAT scans in suspected Alzheimer's disease, *Am. J. Psychiat.*, **141**, 81–3.

Brodal, A. (1981). *Neurological Anatomy*, Oxford University Press, Oxford.

Brody, E.M., Kleban, M.H., Lawton, M.P. and Silverman, H.A. (1971). Excess disabilities of mentally impaired aged: impact of individualized treatment, *Gerontologist*, **11**, 124–32.

Brook, C.P.B., Degun, G. and Mather, M. (1975). Reality orientation, a therapy for psychogeriatric patients: a controlled study, *Br. J. Psychiat.*, **127**, 42–5.

Brooker, C. and Beard, P. (1984). The nursing alternative, *Senior Nurse*, **1**(36), 14–16.

Brown, R.G. and Marsden, C.D. (1984). How common is dementia in Parkinson's disease? *Lancet*, **ii**, 1262–5.

Brown, W.S., Marsh, J.T. and LaRue, A. (1982). Event-related potentials in psychiatry: differentiating depression and dementia in the elderly, *Bull. Los Angeles Neurol. Soc.*, **47**, 91–107.

Bruce, M.E. and Fraser, H. (1981). Effect of route of injection on the frequency and distribution of cerebral amyloid plaques in scrapie mice, *Neuropath. Appl. Neurobiol.*, **7**, 289–98.

Brun, A., Gottfries, C.G. and Roos, B.E. (1971). Studies of the monoamine metabolism in the central nervous system in Jakob-Creutzfeldt disease. *Acta Neurol. Scand.*, **47**, 642–5.

Bucht, G., Adolfsson, R. and Winblad, B. (1984). Dementia of the Alzheimer type and multi-infarct dementia: a clinical description and diagnostic problems, *J. Am. Geriat. Soc.*, **32**, 491–8.

Buckley, C.E. and Roseman, J.M. (1976). Immunity and survival, *J. Am. Geriat. Soc.*, **24**, 241–8.

Buckley, C.E., Buckley, E.G. and Dorsey, F.C. (1974). Longitudinal changes in serum immunoglobulin levels in older humans, *Fed. Proc.*, **33**, 2036–9.

Burch, P.R.J. (1968). *An Enquiry Concerning Growth, Disease and Aging*, Oliver and Boyd, Edinburgh.

215

Busse, E.W., Barnes, R.L., Friedman, E.L. and Kety, E.J. (1956). Psychological functioning of aged individuals with normal and abnormal electroencephalograms, *J. Nerv. Ment. Dis.*, **124**, 135–41.

Butler, A. (1982). Research in the efficacy of alarm systems for the elderly, *Social Work Service*, **29**, 53–6.

Cady, E.B., Dawson, M.J., Hope, P.L., Tofts, P.S., Costello, A.M.deL., Delpy, D.T., Reynolds, E.O.R. and Wilkie, D.R. (1983). Non-invasive investigation of cerebral metabolism in newborn infants by phosphorus nuclear magnetic resonance spectroscopy, *Lancet*, **i**, 1059–62.

Caird, W.K. and Sanderson, R.E. and Inglis, J. (1962). Cross validation of a learning test for use with elderly psychiatric patients, *J. Ment. Sci.*, **108**, 268–70.

Callard, R.E. and Basten, A. (1977). Immune function in aged mice. I. T-cell responsiveness using phytohemagglutinin as a functional probe, *Cell. Immunol*, **31**, 13–25.

Campbell, A.J., Reinken, J., Allan, B. and Martinez, G. (1981). Falls in old age: a study of frequency and related clinical factors, *Age Ageing*, **10**, 264–70.

Campbell, A.J., Reinken, J. and McCosh, L. (1985). Incontinence in the elderly: prevalence and prognosis, *Age Ageing*, **14**, 65–70.

Cardozo, L.D. and Stanton, S.L. (1979). An objective comparison of the effects of parenterally administered drugs in patients suffering from detrusor instability, *J. Urol.*, **122**, 58–9.

Ceder, G. and Schuberth, J. (1977). In vivo formation and post-mortem changes of choline and acetylcholine in the brain of mice, *Brain Res.*, **128**, 580–4.

Chandler, J.H. (1966). EEG in prediction of Huntingdon's chorea. An eighteen-year follow-up, *Electroenceph. Clin. Neurophysiol.*, **21**, 79–0.

Chaqui, P. and Levy, R. (1982). Fluctuations of free choline levels in plasma of Alzheimer patients receiving lecithin: preliminary observations, *Br. J. Psychiat.*, **140**, 464–9.

Chase, T.N., Durso, R., Fedio, P. and Tamminga, C.A. (1982). Vasopressin treatment of cognitive defects, in *Alzheimer's Disease: A Report of Progress in Research* (Eds. S. Corkin, J.H. Growdon, K.L. Davis, E. Usdin and R.J. Wurtman), Raven Press. New York.

Cheney, D.L., Moroni, F., Malthe-Sorenssen, D. and Costa, E. (1978). Endogenous modulation of acetylcholine turnover rate, in *Cholinergic Mechanisms and Psychopharmacology* (Ed. D.J. Jenden), Plenum Press, New York.

Christenson, R. and Blazer, D. (1984). Epidemiology of persecutory ideation in an elderly population in the community, *Am. J. Psychiat.*, **141**, 1088–91.

Christie, A.B. (1982). Changing patterns in mental illness in the elderly, *Br. J. Psychiat.*, **140**, 154–9.

Christie, A.B. and Train, J.D. (1984). Change in the pattern of care for the demented, *Br. J. Psychiat.*, **144**, 9–15.

Christie, J.E. (1982). Physostigmine and arecoline infusions in Alzheimer's disease, in *Alzheimer's Disease: A Report of Progress in Research* (Eds. S. Corkin, J.H. Growdon, K.L. Davis, E. Usdin and R.J. Wurtman), Raven Press, New York.

Chudnovsky, N. (1979). Community-based management of mild to moderate mental deterioration in older age outpatients. Scientific exhibit, American Academy of Family Physicians, 31st Annual Scientific Assembly, Atlanta.

Clark, A.W., Parhad, I.M., Struble, R.G., Whitehouse, P.J. and Price, D.L. (1983). The nucleus basalis of Meynert (nbM) in Alzheimer's disease/senile dementia of the Alzheimer type (AD/SDAT), *Current Rep. Neurol.*, **6**, 1.

Clarke, M., Hughes, A.O., Dodd, K.J., Palmer, R.L., Brandon, S., Holden, A. and Pearce, D. (1979). The elderly in residential care: patterns of disability, *Health Trends*, **11**, 17–20.

216

Clarke, M., Clarke, S., Odell, A. and Jagger, C. (1984). The elderly at home: health and social status, *Health Trends*, **16**, 3–8.

Cohen, A.S. and Cathcart, E.S. (1974). Amyloidosis and immunoglobulins, *Adv. Intern. Med.*, **19**, 41–55.

Cohen, D. and Eisdorfer, C. (1980a). Serum immunoglobulins and cognitive status in the elderly, I. A population study, *Br. J. Psychiat.*, **136**, 33–9.

Cohen, D. and Eisdorfer, C. (1980b). Serum immunoglobulins and cognitive status in the elderly: II. an immunological–behavioural relationship? *Br. J. Psychiat.*, **136**, 40–5.

Colgan, J. (1985). Regional density and survival in senile dementia: an interim report on a prospective computerised tomographic study, *Br. J. Psychiat.*, **147**, 63–6.

Colgan, J. and Philpot, M. (1985). The routine use of investigations in elderly psychiatric patients, *Age Ageing*, **14**, 163–7.

Collerton, D. and Fairbairn, A. (1985). Alzheimer's disease and the hippocampus, *Lancet*, **8**, 278–9.

Collins, K.J. (1983). *Hypothermia: The Facts*. Oxford University Press, Oxford.

Constantinidis, J. (1978). Is Alzheimer's disease a major form of senile dementia? Clinical, anatomical and genetic data, in *Alzheimer's Disease: Senile Dementia and Related Disorders* (Eds. R. Katzman, R.D. Terry and K.L. Blick), Raven Press, New York.

Cooper, B. and Bickel, H. (1984). Population screening and the early detection of dementing disorders in old age: a review, *Psychol. Med.*, **14**, 81–95.

Copeland, J.R.M., Kelleher, M.J., Kellett, J.M., Barron, G., Cowan, D.W. and Gourlay, A.J. (1975). Evaluation of a psychogeriatric service: the distinction between psychogeriatric and geriatric patients, *Br. J. Psychiat.*, **126**, 21–9.

Corsellis, J.A.N. (1962). *Mental Illness and the Ageing Brain* (Maudsley Monograph), Oxford University Press, Oxford.

Corsellis, J.A.N. (1969). The pathology of dementia, *Br. J. Hosp. Med.*, **2**, 695–604.

Corsellis, J.A.N. (1979). On the transmission of dementia: a personal view of the slow virus problem, *Br. J. Psychiat.*, **134**, 553–9.

Corsellis, J.A.N. and Evans, P.H. (1965). The relation of stenosis of the extracranial cerebral arteries to mental disorders and cerebral degeneration in old age, *Proc. 5th Int. Congr. Neuropath.*, 546–50. Excerpta Medica, Amsterdam.

Corsellis, J.A.N., Bruton, C.J. and Freeman-Browne, D. (1973). The aftermath of boxing, *Psychol. Med.*, **3**, 270–303.

Cosin, L.Z., Mort, P., Post, F., Westrop, C. and Williams, M. (1958). Experimental treatment of persistent senile confusion, *Int. J. Soc. Psychiat.*, **4**, 24–42.

Coughlan, A.K. and Hollows, S.E. (1984). Use of memory tests in differentiating organic disorder from depression, *Br. J. Psychiat.*, **145**, 164–7.

Cowan, D.W., Wright, P.M., Gourlay, A.J., Smith, A., Baron, G., de Gruchy, J., Copeland, J.R.M., Kelleher, M.J. and Kellett, J.M. (1975). A comparative psychometric assessment of psychogeriatric and geriatric patients, *Br. J. Psychiat.*, **14**, 33–41.

Cox, J.R., Pandurangi, V.R. and Wallace, M.G. (1978). Drugs will help if dementing patients are caught early, *Mod. Geriatrics*, **9**(4), 12–15.

Crapper, D.R. and Dalton, A.J. (1973). Aluminium induced neurofibrillary degeneration, brain electrical activity and alterations in acquisitions and retention, *Physiol. Behav.*, **19**, 935–45.

Crapper, D.R. and De Boni, V. (1977). Aluminium and the genetic apparatus in Alzheimer's disease, in *The Aging Brain and Senile Dementia* (Ed. K. Nandy and I. Sherwin), Plenum Press, New York.

Crapper, D.R. and De Boni, V. (1980) Models for the biochemical study of dementia, in *Biochemistry of Dementia* (Ed. P.J. Roberts), Wiley, Chichester.

Crapper, D.R., Krishnan, S.S. and Quitkatt, S. (1976). Aluminium, neurofibrillary degeneration and Alzheimer's disease, *Brain*, **99**, 67–80.

Crapper, D.R., Karlik, S. and De Voni, V. (1978). Aluminium and other metals in senile (Alzheimer) dementia, in *Alzheimer's Disease: Senile Dementia and Related Disorders* (Eds. R. Katzman, R.D. Terry and K.L. Bick), Raven Press, New York.

Craufurd, D.I.O. and Harris, R. (1986). Ethics of predictive testing for Huntingdon's chorea: the need for more information, *Br. Med. J.*, **293**, 249–51.

Creutzfeldt, H.G. (1920). Über eine eigenartige herdformige Erkrankung des Zentral Nervensystems, *Z. Neurol. Psychiat.*, **57**, 1–18.

Crow, T.J., Cross, A.J., Grove-White, I.G. and Ross, D.G. (1982). Central neurotransmitters, memory and dementia, in *Psychopharmacology of Old Age* (Ed. D. Wheatley), Oxford Medical Publications, Oxford.

Cutting, J. (1978). The relationship between Korsakov's syndrome and 'alcoholic dementia', *Br. J. Psychiat.*, **132**, 240–51.

Dahl, D. and Bignami, A. (1978). Immunochemical cross-reactivity of normal neurofibrils and aluminium induced neurofibrillary tangles, *Exp. Neurol.*, **58**, 74–80.

Dall, J.C.L. (1982). in 'Thiamine Drug Cited in Management of the Elderly', *Psychiatric Topics*, **2**, 6.

Dalton, A.J., Crapper, D.R. and Schlotterer, G.R. (1974). Alzheimer's disease in Down's syndrome: visual retention deficits, *Cortex*, **10**, 366–77.

Davidson, E.A. and Robertson, E.E. (1955). Alzheimer's disease with acne rosacea in one set of identical twins, *J. Neurol. Neurosurg. Psychiat.*, **18**, 72–7.

Davies, M., Mawer, E.B., Hann, J.T., Stephens, W.P. and Taylor, J.L. (1985). Vitamin D prophylaxis in the elderly: a simple effective method suitable for large populations, *Age Ageing*, **14**, 349–54.

Davies, P. (1977). Cholinergic mechanisms in Alzheimer's disease, *Br. J. Psychiat.*, **131**, 318–19.

Davies, P., Hollister, L.E., Overall, J., Johnson, A. and Train, K. (1976). Physostigmine: effects on cognition and affect in elderly subjects, *Psychopharmacology*, **51**, 23–7.

Davis, K.L., Mohs, R.C., Davis, B.C., Levy, M.I., Horvath, T.B., Rosenberg, G.S., Ross, A., Rothpearl, A. and Rosen, W. (1982). Cholinergic treatment in Alzheimer's disease: implications for future research, in *Alzheimer's Disease: A Report of Progress in Research* (Eds. S. Corkin, J.H. Growdon, K.L. Davis, E. Usdin, R.J. Wurtman), Raven Press, New York.

Davison, A. (1985). The pathophysiology of dementia, *Practical Reviews in Psychiatry*, **6**, 1–4.

de Alarcon, J.G. (1971). Social causes and social consequences of mental illness in old age, in *Recent Developments in Psychogeriatrics* (Eds. D.W.K. Kay, A. Walk), Royal Medico-Psychological Association, London.

Denham, M.J. and Jefferys, P.M. (1972). Routine mental testing in the elderly, *Mod. Geriat.*, **2**, 275–279.

Department of Health and Social Security (1970). *Psycho-geriatric Assessment Units*, Circular HM(70)11, HMSO, London.

Department of Health and Social Security (1975). *Better Services for the Mentally Ill*, Cmnd. 6233, HMSO, London.

Department of Health Social Security (1979). *Nutrition and Health in Old Age: Report on Health and Social Subjects* No. 16, HMSO, London.

Department of Health and Social Security (1983). *Mental Health Act 1983: Memorandum on Parts I to IV, VIII and X*, HMSO, London.

Department of Health and Social Security (1986). *Neighbourhood Nursing — A Focus for Care* (The Cumberledge Report), HMSO, London.

Department of Health and Social Security and Welsh Office (1977). *Residential Homes for the Elderly: Arrangements for Health Care, A Memorandum of Guidance*, HMSO, London.

218

Department of Health and Social Security and Welsh Office (1978). *A Happier Old Age: A Discussion Document on Elderly People in our Society*, HMSO. London.

Dewhurst, K. (1969). The neurosyphilitic psychoses today: a survey of 91 cases, *Br. J. Psychiat*, **115**, 31–8.

De Wied, D. (1969). Effects of peptide hormones on behavior, in *Frontiers in Neuroendocrinology* (Eds. W.F. Ganong and L. Martini), Oxford University Press, New York.

De Wied, D. (1977). Behavioral effects of neuropeptides related to ACTH, MSH and β-LPH, *Ann. NY Acad. Sci.*, **297**, 263–74.

Dick, J.P., Guiloff, R.J., Stewart, A., Blackstock, J., Bielawski, C., Paul, E.A. and Marsden, C.D. (1984). Mini-mental state examination in neurological patients, *J. Neurol. Neurosurg. Psychiat.*, **47**, 496–9.

Diederichsen, H. and Pyndt, I.C. (1968). Antibodies against neuron in a patient with systemic lupus erythematosus, cerebral palsy and epilepsy, *Brain*, **93**, 407–12.

Dove, A.F. and Dave, S.H. (1968). Elderly patients in the accident department and their problems, *Br. Med. J.*, **292**, 807–9.

Drachman, D.A. and Leavitt, J. (1974). Human memory and the cholinergic system. A relationship to ageing? *Arch Neurol.*, **30**, 113–21.

Dreyfus, P.M. (1974). Diseases of the nervous system in chronic alcoholism, in *The Biology of Alcoholism*, Vol. 3 (Eds. B. Kissin and H. Begleiter), Plenum Press, New York.

Drug and Therapeutics Bulletin (1984). The drug treatment of senile dementia, **22**(25), 98–100.

DSM III (1980). *Diagnostic and Statistical Manual of Mental Disorders*, 3rd end., American Psychiatric Association, Washington DC.

Duckett, S. and Galle, P. (1976). Mise en évidence de l'aluminium dans les plaques séniles de la maladie d'Alzheimer: Étude a la microsonde de Castaing, *C.R. Acad. Sci. (d)*, **282**, 393–5.

Duffy, F., Wolf, J., Collins, G., DeVoe, A.G., Streeten, B. and Cowen, D. (1974). Possible person-to-person transmission of Creutzfeldt-Jakob disease. *N. Engl. J. Med.*, **299**, 692–3.

Dunant, Y. and Israel, M. (1985). The release of acetylcholine, *Sci. Am.*, **254**(4), 40–8.

Dunn, T. and Arie, T. (1973). Mental disturbance in the ill old person, *Br. Med. J.*, **ii**, 413–16.

Eagles, J.M. and Gilleard, C.J. (1984). The demented elderly admitted to a psychogeriatric assessment unit: changes in disability and outcome from 1977–82, *Br. J. Psychiat.*, **144**, 314–16.

Eagles, J.M. and Gilleard, C.J. (1985). Factors affecting admission and discharge placements of demented elderly patients, *J. Clin. Soc. Psychiat.*, **3**, 29–33.

Eastwood, L.M. Hutchison, J.M.S. and Besson, J.A.O. (1985). Nuclear magnetic resonance (NMR). 1. Imaging biochemical change, *Br. J. Psychiat.*, **146**, 26–31.

Edwards, D., Hawker, A., Hensman, C., Peto, J. and Williamson, V. (1973). Alcoholics known or unknown to agencies: epidemiological status in a London suburb, *Br. J. Psychiat.*, **12**, 169–83.

Eley, R. and Middleton, M. (1983). Square pegs, round holes? The appropriateness of providing care for old people in residential settings, *Health Trends*, **15**, 68–70.

Elithorn, A. and Telford, A. (1969). Computer analysis of intellectual skills, *Int. J. Man-Machine Studies*, **1**, 189–209.

Ellis, W.G., McCullough, J.R. and Corley, C.L. (1974). Presenile dementia in Down's syndrome: ultrastructural identity with Alzheimer's disease, *Neurology*, **24**, 101–6.

Enduring Powers of Attorney Act 1985, HMSO, London.

Equal Opportunities Commission (1984). *Carers and Services: A Comparison of Men and Women Caring for Dependent Elderly People*, Equal Opportunities Commission, London.

Essen-Möller, E. (1956). Individual traits and morbidity in a Swedish rural population, *Acta Psychiat. Neurol. Scand.*, Suppl. 100.

Etienne, P., Gauthier, S., Johnson, G., Collier, B., Mendis, T., Dastoor, D., Cole, M. and Muller, H.F. (1979). Clinical effects of choline in Alzheimer's disease, *Lancet*, **i**, 508–9.

Exton-Smith, A.N. (1980). Nutritional status: diagnosis and prevention of malnutrition, in *Metabolic and Nutritional Disorders in the Elderly* (Eds. A.N. Exton-Smith and F.I. Caird), Wright, Bristol.

Exton-Smith, A.N. (1984). Metabolic bone disease and fracture of the femoral neck, in *Aging and Drug Therapy* (Eds. G. Barbagallo-Sangiorgi and A.N. Exton-Smith), Plenum Press, New York.

Exton-Smith, A.N. and Witts, D.J. (1980). A comparison of chlormethiazole and nitrazepam as hypnotics in elderly subjects — with a note on the pharmacokinetics of chlormethiazole, in *Current Trends in Therapeutics in the Elderly* (Ed. A.N. Exton-Smith), Medical Education (Services), Oxford.

Exton-Smith, A.N. McLaren, R. and Norton, D. (1975). *An Investigation of Geriatric Nursing Problems in Hospital*, Churchill Livingstone, Edinburgh.

Exton-Smith, A.N., Murray, N., Moffat, B., Jayne, D., Wallace, M.G. and Simpson, J.M. (1983). Pilot study of the effect of Hydergine on the event-related evoked potential and on psychological and behavioural indices in dementia, *Br. J. Clin. Pract.*, Suppl. 30, 29–32.

Faculty of Community Medicine (1986). *Charter for Action*, Royal College of Physicians, London.

Ferenczi, S. (1922). Psychoanalysis and the mental disorders of general paralysis of the insane, reprinted in *Final Contributions to the Problems and Methods of Psychoanalysis* (Ed. M. Balint), Hogarth Press, London.

Ferris, S.H., Reisberg, B., Cook, T., Friedman, E., Schneck, M., Mir, P., Sherman, K.A., Corwin, J., Gershon, S. and Bartus, R. (1982). Pharmacologic treatment of senile dementia: choline, L-dopa, piracetam, and choline plus piracetam, in *Alzheimer's Disease: A Report of Progress in Research* (Eds. S. Corkin, J.H. Growdon, K.L. Davis, E. Usdin and R.J. Wurtman), Raven Press, New York.

Ferry, G. (1987). The genetic roots of dementia, *New Scientist*, 12.3.87, 20–21.

Fine, C.W., Lewis, D., Villa-Landa, I. and Blakemore, C.B. (1970). The effect of cyclandelate on mental function in patients with arteriosclerotic brain disease, *Br. J. Psychiat.*, **117**, 157–61.

Finkelstein, M.S. (1984). Defences against infection in the elderly: the compromises of aging, *Triangle*, **23**(2), 57–64.

Fisch, M., Goldfarb, A.I., Shahinian, S.P. and Turner, H. (1968). Chronic brain syndrome in the community aged, *Arch. Gen. Psychiat.*, **18**, 739–45.

Fischer, R.H. (1975). The urinary excretion of homovanyllic acid and 4-hydroxy-3-methoxy mandelic acid in the elderly demented, *Geront. Clin.*, **14**, 172–5.

Fish, F. and Williamson, J. (1964). A delirium unit in an acute general hospital, *Geront. Clin.*, **6**, 71–80.

Fisher, C.M. (1962). Concerning recurrent transient cerebral ischaemic attacks, *Can. Med. Ass. J.*, **96**, 1091–9.

Fisher, C.M. (1968). Dementia in cerebral vascular disease, in *Transactions of the Sixth Conference on Cerebral Vascular Disease*, American Neurological Association, Grune and Stratton, New York.

Flament-Durand, J. and Couck, A.M. (1979). Spongiform alterations in brain biopsies of presenile dementia, *Acta Neuropathol.*, **46**, 159–62.

Flint, F.J. and Richards, S.M. (1956). Organic basis of confusional states in the elderly, *Br. Med. J.*, **ii**, 1537–9.

Folsom, J.C. (1967). Intensive hospital therapy for geriatric patients, *Curr. Psychiat. Ther.*, **7**, 209–15.

Folsom, J.C. (1968). Reality orientation for the elderly patient, *J. Geriat. Psychiat.*, **1**, 291–307.

Folstein, M.F., Folstein, S.E. and McHugh, P.R. (1975). 'Mini-Mental State'. A practical method for grading the cognitive state of patients for the clinician, *J. Psychiat. Res.*, **12**, 189–98.

Foster, E.M., Kay, D.W.K. and Bergmann, K. (1976). The characteristics of old people receiving and needing domiciliary services: the relevance of psychiatric diagnosis, *Age Ageing*, **5**, 245–55.

Fox, R.H., Woodward, R.M., Exton-Smith, A.N., Green, M.F., Dennison, D.V. and Wicks, M.A. (1973). Body temperatures in the elderly: a national survey of physiological, social and environmental conditions, *Br. Med. J.*, **i**, 200–6.

Fraser, R.M. (1984). Treatment of depression in the elderly, in *Aging and Drug Therapy* (Eds. G. Barbagallo-Sangiorgi and A.N. Exton-Smith), Plenum Press, New York.

Fraser, R.M. and Glass, I.B. (1980). Unilateral and bilateral ECT in elderly patients, *Acta Psychiat. Scand.*, **62**, 13–31.

Fraser, R.M. and Healy, R. (1986). Psychogeriatric liaison: a service to a district general hospital, *Bull. Roy. Coll. Psychiat.*, **10**, 312–14.

Frey, T.S. and Sjörgen, H. (1959). The electroencephalogram in elderly persons suffering from neuropsychiatric disorder, *Acta Psychiat. Scand.*, **34**, 38–50.

Fries, J.F. (1980). Aging, natural death, and the compression of morbidity, *N. Engl. J. Med.*, **303**, 130–5.

Gaitz, C.M., Varner, R.V. and Overall, J.E. (1977). Pharmacotherapy for organic brain syndrome in late life: evaluation of an ergot derivative vs. placebo, *Arch. Gen. Psychiat.*, **34**, 839–45.

Gadjusek, D.D. (1977). Unconventional viruses and the origin and disappearance of kuru, *Science*, **197**, 943–60.

Gajdusek, D.C. and Zigas, V. (1957). Degenerative disease of the central nervous system in New Guinea. The endemic occurrence of 'kuru' in the native population, *N. Engl. J. Med.*, **257**, 947–8.

Garland, M. and James, M. (1978). Incontinence in the elderly, *Hosp. Update*, **4**, 819–33.

Garruto, R.M., Yanagihara, R. and Gajdusek, D.C. (1985). Disappearance of high-incidence amyotrophic lateral sclerosis and parkinsonism–dementia on Guam, *Neurology*, **35**, 193–8.

Gaspar, D. (1980). Hollymoor Hospital dementia service, *Lancet*, **i**, 1402–5.

Gedye, J.L. and Miller, E. (1970). Developments in automated testing systems, in *The Psychological Assessment of Mental and Physical Handicaps* (Ed. P. Mittler), Methuen, London.

General Household Survey 1980 and 1981 (1982 and 1983). Office of Population Censuses and Surveys, Social Services Division, HMSO, London.

Geschwind, N. (1968). The mechanism of normal pressure hydrocephalus, *J. Neurol. Sci.*, **7**, 481–93.

Gibbs, C.J. Jr, Gajdusek, D.C., Asher, D.M., Alpers, M.P., Beck, E., Daniel, P.M. and Matthews, W.B. (1978). Creutzfeldt-Jakob disease (spongiform encephalopathy): transmission to the chimpanzee, *Science*, **161**, 388–9.

Gibson, A.J. and Kendrick, D.C. (1976). The development of a visual learning test to replace the SLT in the Kendrick Battery, *Bull. Br. Psychol. Soc.*, **29**, 200–1.

Gibson, A.J. and Kendrick, D.C. (1979). *The Kendrick Battery for the Detection of Dementia in the Elderly*, NFER Publishing, Windsor.

Gibson, A.J., Moyes, I.C.A. and Kendrick, D. (1980). Cognitive assessment of the elderly long-stay patient, *Br. J. Psychiat.*, **137**, 551–7.

Gibson, P. and Tomlinson, B.E. (1977). The numbers of Hirano bodies in the hippocampus of normal and demented subjects with Alzheimer's disease, *J. Neurol. Sci.*, **33**, 199–206.

Gilleard, C.J. (1981). Incontinence in the hospitalised elderly, *Health Bull. (Edinburgh)*, **39**, 58–61.

Gilleard, C.J. (1984). *Living with Dementia*, Croom Helm, London.

Gilleard, C.J., Belford, H., Gilleard, E., Whittock, J.E. and Gledhill, K. (1984a). Emotional distress among the supporters of the elderly mentally infirm, *Br. J. Psychiat.*, **145**, 172–7.

Gilleard, C.J., Gilleard, E. and Whittick, J.E. (1984b). Impact of psychogeriatric day hospital care on the patient's family, *Br. J. Psychiat.*, **145**, 487–92.

Ginzberg, R. (1950). Psychology in everyday geriatrics, *Geriatrics*, **5**, 36–43.

Glatt, M. (1982). *Alcoholism*, MTP Press, Lancaster.

Glenner, G.C., Terry, R.D., Harada, M., Iserky, C. and Page, D. (1971). Amyloid fibril protein, *Science*, **172**, 1150–1.

Glenner, G.C., Terry, R.D. and Isersky, C. (1973). Amyloidosis, its nature and pathogenesis, *Semin. Hematol.*, **10**, 65–82.

Godbole, A. and Verinis, J.S. (1974). Brief psychotherapy in the treatment of emotional disorders in psychiatrically ill geriatric patients, *Gerontologist*, **14**, 143–8.

Goldfarb, A.I. and Turner, H. (1953). Psychotherapy of aged persons. II. Utilization and effectiveness of 'brief therapy', *Am. J. Psychiat.*, **109**, 916–21.

Goldstein, K. and Scheerer, M. (1941). Abstract and concrete behavior: an experimental study with special tests, *Psychol. Monogr.*, **53**(2), 151.

Goodfield, J. (1985). *From the Face of the Earth*, Andre Deutsch, London.

Goodin, D.S., Squires, K.C. and Starr, A. (1980). Long latency event-related components of the auditory evoked potential in dementia, *Brain*, **101**, 635–48.

Goodnick, P.J. (1985). Should ergot mesylates be used for treating senile dementia of the Alzheimer type? *Geriat. Med. Today.*, **4**, 109–13.

Goodwin, F.K. (1971). Psychiatric side-effects of levodopa in man, *JAMA*, **218**, 1915–20.

Gostin, L.O. (1975). *A Human Condition* (Ed. A. Ross), MIND Special Report, National Association of Mental Health, London.

Gotestam, K.G. (1980). Behavioral and dynamic psychotherapy with the elderly, in *Handbook of Mental Health and Aging* (Eds. J.E. Birren and R.B. Sloane), Prentice-Hall, Englewood Cliffs, New Jersey.

Gottfries, C.G. (1980). Amine metabolism in normal ageing and in dementia disorders, in *Biochemistry of Dementia* (Ed. P.J. Roberts), Wiley, Chichester.

Gottfries, C.G. and Roos, B.E. (1973). Acid monoamine metabolites in cerebrospinal fluid from patients with presenile dementia (Alzheimer's disease), *Acta Psychiat. Scand.*, **49**, 257–63.

Goudsmit, J., Morrow, C.H., Asher, D.M., Yanagihara, R.T., Masters, C.L., Gibbs, C.J. Jr. and Gajdusek, D.C. (1980). Evidence for and against the transmissibility of Alzheimer disease, *Neurology*, **30**, 945–50.

Graham, W.L. (1954). The aged sick: admission to hospital or care at home? *Lancet*, **i**, 304–6.

Grainger, K. and Mastaglia, F. (1976). Smoking, transient ischaemic attacks and stroke: a temporal association, *Med. J. Aust.*, **2**, 302–3.

Gray, J.A.M. (1980). Section 47, *Age Ageing*, **4**, 205–9.

Green. A.R. and Costain, D.W. (1981). *Pharmacology and Biochemistry of Psychiatric Disorders*, Wiley, Chichester.

Green, J.G. and Timbury, G.C. (1979). A geriatric psychiatry day hospital service: a five year review, *Age Ageing*, **8**, 49–53.

Greer, A., McBride, D.H. and Shenkin, A. (1986). Comparison of the nutritional state of new and long-term patients in a psychogeriatric unit, *Br. J. Psychiat.*, **149**, 738–41.

222

Grosicki, J.P. (1968). Effect of operant conditioning on modification of incontinence in neuropsychiatric geriatric patients, *Nursing Research*, **17**, 304–11.

Gruenberg, E.M. (1954). Community conditions and psychoses of the elderly, *Am. J. Psychiat.*, **110**, 888–96.

Gruenberg, E.M. (1961). A mental health survey of older persons, in *Comparative Epidemiology of the Mental Disorders* (Eds. P.H. Hoch and J. Zubin), Grune and Stratton, New York.

Grundy, E. (1984). Mortality and morbidity among the old, *Br. Med. J.*, **288**, 663–4.

Gurland, B., Kuriansky, J., Sharpe, L., Simon, R., Stiller, P. and Birkett, P. (1978). The comprehensive assessment and referral evaluation (CARE): rationale, development and reliability, *Int. J. Aging Hum. Dev.*, **8**, 9–42.

Gurland, B., Golden, R. and Challop, J. (1982). Unidimensional and multidimensional approaches to the differentiation of depression and dementia in the elderly, in *Alzheimer's Disease: A Report of Progress in Research* (Eds. S. Corkin, J.H. Growdon, K.L. Davis, E. Usdin and R.J. Wurtman), Raven Press, New York.

Hachinski, V.C. (1978). Cerebral blood flow: differentiation of Alzheimer's disease from multi-infarct dementia, in *Alzheimer's Disease: Senile Dementia and Related Disorders* (Eds. R. Katzman, R.D. Terry and K.L. Blick), Raven Press, New York.

Hachinski, V.C., Lassen, N.A. and Marshall, J. (1974). Multi-infarct dementia: a cause of mental deterioration in the elderly, *Lancet*, **ii**, 207–10.

Hachinski, V.C., Iliff, L.D., Zilkha, E., DuBoulay, G.H., McAllister, J., Ross Russell, R.W. and Symon, L. (1975). Cerebral blood flow in dementia, *Arch. Neurol.*, **32**, 632–7.

Hagnell, O. (1970). Disease expectancy and incidence of mental illness among the aged, *Acta Psychiat. Scand.*, Suppl. 219, 83–9.

Hagnell, O., Lanke, J., Rorsman, B. and Öjesjö, L. (1981). Does the incidence of age psychosis decrease? *Neuropsychobiol.*, **7**, 201–11.

Hahn, R.D., Webster, B., Weickhardt, G., Thomas, E., Timberlake, W., Solomon, H., Stokes, J.H., Moore, J.E., Heyman, A., Gammon, G., Gleeson, G.A., Curtis, A.C. and Cutler, J.C. (1959). Penicillin treatment of general paresis (dementia paralytica), *Arch. Neurol. Psychiat.*, **81**, 557–90.

Hakim, I.M. and Mathieson, G. (1979). Dementia in Parkinson's disease: a neuropathologic study, *Neurology*, **29**, 1209–14.

Halgin, R., Riklan, M. and Misiah, H. (1977). Levodopa, parkinsonism, and recent memory, *J. Nerv. Ment. Dis.*, **164**, 269–72.

Hamilton, M. (1960). A rating scale for depression, *J. Neurol. Neurosurg. Psychiat.*, **23**, 56–62.

Hancock, M.R., Hullin, R.P., Ayland, P.R., King, J.R. and Morgan, D.B. (1985). Nutritional status of the elderly on admission to mental hospital, *Br. J. Psychiat.*, **147**, 404–7.

Hanley, I.G., McGuire, R.J. and Boyd, W.D. (1981). Reality orientation and dementia: a controlled trial of two approaches, *Br. J. Psychiat.*, **138**, 10–14.

Harding, G.F.A., Wright, C.E. and Orwin, A. (1985). Primary presenile dementia: the use of the visual evoked potential as a diagnostic indicator, *Br. J. Psychiat.*, **147**, 532–9.

Hardy, T.K. and Wakely, D. (1962). The amnesic properties of hyoscine and atropine in pre-anaesthetic medication, *Anaesthesia*, **17**, 331–6.

Hare, M. (1978). Clinical check-list for diagnosis of dementia, *Br. Med. J.*, **ii**, 266–7.

Harner, R.N. (1975). EEG evaluation of the patient with dementia, in *Psychiatric Aspects of Neurological Disease* (Eds. D.F. Benson and D. Blumer), Grune and Stratton, New York.

Harrison, M.J.G., Thomas, D.J., du Boulay, G.H. and Marshall, J. (1979). Multi-infarct dementia, *J. Neurol. Sci.*, **40**, 97–103.

Hartelius, H. (1972). An Investigation of Mental Morbidity in a Rural County in the

South of Sweden, *Acta Psychiat. Scand.*, Suppl. 228.

Hassall, C., Gath, D. and Cross, K.W. (1972). Psychiatric day-care in Birmingham, *Br. J. Prev. Soc. Med.*, **26**, 112–20.

Hayflick, L. (1983). Perspectives in biogerontology, in *Geropsychiatric Diagnostics and Treatment* (Ed. M. Bergener), Springer, New York.

Hazzard, W. (1984). Paper at Conference on Sex Differentials in Aging, Johns Hopkins School of Medicine, Baltimore.

Health Advisory Service (1982). *The Rising Tide*, Health Advisory Service, London.

Heath, R.G. and Krupp, I.M. (1967). Schizophrenia as an immunologic disorder, *Arch. Gen. Psychiat.*, **16**, 1–9.

Helgason, T. (1977). Psychiatric Services and Mental Illness in Iceland, *Acta Psychiat. Scand.*, Suppl. 268.

Hendrickson, E., Levy, R. and Post, F. (1979). Averaged evoked responses in relation to cognitive and affective state of elderly psychiatric patients, *Br. J. Psychiat.*, **134**, 494–501.

Herbst, K.R.G. (1982). Deafness, dementia and depression, in *Psychopharmacology of Old Age* (Ed. D. Wheatley), Oxford Medical Publications, Oxford.

Heston, L.L. (1984). Down's syndrome and Alzheimer's disease: defining an association, *Psychiat. Dev.*, **4**, 287–294.

Heston, L.L. Mastri, R., Anderson, V.W. and White, J. (1981). Dementia of the Alzheimer type, *Arch. Gen. Psychiat.*, **38**, 1085–90.

Hewitt, K.E., Carter, G. and Jancar, J. (1985). Ageing in Down's syndrome, *Br. J. Psychiat.*, **147**, 58–62.

Heyman, A., Wilkinson, W.E., Hurwitz, B.J., Schmechel, D., Sigmon, A.H., Weinberg, T., Helms, M.J. and Swift, M. (1983). Alzheimer's disease: genetic aspects and associated clinical disorders, *Ann. Neurol.*, **14**, 507–15.

Hirano, A. (1965). Slow, latent and temporate virus infections, in *Monograph No. 2, Nat. Inst. of Health* (Eds. D.C. Gajdusek and C.J. Gibbs, Jr).

Hodkinson, H.M. (1972). Evaluation of a mental test score for assessment of mental impairment in the elderly, *Age Ageing*, **1**, 233–8.

Hodkinson, H.M. (1973). Mental impairment in the elderly, *J. Roy. Coll. Phycns*, **7**, 305–17.

Holden, U.P. and woods, R.T. (1982). *Reality Orientation: Psychological Approaches to the 'Confused' Elderly*, Churchill Livingstone, Edinburgh.

Hollister, L.E. (1983). Clinical trials of a co-dergocrine in senile dementia, *Br. J. Clin. Pract.*, Suppl. 30, 41–45.

Holt, R. (1984). *Hansard*, April 9.

Howard, R.C., Fenton, F.W. and Fenwick, P.B.C. (1984). The contingent negative variation, personality and antisocial behaviour, *Br. J. Psychiat.*, **144**, 463–474.

Huber, S.J. and Paulson, G.W. (1985). The concept of subcortical dementia, *Am. J. Psychiat.*, **142**, 1312–16.

Hughes, C.P. and Gado, M. (1984). Recognition of hydrocephalus as a cause of dementia in the elderly, *Geriat. Med. Today*, **3**, 108–22.

Hughes, C.P., Berg, L., Danziger, W.L., Coben, L.A. and Martin, R. (1982). A new clinical scale for the staging of dementia, *Br. J. Psychiat.*, **140**, 566–72.

Hulicka, I.M. (1966). Age differences in Wechsler Memory Scale scores, *J. Genet. Psychol.*, **109**, 135–45.

Hunt, L.B. (1985). Implementation of policies for community care — the DHSS contribution, *Health Trends*, **17**, 4–5.

Hunter, R. Dayan, A.D. and Wilson, J. (1972). Alzheimer's disease in one monozygotic twin, *J. Neurol. Neurosurg. Psychiat.*, **35**, 707–10.

Hyman, B.T., Van Hoesen, G.W., Damasio, A.R. and Barnes, C.L. (1984). Alzheimer's disease: cell-specific pathology isolates the hippocampal formation, *Science*, **225**, 1168–70.

224

Inglis, J. (1959). A paired associate learning test for use with elderly psychiatric patients, *J. Ment. Sci.*, **105**, 440–8.

Ingvar. D.H., Brun, A., Hagberg, B. and Gustafson, L. (1978). Regional cerebral blood flow in the dominant hemisphere in confirmed cases of Alzheimer's disease, Parkinson's disease and multi-infarct dementia: relationship to clinical symptomatology and neuropathological findings, in *Alzheimer's Disease: Senile Dementia and Related Disorders* (Eds. R. Katzman, R.D. Terry and K.L. Blick), Raven Press, New York.

Irving, G., Robinson, R.A. and McAdam, W. (1970). The validity of some cognitive tests of dementia, *Br. J. Psychiat.*, **117**, 149–56.

Iversen, L.L. (1979). The chemistry of the brain, in *The Brain: A Scientific American Book*, Freeman, San Francisco.

Iversen, L.L., Rossor, M.N., Reynolds, G.P., Hills, R., Roth, M., Mountjoy, C.Q., Foote, S.L., Morrison, J.H. and Bloom, F.E. (1983). Loss of pigmented dopamine-beta-hydroxylase positive cells from locus coeruleus in senile dementia of Alzheimer's type, *Neurosci. Lett.*, **39**, 95–100.

Jacoby, R.J., Levy, R. and Dawson, J.M. (1980a). Computerised tomography in the elderly. 1. The normal population, *Br. J. Psychiat.*, **136**, 249–55.

Jacoby, R.J., Levy, R. and Dawson, J.M. (1980b). Computerised tomography in the elderly. 2. Senile dementia — diagnosis and functional impairment, *Br. J. Psychiat.*, **136**, 256–69.

Jacoby, R.J., Dolan, R.J., Levy, R. and Baldy, R. (1983). Quantitative computerised tomography in elderly depressed patients, *Br. J. Psychiat*, **143**, 124–7.

Jakob, A. (1921). Über eigenartige Erkrankung des Zentralnerven systems mit bemerkenswertem anatomischen Befunde (Spastiche Pseudosklerose-Encephalomyelopathis mit dissemimerten Degenerationsherden). *Dtsch Z. Nervenheilkunde*, **70**, 132–46.

Jamada, M. and Mehraein, P. (1968). Über die Haufigkeit der Zerebralen Arteriosklerose bei Morbus Alzheimer und seniler Dementia, *Arzneimittel-Forsch.*, **22**, 133–6.

Janowsky, D.S., Risch, S.C., Huey, L.Y., Kennedy, B. and Ziegler, M. (1985). Effects of physostigmine on pulse, blood pressure, and serum epinephrine levels, *Am. J. Psychiat.*, **142**, 738–40.

Jarvis, G.J. and Miller, D.R. (1980). Controlled trial of bladder drill for detrusor instability, *Br. Med. J.*, **ii**, 1322.

Jervis, G.A. (1971). Pick's disease, in *Pathology of the Nervous System* (Ed. J. Minckler), McGraw-Hill, New York.

Jones, D.A. and Vetter, N.J. (1985). Formal and informal support received by carers of elderly dependents, *Br. Med. J.*, **281**, 643–5.

Jones, I.G. and Munbodh, R. (1982). An evaluation of a day hospital for the demented elderly, *Health Bull. (Edinburgh)*, **40**, 10–15.

Jonker, C., Eikelenboom, P. and Tavernier, P. (1982). Immunological indices in the cerebrospinal fluid of patients with presenile dementia of the Alzheimer type, *Br. J. Psychiat.*, **140**, 44–9.

Judge, I.G. (1968). Hypokalaemia in the elderly, *Geront. Clin.*, **10**, 102–7.

Junod, J.-P. (1981). *Médicine et Hygiene, 1967 à 1981*, Institutions de Gériatrie, Geneva.

Kahana, E., Alter, M., Brahman, J. and Sofer, D. (1974). Creutzfeldt-Jakob disease: focus among Libyan Jews in Israel, *Science*, **183**, 90–1.

Kallmann, F.J. (1950). The genetics of psychoses — an analysis of 1232 index families, *Congrès Internationale de Psychiatrie*, Vol. 6, Hermann et Cie, Paris.

Kalter, S. and Kelly, S. (1975). Alzheimer's disease: evaluation of immunological indices, *NY State J. Med.*, **75**, 1221–5.

Kaneko, Z. (1969). Abstract 284, *Proc. 8th Int. Congress of Gerontology*, Washington DC.

225

Kang, J., Lemaire, H.-G., Unterbeck, A., Salbaum, J.M., Masters, C.L., Grzeschik, K-H, Multaup, G., Beyreuther, K. and Müller-Hill, B. (1987). The precursor of Alzheimer's disease amyloid A4 protein resembles a cell-surface receptor, *Nature*, **325**, 733–736.

Katzman, R. (1978). Normal pressure hydrocephalus, in *Alzheimer's Disease: Senile Dementia and Related Disorders* (Eds. R. Katzman, R.D. Terry and K.L. Blick), Raven Press, New York.

Kay, D.W.K. and Bergmann, K. (1980). Epidemiology of mental disorders amongst the aged in the community, in *Handbook of Mental Health and Aging* (Eds. J.E. Birren and R.B. Sloane), Prentice-Hall, New Jersey.

Kay, D.W.K. and Roth, M. (1955). Physical accompaniments of mental disorder in old age, *Lancet*, **ii**, 740–5.

Kay, D.W.K., Beamish, P. and Roth, M. (1964a). Old age mental disorders in Newcastle upon Tyne. I.A. study of prevalence, *Br. J. Psychiat.*, **110**, 146–58.

Kay, D.W.K., Beamish, P. and Roth, M. (1964b). Old age mental disorders in Newcastle upon Tyne. II. A study of possible social and medical causes, *Br. J. Psychiat.*, **110**, 668–82.

Kay, D.W.K., Bergmann, K., Foster, E.M., McKechnie, A.A. and Roth, M. (1970). Mental illness and hospital usage in the elderly: a random sample followed up, *Comp. Psychiat.*, **11**, 26–35.

Kay, M.M.B. (1985). Immunological changes associated with normal aging, *Geriat. Med. Today*, **4**, 30–37.

Kaye, W.H., Weingartner, H., Gold, P., Ebert, M.H., Gilin, J.C., Sitaram, N. and Smallberg, S. (1982). Cognitive effects of cholinergic and vasopressin-like agents in patients with primary degenerative dementia, in *Alzheimer's Disease: A Report of Progress in Research* (Eds. S. Corkin, J.H. Growdon, K.L. Davis, E. Usdin and R.J. Wurtman), Raven Press, New York.

Kellett, J.M., Copeland, J.R.H. and Kelleher, M.J. (1975). Information leading to accurate diagnosis in the elderly, *Br. J. Psychiat.*, **126**, 423–30.

Kelley, A.A., Stinus, L. and Iversen, S.D. (1979). Behavioural activation induced in the rat by substance P infusion into the ventral tegmental area: implication of dopaminergic A10 neurones, *Neurosci. Lett.*, **11**, 335.

Kendrick, D.C. (1965). Speed in learning in the diagnosis of diffuse brain pathology in elderly subjects: a bayesian statistical approach. *Br. J. Soc. Clin. Psychol.*, **4**, 141–8.

Kendrick, D.C. (1967). A cross validation of the SLT and DCT in screening for diffuse brain pathology in elderly patients, *Br. J. Med. Psychol.*, **40**, 173–8.

Kennes, B., Dumont, I., Brohee, D., Hubert, C. and Neve, P. (1983). Effect of vitamin C supplements on cell-mediated immunity in old people, *Gerontol.*, **29**, 305–10.

Kirschbaum, W.R. (1968). *Jakob-Creutzfeldt Disease*, Elsevier, New York.

Kirshner, H.S. (1984). Language disturbance: an initial symptom of cortical degeneration and dementia, *Arch. Neurol.*, **41**, 491–6.

Klonoff, H. and Kennedy, M. (1965). Memory and perceptual functioning in octogenarians and nonagenarians in the community. *J. Geront.*, **20**, 328–33.

Klonoff, H. and Kennedy, M. (1966). A comparative study of cognitive functioning in old age, *J. Geront.*, **21**, 239–43.

Knuttson, E. and Lying-Tunnell, V. (1985). Gait apraxia in normal-pressure hydrocephalus: pattern of movement and muscle inactivation, *Neurology*, **35**, 155–60.

Kopelman, M.D. (1986). Clinical tests of memory, *Br. J. Psychiat.*, **148**, 517–25.

Kraepelin, E. (1893). *Psychiatrie*, 4th ed., Meiner, Leipzig.

Kraepelin, E. (1910). *Psychiatrie*, 8th ed., vol. 2., Barth, Leipzig.

Kraepelin, E. (1912). *Psychiatrie*, 7th ed., abstr. by A.R. Diefendorf, Macmillan, London.

Kral, V.A. (1962). Senescent forgetfulness: benign and malignant, *Can. Med. Ass. J.*, **86**, 257–60.

226

Kramer, M. (1980). The rising pandemic of mental disorders and associated chronic diseases and disabilities, in *Epidemiological Research as Basis for the Organisation of Extramural Psychiatry* (eds. E. Strömgren, A. Dupont and J.A. Nielsen), *Acta Psychiat. Scand.*, **62**, Suppl. 285, 382–97.

Kristensen, V., Olsen, N. and Thielgaard, A. (1977). Levodopa treatment of presenile dementia, *Acta Psychiat. Scand.*, **55**, 41–51.

Krnjević, K., Reinhardt, W. and Ropert, N. (1982). Choline as an acetylcholine agonist in the mammalian neocortex and hippocampus, in *Alzheimer's Disease: A Report of Progress in Research* (Eds. S. Corkin, J.H. Growdon, K.L. Davis, E. Usdin and R.J. Wurtman), Raven Press, New York.

Kugler, J., Oswald, W.D., Herzfeld, U., Suens, R., Pingel, J. and Wetzel, D. (1978). Langzeittherapie altersbedingter Insuffizienzerscheinungen des Gehirns, *Detsch. Med. Wschr.*, **103**, 456–62.

Kuhar, M.J. and Atweh, S.F. (1978). Distribution of some suspected neurotransmitters in the central nervous system, *Rev. Neurosci.*, **3**, 35–86.

Lafora, G.R. (1911). Beitrag zur Kenntnis der Altzheimereschen Krankheit oder prasenilen Demenz mit Herdsymptomen, *Z. ges. Neurol. Psychiat.*, **6**, 15–20.

Lapresle, J., Duckett, S., Galle, P. and Cartier, L. (1975). Documents cliniques, anatomiques et biophysiques dans une encéphalopathie avec présence de dépôts d'aluminium, *C.R. Soc. Biol.*, **169**, 282–5.

Larsson, T., Sjörgen, T. and Jacobson, G. (1963). Senile Dementia: a Clinical, Sociomedical and Genetic Study, *Acta Psychiat. Scand.*, Suppl. 167.

Laslett, P. (1977). *Family Life and Illicit Love in Earlier Generations*, Cambridge University Press, Cambridge.

Lauter, H. and Meyer, J.E. (1968). Clinical and nosological concepts of senile dementia, in *Senile Dementia: Clinical and Therapeutic Aspects* (Eds. C.H. Müller and L. Compi), Huber, Bern.

Law Commission, (1976). The Incapacitated Principal, Working Paper No. 69, HMSO, London.

Law Commission (1983). *The Incapacitated Principal*, Cmnd. 8977, HMSO, London.

Leading Article (1979a). Planning for the old and very old, *British Medical Journal*, **ii**, 952.

Leading Article (1979b). Vasodilators in senile dementia, *British Medical Journal*, **ii**, 511–12.

Learoyd, B.M. (1972). Psychotropic drugs and the elderly patient, *Med. J. Aust.*, **1**, 1131.

Legros, J.L., Gilot, P., Seron, X., Claessens, J., Adam, A., Moeglen, J.M., Audibert, A. and Berchier, P. (1978). Influence of vasopressin on learning and memory, *Lancet*, **i**, 41–2.

Levy, R. (1978). Choline in Alzheimer's disease, *Lancet*, **ii**, 944–5.

Levy, R. (1985). Rational drug treatment of dementia? *Br. Med. J.*, **291**, 139.

Lewis, C., Balinger, B.R. and Presly, A.S. (1978). Trial of levodopa in senile dementia, *Br. Med. J.*, **i**, 550.

Lieberman, A.N. (1983). Parkinsonian dementia and Alzheimer's dementia: clinical and epidemiological associations, in *Alzheimer's Disease: The Standard Reference* (Ed. B. Reisberg), Free Press, New York.

Linnoila, M. and Viukari, M. (1976). Efficacy and side effects of nitrazepam and thioridazine as sleeping aids in psychogeriatric in-patients, *Br. J. Psychiat.*, **128**, 566–9.

Lipowski, Z.J. (1983). The need to integrate liaison psychiatry and geropsychiatry, *Am. J. Psychiat.*, **140**, 1001–5.

Lipsey, J.R., Pearlso, G.D., Robinson, R.G., Rao, K. and Price, T.R. (1984). Nortriptyline treatment of post-stroke depression: a double-blind study, *Lancet*, **i**, 297–300.

Lishman, W.A. (1981). Cerebral disorder in alcoholism, *Brain*, **104**, 1–20.

Lishman, W.A. (1978). *Organic Psychiatry*, Blackwell Scientific, Oxford.

Little, A., Chaqui-Kidd, P. and Levy, R. (1984). Early results from a double-blind placebo controlled trial of high dose lecithin in Alzheimer's disease: psychometric test performance, plasma choline levels and the effects of drug compliance, in *Alzheimer's Disease: Advances in Basic Research and Therapies* (Eds. R.J. Wurtman, S.H. Larkin and J.H. Growdon), Center for Brain Sciences and Metabolism Charitable Trust, Cambridge, Mass.

Lloyd, C.M. (1970). *Royal College of Physicians Study of Mental Impairment in the Elderly*. Report of finding of pilot study, Royal College of Physicians, London.

Loew, D.M. (1980). Pharmacologic aspects to the treatment of senile dementia, in *Aging of the Brain and Dementia* (Eds. L. Amaducci, A.N. Davison and P. Antuono), Raven Press, New York.

Lowenthal, M.F. and Berkman, P. (1967). *Aging and Mental Disorders in San Francisco*, Jossey-Bass, San Francisco.

Lye, M. (1985). Clinical recognition of hypothermia in the elderly, *Geriat. Med. Today*, **4**(3), 63–6.

McCarthy, R. and Gresty, M. (1985). Parkinson's disease and dementia, *Lancet*, **i**, 407.

McDermott, J.R., Smith, A.I., Iqbal, K. and Wisniewski, H.M. (1979). Brain aluminium in aging and Alzheimer disease, *Neurology*, **29**, 809–14.

MacDonald, M.L. and Butler, A.K. (1974). Reversal of helplessness: producing walking behavior in nursing home wheelchair residents using behavior modification procedures, *J. Geront.*, **29**, 97–101.

McDonald, R.J. (1982). Drug treatment of senile dementia, in *Psychopharmacology of Old Age* (Ed. D. Wheatley), Oxford Medical Publications, Oxford.

MacFarlane, A.B. (1985). Medical evidence in the Court of Protection, *Bull. Roy. Coll. Psychiat.*, **9**, 26–8.

McFarlane, P. (1983). Compulsory restraint, in *Advanced Geriatric Medicine* (Eds. J.G. Grimley-Evans and F.I. Caird), Pitman, London.

MacKay, I.R. (1972). Ageing and immunological function in man, *Gerontology*, **18**, 285–304.

McDonald, C. (1969). Clinical heterogenicity in senile dementia, *Br. J. Psychiat.*, **115**, 267–71.

McLaren, S.M., McPherson, F.M., Sinclair, F. and Ballinger, B.R. (1981). Prevalence and severity of incontinence among hospitalised female psychogeriatric patients, *Health Bull. (Edinburgh)*, **39**, 157–61.

McLaughlin, A.I.G., Kazanthis, G., King, E., Teare, D., Porter, R.J. and Owen, R. (1962). Pulmonary fibrosis and encephalopathy associated with the inhalation of aluminium dust, *Br. J. Industr. Med.*, **19**, 253–63.

Macmillan, D. (1960). Preventive geriatrics: opportunities of a community mental health service, *Lancet*, **ii**, 1439–41.

Mahendra, B. (1984). *Dementia: A Survey of the Syndrome of Dementia*, MTP Press, Lancaster.

Malamud, N. (1972). Neuropathology of organic brain syndromes associated with ageing, in *Ageing and the Brain* (Ed. C.M. Gaitz), Plenum Press, New York.

Malamud, N. and Skillicorn, S.A. (1956). Relationship between the Wernicke and the Korsakoff syndrome, *Arch. Neurol. Psychiat.*, **56**, 586–96.

Malone-Lee, J. (1984). The pharmacology of urinary incontinence, in *Aging and Drug Therapy* (Eds. Barbagallo-Sangiorgi and A.N. Exton-Smith), Plenum Press, New York.

Mann, A.H., Graham, N. and Ashby, D. (1984a). Psychiatric illness in residential homes for the elderly: a survey in one London borough, *Age Ageing*, **13**, 257–65.

Mann, A.H., Wood, K., Cross, P., Gurland, B., Scheiber, P. and Hafner, H. (1984b).

Institutional care of the elderly: a comparison of the cities of New York, London and Mannheim, *Soc. Psychiat.*, **19**, 97–102.

Mann, D.M.A. and Sinclair, K.G.A. (1978). The quantitative assessment of lipofuscin pigment, cytoplasmic RNA, and nucleolar volume in senile dementia, *Neuropath. Appl. Neurobiol.*, **4**, 129–35.

Mann, D.M.A., Lincoln, J., Yates, P.O., Stamp, J.E. and Toper, S. (1980). Changes in the monoamine containing neurones of the human CNS in senile dementia, *Br. J. Psychiat.*, **136**, 533–41.

Mann, D.M.A. and Yates, P.O. (1982). Is the loss of cerebral cortical choline acetyl transferase activity in Alzheimer's disease due to degeneration of ascending cholinergic nerve cells? *J. Neurol. Neurosurg. Psychiat.*, **45**, 936–43.

Mann, D.M.A., Yates, P.O. and Marcynuik, B. (1984). Age and Alzheimer's disease, *Lancet*, **i**, 281–2.

Marks, R., Dudley, F. and Wan, A. (1978). Trimethylamine metabolism in liver disease, *Lancet*, **i**, 1106–7.

Marr, J. (1983). The capacity for joy, *Nursing Times*, **1983**, Sept., 56–61.

Marsden, C.D. (1984). Neurological causes of dementia other than Alzheimer's disease, in *Handbook of Studies on Psychiatry and Old Age* (Eds. D.W.K. Kay and G.D. Burrows), Elsevier, Amsterdam.

Marsden, C.D. and Harrison, M.J.G. (1972). Outcome of investigations of patients with presenile dementia, *Br. Med. J.*, **ii**, 249–52.

Masters, C.L. and Gajdusek, D.C. (1982). The spectrum of Creutzfeldt-Jakob disease and the virus-indiced spingiform encephalopathies, in *Recent Advances in Neuropathology*, Vol. 2 (Eds. W.T. Smith and J.B. Cavanagh), Churchill Livingstone, Edinburgh.

Masters, C.L., Harris, J.O., Gajdusek, D.C., Gibbs, C.J. Jr. Bernouilli, C. and Asher, C.M. (1979). Creutzfeldt-Jakob disease: patterns of world-wide occurrence and the significance of familial and sporadic clustering, *Ann. Neurol.*, **5**, 177–88.

Masters, C.L., Gajdusek, D.C. and Gibbs, C.J. Jr (1981). The familial occurrence of Creutzfeldt-Jakob disease and Alzheimer's disease, *Brain*, **104**, 535–58.

Matthews, W.B. (1985). Creutzfeldt-Jakob disease, *Br. Med. J.*, **291**, 483.

May, W.W. (1968). Creutzfeldt-Jakob disease, *Acta Neurol. Scand.*, **44**, 1–32.

Mayer, P.P., Chughtai, M.A. and Cape, R.D.T. (1976). An immunological approach to dementia in the elderly, *Age Ageing.*, **5**, 164–70.

Mayeux, R., Stern, Y., Rosen, G. and Leventhal, J. (1981). Depression, intellectual impairment, and Parkinson's disease, *Neurology*, **31**, 645–9.

Meacher, M. (1972). *Taken for a Ride: Special Residential Homes for Confused Old People*, Longmans, London.

Meaney, T.F. and Weinstein, M.A. (1986). Digital subtraction angiography, in *Diagnostic Radiology*, Churchill Livingstone, London.

Meier-Ruge, W., Emmenegger, H., Enz, A., Gygax, P., Iwangoff, P. and Wiernsperger, N. (1978). Pharmacological aspects of dihydrogenated ergot alkaloids in experimental brain research, *Psychopharmacology*, **16**, Suppl. 1, 45–62.

Mellstrom, D., Rundgren, A. and Svanborg, A. (1981). Previous alcohol consumption and its consequences for aging, morbidity and mortality in men aged 70 to 75, *Age Ageing*, **10**, 277–86.

Mental Health Act 1983, HMSO, London.

Mental Health Act Commission (1985a) *Consent to Treatment: discussion paper*, Mental Health Act Commission, London.

Mental Health Act Commission (1985b). *The First Biennial Report of the Mental Health Act Commission*, HMSO, London.

Millard, P.H. (1984). Treatment for ageing brains, *Br. Med. J.*, **289**, 1094.

Millard, P.H., Peel, E. and Thomas, S. (1984). Nutrition of elderly patients in long-stay wards, in *Aging and Drug Therapy* (Eds. G. Barbagallo-Sangiorgi and A.N. Exton-Smith), Plenum Press, New York.

Miller, E. (1968). A case for automated clinical testing, *Bull. Br. Psychol. Soc.*, **21**, 75–8.

Miller, E. (1977). *Abnormal Ageing: The Psychology of Senile and Presenile Dementia*, Wiley, London.

Milner, B. (1970). Memory and the medial temporal region of the brain, in *Biology of Memory* (Eds. K.H. Pribram and D.E. Broadbent), Academic Press, New York.

Moffatt, W.R., Siddiqui, A.R. and McKay, D.N. (1970). The use of sulthiame with mentally disturbed subnormal patients, *Br. J. Psychiat.*, **117**, 673–8.

Mohs, R.C., Rosen, W.G. and Davis, K.L. (1982). Defining treatment efficacy in patients with Alzheimer's disease, in *Alzheimer's Disease: A Report of Progress in Research* (Eds. S. Corkin, J.G. Growdon, K.L. Davis, E. Usdin, R.J. Wurtman), Raven Press, New York.

Montgomery, S.A. (1982). Treatment of depression in old age, in *Psychopharmacology of Old Age* (Ed. D. Wheatley), Oxford Medical Publications, Oxford.

Moore, V. and Wyke, M.A. (1984). Drawing disability in patients with senile dementia, *Psychol. Med.*, **14**, 97–105.

Morgan, D.B. (1981). Hypokalaemia and diuretics, in *Arrhythmias and Myocardial Infarction: The Role of Potassium, Royal Society of Medicine International Congress and Symposium Series*, **44**, 3–8.

Morgan, R.F. (1965). Note on the psychopathology of senility: senescent defence against the threat of death, *Psychol. Rep.*, **17**, 305–6.

Motycka, A. and Jandová, Z. (1975). Autoantibodies and brain ischaemic topography, Casopis Lekarv Ceskych (Pratia), **114**, 1455–7.

Munro, H.N. (1982). Overview: nutritional status of the aged, in *Alzheimer's Disease: A Report of Progress in Research* (Ed. S. Corkin, J.H. Growdon, K.L. Davis, E. Usdin and R.J. Wurtman), Raven Press, New York.

Murphy, E. (1985). The GP and the psychogeriatrician, *Geriat. Med.*, **15**(5), 1.

Muslin, H. and Epstein, L.J. (1980). Preliminary remarks on the rationale for psychotherpay of the aged, *Comprehens. Psychiat.*, 21, 1–12.

Naguib, M. and Levy, R. (1982a). Prediction of outcome of senile dementia — a computerised tomography study, *Br. J. Psychiat.*, **140**, 263–7.

Naguib, M. and Levy, R. (1982a). CT scanning in senile dementia: a follow-up of survivors, *Br. J. Psychiat.*, **141**, 618–20.

Nandy, K. (1975). Significance of brain-reactive antibodies in aging and Alzheimer's disease, in *Alzheimer's Disease: Senile Dementia and Related Disorders* (Eds. R.D. Terry, R. Katzman and K.L. Blick), Raven Press, New York.

Nathanson, C. (1984). Paper at Conference on Sex Differentials in Aging, Johns Hopkins School of Medicine, Baltimore.

National Assistance Act 1948, HMSO, London.

National Assistance (Amendment) Act 1951, HMSO, London.

Nayal, S., Castleden, C.M., George, C.F. and Marcer, D. (1978). The effect of an hypnotic with a short half-life on hangover effect in old patients, *Age Aging*, 7, Suppl., 50–4.

Neilsen, J. (1962). Geronto-psychiatric period-prevalence: investigation in a geographically delimited population, *Acta Psychiat. Scand.*, **38**, 307–30.

New York Department of Mental Hygiene (1961). *A Mental Health Survey of Older People*, State Hospitals Press, Utica, New York.

Nikaido, T., Austin, J., Rinehart, R., Trueb, L., Hutchinson, J., Stukenbrok, H. and Miles, B. (1971). Studies in ageing of the brain. 1. Isolation and preliminary characterization of Alzheimer plaques and cores, *Arch. Neurol.*, **25**, 198–211.

Niklowitz, W.J. and Mandybur, T.I. (1975). Neurofibrillary changes following childhood lead encephalopathy, *J. Neurolpathol. Exp. Neurol.*, **34**, 445–55.

Norman, A.J. (1980). Compulsory care, in *Rights and Risk*, National Corporation for the Care of Old People, London.

Nott, P.N. and Fleminger, J.J. (1975). Presenile dementia. The difficulties of early diagnosis, *Acta Psychiat. Scand.*, **51**, 210–17.

Nyström, S. (1967). On relation between clinical features and efficacy of ECT in depression, *Acta. Psychiat. Scand.*, Suppl. 181, 115–18.

Oakley, D.P. (1965). Senile dementia — some aetiological factors, *Br. J. Psychiat.*, **111**, 414–19.

O'Connor, K.P., Shaw, J.C. and Ongley, C.O. (1979). The EEG and differential diagnosis in psychogeriatrics, *Br. J. Psychiat.*, **135**, 156–62.

Office of Health Economics (1980). *Huntingdon's Chorea*, Office of Health Economics, London.

Office of Population Censuses and Surveys (1983). *Social Trends*, 12, HMSO, London.

Oliver, J.E. (1970). Huntingdon's chorea in Northamptonshire, *Br. J. Psychiat.*, **116**, 241–53.

Opit, L.J. and Shaw, S.M. (1976). Care of the elderly sick at home. Whose responsibility is it? *Lancet*, **ii**, 1127–9.

Orwin, A., Wright, C.E., Harding, G.F.A., Rowan, D.C. and Rolfe, E.B. (1986). Serial visual evoked potential recordings in Alzheimer's disease, *Br. Med. J.*, **293**, 9–10.

Outram, G.W. (1980). Mouse scrapie: black box models in slow encephalopathies, in *Animal Models of Neurological Disease* (Eds. F.C. Rose and P.O. Behan), Pitman Medical, Tunbridge Wells.

Overstall, P.W. (1982) Treatment of sleep disturbance in the elderly, in *Psychopharmacology of Old Age* (Ed. D. Wheatley), Oxford Medical Publications, Oxford.

Overstall, P.W. (1984). Pathophysiology of urinary incontinence, in *Ageing and Drug Therapy* (Eds. G. Barbagallo-Sangiori and A.N. Exton-Smith), Plenum Press, New York.

Overstall, P.W., Rounce, K. and Palmer, J.H. (1980). Experience with an incontinence clinic, *J. Am. Geriat. Soc.*, **28**, 535–8.

Paffenberger, R.G. and Wing, A.L. (1971). Chronic disease in former college students. XI. Early precursors of nonfatal stroke, *Am. J. Epidemiol.*, **94**, 524–30.

Pandit, S.K. and Dundee, J.W. (1970). Pre-operative amnesia, *Anaesthesia*, **26**, 493–9.

Pannese, E. (1963). Investigations on the ultrastructural changes of the spinal ganglion neurons in the course of axon regeneration and cell hypertrophy, *Z. Zellforsch.*, **60**, 711–40.

Parfitt. A.M. (1983). Dietary risk factors for age-related bone loss and fractures, *Lancet*, **ii**, 1181–4.

Parkes, J.E., Marsden, C.D., Rees, J.E., Curzon, G., Katamaneni, B.E., Knill-Jones, R., Akbar, A., Das, S. and Kataria, M. (1974). Parkinson's disease, cerebral arteriosclerosis, and senile dementia, *Quart. J. Med. (New Series)*, **28**, 49–61.

Parsons, P.L. (1965). Mental health of Swansea's old folk, *Br. J. Prev. Soc. Med.*, **19**, 43–58.

Pasker, P., Thomas, J.P.R. and Ashley, J.S.A. (1976). The elderly mentally ill — whose responsibility? *Br. Med. J.*, **ii**, 164–6.

Passeri, M. and Palummeri, E. (1984). The prophylaxis of senile osterporosis, in *Aging and Drug Therapy* (Eds. G. Barbagallo-Sangiorgi and A.N. Exton-Smith), Plenum Press, New York.

Patterson, J.A., Michalewski, H.J., Thompson, L.W. and Reisberg, B. (1983). Averaged evoked potentials in dementia, in *Alzheimer's Disease: The Standard Reference* (Ed. B. Reisberg), Free Press, New York.

Patterson, R.M., Bagchi, B.K. and Test, A. (1948). The prediction of Huntingdon's chorea. An electroencephalographic and genetic study, *Am. J. Psychiat.*, **104**, 786–97.

Pattie, A.H. and Gilleard, C.J. (1976). The Clifton Asssessment Scale — further validation of a psychogeriatric assessment schedule, *Br. J. Psychiat.*, **129**, 68–72.

Pattie, A.H. and Gilleard, C.J. (1978a). Admission and adjustment of residents in homes for the elderly, *J. Epid. Comm. Health*, **32**, 212–14.

Pattie, A.H. and Gilleard, C.J. (1978b). The two year predictive validity of the Clifton Assessment Schedule and the shortened Stockton Geriatric Rating Scale, *Br. J. Psychiat.*, **133**, 457–60.

Pattie, A.H. and Gilleard, C.J. (1981). *Clifton Assessment Procedures for the Elderly*, Hodder and Stoughton Educational, Sevenoaks.

Pearce, J. (1974). The extrapyramidal disorder of Alzheimer's disease, *Eur. Neurol.*, **12**, 94–103.

Pearce, J.M.S. (1984). *Dementia: A Clinical Approach*, Blackwell Scientific, Oxford.

Peck, A., Wolloch, L. and Rodstein, M. (1978). Mortality of the aged with chronic brain syndrome: further observations in a five-year study, *J. Am. Geriat. Soc.*, **26**, 170–6.

Penfield, W. and Mathieson, G. (1974). Autopsy findings and comments on the role of the hippocampus in experiential recall, *Arch. Neurol.*, **31**, 145–54.

Perkin, G.D. and Handler, C.E. (1983). Wernicke–Korsakoff syndrome, *Br. J. Hosp. Med.*, **20**, 331–4.

Perry, E.K. and Perry, R.H. (1977). Cholinergic and GABA systems in dementia and old age, *Br. J. Psychiat.*, **131**, 319.

Perry, E.K. and Perry, R.H. (1980). The cholinergic system in Alzheimer's disease, in *Biochemistry of Dementia* (Ed. P.J. Roberts), Wiley, Chichester.

Perry, E.K., Tomlinson, B.E., Blessed, G., Bergmann, K., Gibson, P.H. and Perry, R.H. (1978). Correlation of cholinergic abnormalities with senile plaques and mental test scores in senile dementia, *Br. Med. J.*, **ii**, 1457–9.

Perry, R.H. (1984). Neuropathology of dementia, in *Dementia: A Clinical Approach* (Ed. J.M.S. Pearce), Blackwell Scientific, Oxford.

Perry, R.H., Blessed, G., Perry, E.K. and Tomlinson, B.E. (1980). Histochemical observations on cholinesterase activities in the brains of elderly normal and demented (Alzheimer-type) patients, *Age Ageing*, **9**, 9–16.

Pert, C.B. and Snyder, S.H. (1973). Opiate receptor: demonstration in nervous tissue, *Science*, **179**, 1011.

Peters, B.H. and Levin, H.S. (1979). Effects of physostigmine and lecithin on memory in Alzheimer disease, *Ann. Neurol*, **6**, 219–21.

Pick, A. (1982). Über die Beziehungen der senilen Hirnatrophie zur Aphasie, *Prog. Med. Wschr.*, **17**, 165–7.

Pigache, R.M. (1982). A peptide for the aged? Basic and clinical studies, in *Psychopharmacology of Old Age* (Ed. D. Wheatley), Oxford Medical Publications, Oxford.

Pigache, R.M. and Rigter, H. (1981). Effects of peptides related to ACTH on mood and vigilance in man, in *Frontiers of Hormone Research. ACTH and LPH in Health and Siease* Vol. 8, (Eds. Tj.B. Van Wimersma, Greidanus and L.H. Rees), Karger, Basel.

Pinsker, H. and Suljaga-Petchel, K. (1984). Use of benzodiazepines in primary-care geriatric patients, *J. Am. Geriat. Soc.*, **32**, 595–7.

Post, F. (1975). Diagnosis of depression in geriatric patients and treatment modalities appropriate for the population, in *Depression: Behavioral, Biochemical, Diagnostic and Treatment Concepts* (Eds. D.M. Gallant and G.M. Simpson), Spectrum Publications, New York.

Powell-Jackson, J., Kennedy, P., Whitcombe, E.M., Weller, R.O., Preece, M.A. and Newson-Davis, J. (1985). Creuzfeldt-Jakob disease after administration of human growth hormone, *Lancet*, **ii**, 244–6.

Powers of Attorney Act 1971, HMSO, London.

Prudham, D. and Grimley-Evans, J. (1981). Factors associated with falls in the elderly: a community study, *Age Ageing*, **10**, 141–6.

Prusiner, S.B. (1982a). Novel proteinaceous infectious particles cause scrapie, *Science*, **216**, 136–44.

Prusiner, S.B. (1982b). Research on scrapie, *Lancet*, **ii**, 494–5.

Rabins, P.V., Starr, L.B. and Price, T.R. (1984). A two-year longitudinal study of mood disorders following stroke: prevalence and duration at six months follow-up, *Br. J. Psychiat.*, **144**, 488–92.

Ramsay, R.E. (1984). Brain metabolism and PET scanning, *Curr. Rep. Neurol.*, **6**(2), 7–8.

Redlich, E. (1898). Über miliare Sklerose der Hirnrinde bei seniler Atrophie, *Jahrb. Psychiat. Neurol.*, **17**, 208–21.

Reichenfeld, H.F. (1983). The psychogeriatric day hospital: a specific treatment modality in a multidisciplinary network, in *Geropsychiatric Diagnostics and Treatment* (Ed. M. Bergener), Springer, New York.

Reisberg, B., Ferris, S.H. and Crook, T. (1982). Signs, symptoms and course of age-associated cognitive decline, in *Alzheimer's Disease: A Report of Progress in Research* (Eds. S. Corkin, J.H. Growdon, K.L. Davis, E. Usdin and R.J. Wurtman), Raven Press, New York.

Reisine, T.D., Yamamura, H.I., Bird, E.D., Spokes, E. and Enna, S.J. (1978). Pre- and post-synaptic neurochemical alterations in Alzheimer's disease, *Brain Res.*, **159**, 477–80.

Rentoul, E. and Smith, H. (1973). *Glaister's Medical Jurisprudence and Toxicology*, Churchill Livingstone, London.

Renvoise, E.B., Gaskell, R.K. and Klar, H.M. (1985a). The value of routine X-rays in dementia, *Br. J. Psychiat.*, **146**, 560.

Renvoise, E.B., Gaskell, R.K. and Klar, H.M. (1985b). Results of investigations in 150 demented patients consecutively admitted to a psychiatric hospital, *Br. J. Psychiat.*, **147**, 204–5.

Richter, J.A., Perry, E.K. and Tomlinson, B.E. (1980). Acetylcholine and choline levels in postmortem brain tissue: preliminary observations in Alzheimer's disease, *Life Sci.*, **26**, 1683–9.

Rigter, H. (1982). A peptide for the aged? Animal studies, in *Psychopharmacology of Old Age* (Ed. D. Wheatley), Oxford Medical Publications, Oxford.

Robbins, S.L. and Cottran, R.S. (1979). *Pathologic Basis of Disease*, 3rd ed., Saunders, Philadelphia.

Roberts, A.H. (1969). *Brain Damage in Boxers: A Study of the Prevalence of Traumatic Encephalopathy among Ex-Boxers*, Pitman, London.

Roberts, J.K.A. (1984). *Differential Diagnosis in Neuropsychiatry*, Wiley, Chichester.

Roberts, J.K.A. and Lishman, W.A. (1984). The use of the CAT head scanner in clinical psychiatry, *Br. J. Psychiat.*, **145**, 152–8.

Roberts, M.A., McGeorge, A.P. and Caird, F.I. (1978). Electroencephalography and computerised tomography: vascular and non-vascular dementia, *J. Neurol. Neurosurg. Psychiat.*, **41**, 903–6.

Rogers, R.L., Meyer, J.S., Shaw, T.G., Martel, K.F., Hardenberg, J.P. and Ziad, M.D. (1983). Cigarette smoking decreases cerebral blood flow suggesting increased risk for stroke, *JAMA*, **250**, 2796–800.

Rohwer, R.G. (1984). Scrapie infectious agent is virus-like in size and susceptibility to inactivation, *Nature*, **308**, 658–62.

Ron, M.A., Toone, B.K., Garralda, M.E. and Lishman, W.A. (1979). Diagnostic accuracy in presenile dementia, *Br. J. Psychiat.*, **134**, 161–8.

Ron, M., Acker, W. and Lishman, W.A. (1983). Morphological abnormalities in brains of chronic alcoholics. A clinical, psychological and computerised axial tomographic study, *Acta. Psychiat. Scand.*, **134**, 161–8.

Rosen, W.G. and Mohs, R.C. (1982). Evolution of cognitive decline in dementia, in *Alzheimer's Disease: A Report of Progress in Research* (Eds. S. Corkin, J.H. Growdon, K.L. Davis, E. Usdin and R.J. Wurtman), Raven Press, New York.

Rosenberg, R.N. (1983). Recombinant DNA and neurologic disease: the coming of a new age, *Neurology*, **33**, 622–5.

Rosenmayr, L. (1983). On the social constitution of the life course and of aging: elements of a multidisciplinary gerontological perspective, in *Geropsychiatric Diagnostics and Treatment* (Ed. M. Bergener), Springer, New York.

Rossor, M.N., Emson, P.C., Iversen, L.L., Mountjoy, C.Q., Roth, M., Hawthorn, J., Ang, V.T.Y., Jenkins, J.S. and Fahrenberg, J. (1981). Neuropeptides in senile dementia of Alzheimer type: studies on somatostatin, vasoactive intestinal polypeptides and vasopressin, in *Metabolic Disorders of the Nervous System* (Ed. F.C. Rose), Pitman Medical, London.

Rossor, M.N., Iversen, L.L., Reynolds, G.P., Mountjoy, C.Q. and Roth, M. (1984). Early and late types of Alzheimer's disease are neurochemically distinct, *Br. Med. J.*, **288**, 961–4.

Roth, M. (1955). The natural history of mental disorder in old age, *J. Ment. Sci.*, **101**, 281–301.

Roth, M. (1971). Classification and aetiology in mental disorders of old age: some recent developments, in *Recent Developments in Psychogeriatrics* (Eds. D.W.K. Kay and A. Walk), *Br. J. Psychiat.* Spec. Publ. No. 6, Royal Medico-Psychological Association, London.

Roth, M. (1983). Multidimensional diagnosis in gerontopsychiatry, in *Geropsychiatric Diagnostics and Treatment* (Ed. M. Bergener), Springer, New York.

Roth, M., Tomlinson, B.E. and Blessed, G. (1966). Correlation between scores for dementia and counts of 'senile plaques' in cerebral grey matter of elderly subjects, *Nature*, **209**, 109.

Roth, M., Tomlinson, B.E. and Blessed, G. (1967). The relationship between quantitative measures of dementia and of degenerative changes in the cerebral grey matter of elderly subjects, *Proc. Roy. Soc. Med.*, **60**, 254–9.

Rothschild, D. (1937). Pathologic changes in senile psychoses and their psychobiologic significance, *Am. J. Psychiat.*, **93**, 757–84.

Rothschild, D. (1942). Neuropathological changes in arteriosclerotic psychoses and their psychiatric significance, *Arch. Neurol. Psychiat.*, **48**, 417–36.

Royal College of Physicians (1981). *Organic Mental Impairment in the Elderly: A Report of the Royal College of Physicians by the College Committee on Geriatrics*, Royal College of Physicians, London.

Royal College of Psychiatrists (1985a). Medical assessment for elderly people prior to a move to residential accommodation, Division of Old Age Psychiatry: Discussion paper.

Royal College of Psychiatrists (1985b). Report on the Court of Protection, *Bull. Roy. Coll. Psychiat.*, **9**, 144–6.

Ruben, R.J. and Kruger, B. (1983). Hearing loss in the elderly, *The Neurology of Aging* (Eds. R. Katzman and R.D. Terry), Contemporary Neurology series, F.A. Davis, Philadelphia.

St. Clair, D.M., Blackwood, D.H.R. and Christie, J.E. (1975). P3 and other long latency evoked potentials in presenile dementia Alzheimer type and alcoholic Korsakoff syndrome, *Br. J. Psychiat.*, **147**, 702–6.

Salonen, J.T., Puska, P., Tuomilehto, J. and Homan, K. (1982). Relation of blood pressure, serum lipids and smoking to the risk of cerebral stroke, *Stroke*, **13**, 327–33.

Sampson, A. and Sampson, S. (1983). *The Oxford Book of Ages*, Oxford University Press, Oxford.

Sanders, J., Schenk, V.W.D. and Van Veen, P. (1939). A family with Pick's disease, *Verh. Kon. Nederl. Akad. Wetenschlappen*, **2**, 124–8.

Sanders, S.C. (1984). Testamentary capacity, in *Advanced Geriatric Medicine*, (Eds. J.G. Grimley-Evans and F.I. Caird), Pitman, London.

Sanders, W.L. and Dunn, T.L. (1973). Creutzfeldt-Jakob disease treated with amantidine, *J. Neurol. Neurosurg. Psychiat.*, **36**, 581–4.

Sandoz Products Limited (1978). *Can Dementia be Reversed?* Sandoz Products Limited, Feltham.

Sanford, J.R.A. (1975). Tolerance of debility in elderly dependants by supporters at home: its significance for hospital practice, *Br. Med. J.*, **iii**, 471–5.

Scharfetter, C. (1975). The historical development of the concept of schizophrenia, in *Studies of Schizophrenia* (Ed. M.H. Lader), World Psychiatric Association and Royal College of Psychiatrists, London.

Scheinberg, M.A. and Cathcart, E.S. (1976). Comprehensive study of humoral and cellular immune abnormalities in 26 patients with systemic amyloidosis, *Arthr. Rheum.*, **19**, 173–82.

Schiebel, M.E. and Schiebel, A.B. (1976). Structural changes in the aging brain, in *Aging, Clinical, Morphological and Neurochemical Aspects of the Aging Central Nervous System*, Vol. 1 (Eds. H. Brody, D. Harmon and J.M. Ordy), Raven Press, New York.

Schlaepfer, W.W. and Lynch, R.G. (1976). Immunofluorescent studies of neurofilaments in the peripheral and central nervous systems of rats and humans (Abstr.) *J. Neuropath. Exp. Neurol.*, **35**, 345.

Schneider, E.L. and Brody, J.A. (1983). Aging, natural death, and the compression of morbidity: another view, *N. Engl. J. Med.*, **309**, 854–5.

Schnitzler, J.G. (1911). Zur Abgrenzung der sog. Alzheimeren Krankheit, *Z. Neurol. Psychiat.*, **7**, 34.

Schorah, C.J. and Morgan, D.B. (1985). Nutritional deficiencies in the elderly, *Hospital Update*, May, 353–60.

Schuberth, J. and Jenden, D.J. (1975). Transport of choline from plasma to CSF in the rabbit with reference to the origin of choline and acetylcholine metabolism in brain, *Brain Res.*, **84**, 245–56.

Scott, D. (1972). *Understanding EEG*, Duckworth, London.

Seitelberger, F. (1983). Normal and pathological aging of the brain, in *Geropsychiatric Diagnostics and Treatment* (Ed. M. Bergener), Springer, New York.

Selecki, B.R. (1965). Intracranial space-occupying lesions among patients admitted to mental hospitals, *Med. J. Aust.*, **1**, 383–90.

Shader, R.I., Harmatz, J.S. and Saltzman, C. (1974). A new scale for clinical assessment in geriatric populations: Sandoz Clinical Assessment — Geriatric (SCAG), *J. Am. Geriat. Soc.*, **22**, 107–13.

Shader, R.I., Harmatz, J.S. and Tammerk, H.A. (1979). Towards an observation structure for rating dysfunction and pathology in ambulatory geriatrics, in *CNS Aging and its Neuropharmacology*, Vol. 15 (Ed. W. Meier-Ruge), Karger, Basel.

Shah, K.V., Banks, G.D. and Merskey, H. (1969). Survival in atherosclerotic and senile dementia, *Br. J. Psychiat.*, **15**, 1283–6.

Sharma, V.K., Harik, S.I. and Ganapathi, M. (1979). Locus coeruleus lesion and chronic reserpine treatment: effect on adrenergic and cholinergic receptors in cerebral cortex and hippocampus, *Exp. Neurol.*, **65**, 685–9.

Sharman, M.G., Watt, D.C., Janota, I. and Carrasco, L.H. (1979). Alzheimer's disease in a mother and identical twin sons, *Psychol. Med.*, **9**, 771–4.

Shaw, D.M., Kellam, A.M.P. and Mottram, R.F. (1982). *Brain Sciences in Psychiatry*, Butterworth Scientific, London.

Shepherd, M. (1984). Psychogeriatrics and the neo-epidemiologists, *Psychol. Med.*, **14**, 1–4.

Shulman, K. and Arie, T. (1978). Fall in admission rate of old people to psychiatric units, *Br. Med. J.*, **i**, 156–8.

Shulman, R.G. (1983). NMR spectroscopy of living cells, *Sci. Am.*, **248**, 86–93.

Signoret, J.L., Whitelet, A. and Lhermitte, F. (1978). Influence of choline on amnesia in early Alzheimer's disease, *Lancet*, **ii**, 837.

Simpson, J.M. and Linney, A.D. (1983). The use of computer automated psychological tests to assess mentally impaired old people. Paper at the symposium 'Research Progress in Dementia', Charing Cross Hospital Medical School, London.

Simpson, J.M., Van der Cammen, T., Fraser, R.M., Exton-Smith, A.N. (1984). The role of the memory clinic, in *Promoting the Wellbeing of the Elderly* (Eds. M.F. Collen and H.R. Oldfield), International Health Evaluation Association and BUPA Medical Research, London.

Sitaram, N., Weingartner, H., Carne, E.D. and Gillin, J.C. (1978). Choline: selective enhancement of serial learning and encoding low imagery words in man, *Life Sci.*, **22**, 1555–63.

Sjörgen, T., Sjörgen, H. and Lindgren, A.C.H. (1952). Morbus Alzheimer and Morbus Pick. A Genetic, Clinical and Patho–Anatomical Study, *Acta Psychiat. Neurol. Scand.*, Suppl. 82.

Skelton-Robinson, M. and Jones, S. (1984). Nominal dysphasia and the severity of senile dementia, *Br. J. Psychiat.*, **145**, 168–71.

Skidmore, D. (1985). More than chalk and talk, *Community Outlook*, September, 11–13.

Slaets, J. and Fortgens, C. (1984). On the value of P300 event-related potentials in the differential diagnosis of dementia, *Br. J. Psychiat.*, **145**, 652–6.

Smith, C.M., Swash, M., Exton-Smith, A.N., Phillips, M.J., Overstall, P.W., Piper, M.E. and Bailey, M.R. (1978). Choline therapy in Alzheimer's disease, *Lancet*, **ii**, 318.

Smith, C.M., Temple, S.A. and Swash, M. (1982). Effects of physostigmine on responses in memory tests in patients with Alzheimer's disease, in *Alzheimer's Disease: A Report of Progress in Research* (Eds. S. Corkin, J.H. Growdon, K.L. Davis. E. Usdin and R.J. Wurtman), Raven Press, New York.

Smith, N.K.G. and Powell, R.J. (1985). Immunological tests and the diagnosis of dementia in elderly women, *Age Ageing*, **14**, 91–5.

Sneath, P., Chanarin, I., Hodkinson, H.H., McPherson, C.K. and Reynolds, E.H. (1973). Folate status in a geriatric population and its relation to dementia, *Age Ageing*, **2**, 177–82.

Soininen, H. (1983). Electroencephalographic signs of senile dementia, *Geriat. Med. Today*, **2**(10), 39–47.

Soininen, H., Puranen, M. and Riekkinen, P.J. (1982). Computed tomography findings in senile dementia and normal aging, *J. Neurol. Neurosurg. Psychiat.*, **45**, 50–4.

Somerville, R.A. (1985). Ultrastructural links between scrapie and Alzheimer's disease, *Lancet*, **i**, 504–6.

Sommer, R. and Ross, H. (1958). Social interaction on a geriatric ward, *Int. J. Soc. Psychiat.*, **4**, 128–33.

Sourander, P. and Sjörgen, H. (1970). The concept of Alzheimer's disease and its clinical implications, in *Alzheimer's Disease and Related Conditions* (Eds. G.E.W. Wolstenholme and M.E. O'Connor), Ciba Foundation Symposium, Churchill, London.

Speller, S.R. (1971). *Mentally Disordered Patients in Law Relating to Hospitals and Kindred Institutions*, Lewis, London.

Stefoski, D., Bergen, R., Fox, J., Morrell, F., Huckmans, A. and Ramsay, R. (1976). Correlation between diffuse EEG abnormalities and cerebral atrophy in senile dementia, *J. Neurol. Neurosurg. Psychiat.*, **39**, 751–5.

Stirling, E. (1985). Paper at seminar: 'Local Services for Elderly People with Severe

236

Psychiatric Disabilities' — Lessons from the Newcastle Experience, King's Fund Centre, London.

Stone, C.P., Girdner, J. and Albrecht, R. (1946). Alternative form of Wechsler's memory scale, *J. Psychol.*, **22**, 199–206.

Strömgren, L.L., Christensen, A.-L. and Fromholt, P. (1976). The effects of unilateral brief-interval ECT on memory, *Acta Psychiat. Scand.*, **54**, 336–46.

Swift, C. (1982). Hypnotic drugs, in *Recent Advances in Geriatric Medicine* (Ed. B. Isaacs), Churchill Livingstone, London.

Sylvester, P.E. (1983). Aging in the mentally retarded, in *First European Symposium on Scientific Studies in Mental Retardation*, Royal Society of Medicine, London.

Taylor, T.V., Dymock, I.W. and Torrance, B. (1974a). The role of vitamin C in the treatment of pressure sores in surgical patients, *Br. J. Surg.*, **61**, 921.

Taylor, T.V., Rimmer, S., Day, B., Butcher, J. and Dymock, I.W. (1974b). Ascorbic acid supplementation in the treatment of pressure sores *Lancet*, **ii**, 544–6.

Tecce, J.J., Cattanach, L., Boehner-Davis, M.B., Branconnier, R.J. and Cole, J.O. (1983). CNV rebound, attention performance, and Hydergine treatment in Alzheimer patients, *Br. J. Clin. Pract.*, Suppl. 30, 19–22.

Termine, J.D., Eanes, E.D. and Ein, D. (1972). Infrared spectroscopy of human amyloid fibrils and immunoglobulin proteins, *Biopolymers*, **11**, 1103.

Terry, R.D. (1963). The fine structure of neurofibrillary tangles in Alzheimer's disease, *J. Neuropath. Exp. Neurol.*, **22**, 629–42.

Terry, R.D. (1978). Aging, senile dementia and Alzheimer's disease, in *Alzheimer's Disease: Senile Dementia and Related Disorders* (Eds. R. Katzman, R.D. Terry and K.L. Blick), Raven Press, New York.

Terry, R.D. and Wisniewski, H.M. (1970). The ultrastructure of the neurofibrillary tangle and the senile plaque, in *Alzheimer's Disease and Related Conditions* (Eds. G.E.M. Wolstenholme and M.E. O'Connor), Ciba Foundation Symposium, Churchill, London.

Terry, R.D., Fitzgerald, C., Pack, A., Millner, J. and Farmer, P. (1977). Cortical cell counts in senile dementia (Abstr). *J. Neuropath. Exp. Neurol.*, **36**, 633.

Thal, L.J. (1984). Current concepts of the pathogenesis of senile dementia of the Alzheimer type, *Geriat. Med. Today*, 3(1), 86–9.

Thompson, L.W. (1976). *Neurobiology of Aging*, Raven Press, New York.

Thompson, M.K. (1985). Myths about the care of the elderly, *Lancet*, **i**, 523.

Tinker, G. (1979). Accidents in geriatric departments, *Age Ageing*, **8**, 196–9.

Tinklenberg, J.R., Pigache, R., Pfefferbaum, A. and Berger, P.A. (1982). Vasopressin peptides and dementia, in *Alzheimer's Disease: A Report of Progress in Research* (Eds. S. Corkin, J.H. Growdon, K.L. Davis, E. Usdin and R.J. Wurtman), Raven Press, New York.

Tobin, G.W. and Brocklehurst, J.C. (1986). Faecal incontinence in residential homes for the elderly: prevalence, aetiology and management, *Age Ageing*, **15**, 41–6.

Tomlinson, B.E. (1972). Morphological brain changes in non-demented old people, in *Aging of the Central Nervous System* (Eds. H.M. von Praag and A.F. Kalverboer), De Ervon F. Bohn, New York.

Tomlinson, B.E. (1980). The structural and quantitative aspects of the dementias, in *Biochemistry of Dementia* (Ed. P.J. Roberts), Wiley, Chichester.

Tomlinson, B.E. and Henderson, G. (1976). Some quantitative cerebral findings in normal and demented old people, in *Neurobiology of Aging* (Eds. R.D. Terry and S. Gershon), Raven Press, New York.

Tomlinson, B.E. Blessed, G. and Roth, M. (1968). Observations on the brains of non-demented old people, *J. Neurol. Sci.*, **7**, 331–56.

Tomlinson, B.E., Blessed, G. and Roth, M. (1970). Observations on the brains of demented old people, *J. Neurol. Sci.*, **11**, 205–42.

Tomonaga, M.)1984). Neuropathology of locus coeruleus in the elderly, *Curr. Rep. Neurol*, **6**, 6.
Torak, R.M. (1978). *The Pathologic Physiology of Dementia*, Springer, Berlin.
Townsend, P. (1957). *The Family Life of Old People*, Penguin, Harmondsworth.
Traub, R., Gajdusek, D.C. and Gibbs, C.J. Jr (1977). Transmissible virus dementia: the relation of transmissible spongiform encephalopathy to Creutzfeldt–Jakob disease, in *Aging and Dementia*, Spectrum Publications, New York.
Truswell, A.S. (1985). ABC of nutrition: vitamins II, *Br. Med. J.*, **291**, 1103–5.
Tuček, S. (1978). *Acetylcholine Synthesis in Neurons*, Chapman and Hall, London.
Van der Cammen, T.J., Simpson, J.M., Fraser, R.M., Preker, A.S. and Exton-Smith, A.N. (1987). The memory clinic: a new approach to the detection of dementia, *Br. J. Psychiat.* (in press).
Vestal, R.E., McGuire, E.A., Tobin, J.D., Andres, R., Norris, A.H. and Mezey, E. (1977). Aging and ethanol metabolism, *Clin. Pharmacol. Ther.*, **21**, 343–54.
Victor, M. and Banker, B.Q. (1978). Alcohol and dementia, in *Alzheimer's Disease: Senile Dementia and Related Disorders* (Eds. R. Katzman, R.D. Terry and K.L. Blick), Raven Press, New York.
Victor, M., Adams, R.D. and Collins, G.H. (1971). *The Wernicke– Korsakoff Syndrome*, Blackwell Scientific, Oxford.
Victoratos, G.C., Lenman, J.A.R. and Herzberg, L. (1977). Neurological investigation of dementia, *Br. J. Psychiat.*, **130**, 131–3.
Visser, H. (1983). Gait and balance in senile dementia of Alzheimer's type, *Age Ageing*, **12**, 296–301.
Walford, R.L. (1970). *Immunologic Theory of Ageing*, Williams and Wilkins, Baltimore.
Walker, W.J. (1976). Success story: the program against major cerebrovascular risk factors, *Geriatrics*, **1976**, March, 97–104.
Walter, W.G., Cooper, R., Aldridge, V.J., McCallum, W.C. and Winter, A.L. (1964). Contingent negative variation: an electric sign of sensorimotor association and expectancy in man, *Nature*, **203**, 380–4.
Wattis, J.P. (1983). Alcohol and old people, *Br. J. Psychiat.*, **143**, 306–7.
Wattis, J.P., Wattis, L. and Arie, T. (1981). Psychogeriatrics: a national survey of a new branch of psychiatry, *Br. Med. J.*, **282**, 1529–33.
Whalley, L.J., Carothers, A.D., Collyer, S., DeMay, R. and Frackiewicz, A. (1982). A study of familial factors in Alzheimer's disease, *Br. J. Psychiat.*, **140**, 249–56.
Whitehead, A. (1977). Changes in cognitive functioning in elderly psychiatric patients, *Br. J. Psychiat.*, **130**, 605–8.
Whitehead, A. (1982). Measurement of change in the elderly, in *Psychopharmacology of Old Age* (Ed. D. Wheatley), Oxford Medical Publications, Oxford.
Wilkins, R.H. and Brody, I.A. (1969). Alzheimer's disease, *Arch. Neurol.*, **21**, 108–10.
Will, R.G. and Matthews, W.B. (1982). Evidence for case-to-case transmission of Creutzfeldt–Jakob disease, *J. Neurol. Neurosurg. Psychiat.*, **45**, 235–8.
Williams, M. (1968). The measurement of memory in clinical practice, *Br. J. Soc. Clin. Psychol.*, **7**, 19–34.
Williamson, J., Gray, S., Stokoe, I.H., Fisher, M., Smith, A., McGhee, A. and Stephenson, E. (1964). Old people at home: their unreported needs, *Lancet*, **i**, 1117–20.
Wilson, D.C. (1955). The pathology of senility, *Am. J. Psychiat*, **111**, 902–6.
Winblad, B., Adolfsson, R., Carlsson, A. and Gottfries, C.G. (1982). Biogenic amines in brains of patients with Alzheimer's disease, in *Alzheimer's Disease: A Report of Progress in Research* (Eds. S. Corkin, J.H. Growdon, K.L. Davis, E. Usdin and R.J. Wurtman), Raven Press, New York.
Wisniewski, H.M. (1975). Personal communication, cited in R.M. Torak (1978). *The*

238

Pathologic Physiology of Dementia, Springer-Verlag, Berlin.

Wisniewski, H.M. and Terry, R.D. (1973). Reexamination of the pathogenesis of the senile plaque, in *Progress in Neurology*, Vol. 2, (Ed. H.M. Zimmerman), Grune and Stratton, New York.

Wisniewski, H.M., Johnson, A.B., Raine, C.S., Kay, W.J. and Terry, R.D. (1970). Senile plaques and cerebral amyloidosis in aged dogs, *Lab. Invest.*, **23**, 287–96.

Wisniewski, K., Howe, J., Williams, D.G. and Wisniewski, H.M. (1978). Precocious aging and dementia in patients with Down's syndrome, *Biol. Psychiat.*, **5**, 619–27.

Wolff, H.H. (1973). Psychotherapy: its place in psychosomatic management, *Psychother. Psychosom.*, **22**, 233–49.

Wolff, K. (1963). Individual psychotherapy with geriatric patients. *Dis. Nerv. Syst.*, **24**, 688–91.

Wood, R.A. (1984). Clinical algorithms: memory loss, *Br. Med. J.*, **288**, 1443–47.

Woods, R.T. (1979). Reality orientation and staff attention: a controlled study, *Br. J. Psychiat.*, **134**, 502–7.

Woods, R.T. and Britton, P.G. (1985). *Clinical Psychology with the Elderly*, Croom Helm, London.

World Health Organization (1969). *Mental Health Problems of Aging and the Aged*, Technical Report Series No. 171, WHO, Geneva.

Worm-Petersen, J. and Pakkenberg, H. (1967). Atherosclerosis of cerebral arteries, pathological and clinical correlations, *Acta Neurol. Scand.*, **43**, Suppl. 31.

Wright, A.F. and Whalley, L.J. (1984). Genetics, ageing and dementia, *Br. J. Psychiat.*, **141**, 20–38.

Wurtman, R.J. (1982). Forecast, in *Alzheimer's Disease: A Report of Progress in Research* (Eds. S. Corkin, J.H. Growdon, K.L. Davis, E. Usdin and R.J. Wurtman), Raven Press, New York.

Wurtman, R.J. (1983). Nutrients that modify brain function, *Sci. Am.*, **246**(4), 42–51.

Wurtman, R.J. (1985). Alzheimer's disease, *Sci. Am.*, **252**(2), 48–56.

Wurtman, R.J. and Fernstrom, J.D. (1976). Control of brain neurotransmitter synthesis by precursor availability and nutritional state, *Biochem. Pharmacol.*, **25**, 1691–6.

Wurtman, R.J., Hirsch, M.J. and Growdon, J.H. (1977). Lecithin consumption raises serum-free choline levels, *Lancet*, **ii**, 68–9.

Yakovlev, P.I. (1947). Paraplegias of hydrocephalus, *Am. J. Ment. Def.*, **51**, 561–76.

Yates, C.M., Blackburn, I.A., Christie, J.E., Glen, A.I.M., Shering, A., Simpson, J., Whalley, L.J. and Ziesel, S. (1980). Clinical and biochemical studies in Alzheimer's disease, in *Biochemistry of Dementia* (Ed. P.J. Roberts), Wiley, Chichester.

Yesavage, J.A., Tinklenberg, J.J., Hollister, L.E. and Berger, P.A. (1979). Vasodilators in senile dementia: a review of the literature, *Arch. Gen. Psychiat.*, **36**, 220–3.

Young, J., Hall, P. and Blakemore, C. (1974). Treatment of the cerebral manifestations of arteriosclerosis with cyclandelate, *Br. J. Psychiat.*, **124**, 177–80.

Index

240